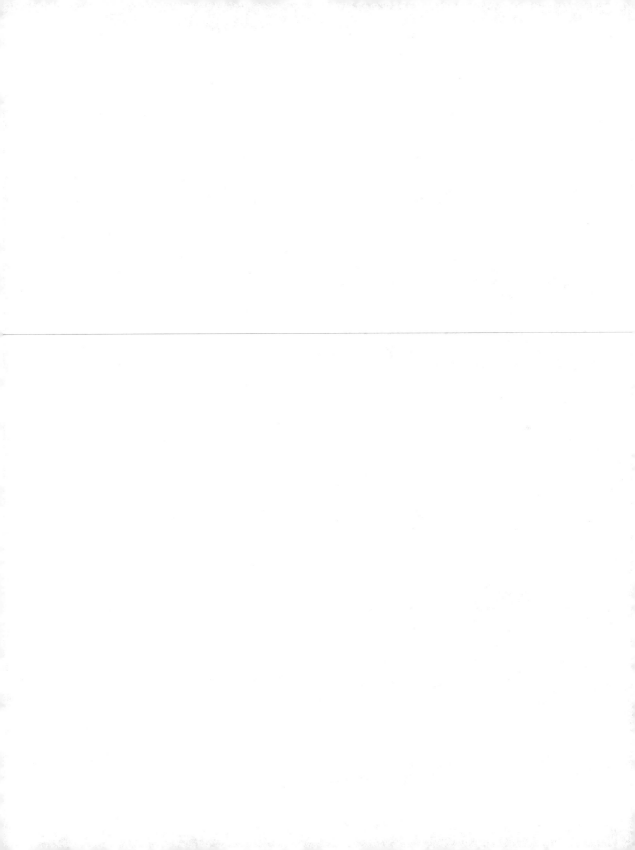

Faith Community Nursing

Janet S. Hickman, EdD, RN
Professor
Department of Nursing
West Chester University
West Chester, Pennsylvania

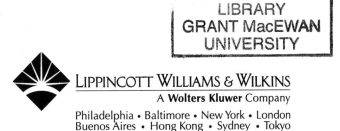

LIPPINCOTT WILLIAMS & WILKINS
A **Wolters Kluwer** Company

Philadelphia • Baltimore • New York • London
Buenos Aires • Hong Kong • Sydney • Tokyo

Acquisitions Editor: Margaret Zuccarini
Managing Editor: Betsy Gentzler
Editorial Assistant: Delema Caldwell-Jordan
Production Project Manager: Cynthia Rudy
Director of Nursing Production: Helen Ewan
Senior Managing Editor / Production: Erika Kors
Art Director: Joan Wendt
Manufacturing Coordinator: Karin Duffield
Production Services / Compositor: Schawk, Inc.
Printer: R. R. Donnelley–Crawfordsville

9 8 7 6 5 4 3 2 1

Library of Congress Cataloging-in-Publication Data

Hickman, Janet Susan.
   Faith community nursing / Janet S. Hickman.
      p. ; cm.
   Includes bibliographical references and index.
   ISBN 0-7817-5457-7 (alk. paper)
   1. Parish nursing—Philosophy. 2. Community health nursing—Philosophy. I. Title.
     [DNLM: 1. Community Health Nursing—methods. 2. Spirituality. 3. Holistic Nursing—methods. 4. Nurse's Role. 5. Pastoral Care. WY 87 H628f 2006]
   RT120.P37H44 2006
   610.73'43—dc22

                                             2005021578

LWW.com

About the Author

Janet S. Hickman, EdD, RN, is Professor of Nursing at West Chester University, West Chester, Pennsylvania. Dr. Hickman developed and implemented the Master's in Community Health Nursing Program at WCU. Her areas of professional interest include parish and community health nursing, higher education and nursing curricula, administration, and nursing theory. Before coming to WCU, Dr. Hickman was the Associate Dean for Health Sciences and Chair of the Department of Nursing at Eastern College (now Eastern University), St. Davids, Pennsylvania.

Dr. Hickman has authored book chapters and articles on nursing theory, critical thinking and clinical judgment, and family assessment.

Dedication

This book is dedicated to my parents, Frances and Richard Liberth, my husband Kennedy, my son Kennedy, and my daughter-in-law Patty. Without their love and encouragement this book would not have been a reality.

Contributors

Linda Clay, RN, MSN

Instructor
Center for Arts and Technology
Coatesville, Pennsylvania
and
Congregational/Parish Nurse
Church of the Loving Shepherd
West Chester, Pennsylvania

Julia P. George, RN, PhD

Professor Emeritus
California State University, Fullerton
Fullerton, California

Polly Sue Gockley, RN, MSN

Instructor
Harrisburg Area Community College
Lancaster, Pennsylvania
and
Congregational Nurse
Zion Lutheran Church
East Petersburg, Pennsylvania

Charlotte H. Mackey, RN, MSN, EdD

Associate Professor of Nursing
West Chester University
West Chester, Pennsylvania

Susan Metzger, RN, MSN

Project Manager
Pulmonary, Allergy, and Critical Care
School of Medicine
University of Pennsylvania
Philadelphia, Pennsylvania

Susan C. Slaninka, RN, EdD

Adjunct Faculty
Villanova University
Villanova, Pennsylvania

Reviewers

Norma Anderson, PhD, RN-C
Associate Professor of Nursing
Saint Louis University School of Nursing
St. Louis, Missouri

Carol Cherry, RN, MSN
Associate Professor
Marian College
Indianapolis, Indiana

Carol Harrison, RN, EdD
Chair and Professor
Spring Hill College
Mobile, Alabama

Norma Krumwiede, EdD, MEd, MN, RN
Associate Professor
Minnesota State University, Mankato
Mankato, Minnesota

Gretchen McDaniel, DSN, RN
Professor, Director of NurCE
Ida V. Moffett School of Nursing
Samford University
Birmingham, Alabama

Margaret Miller, PhD, RN
Professor, MSN Program
Donna and Allan Lansing School of Nursing
and Health Sciences
Bellarmine University
Louisville, Kentucky

Sylvia Miller, RN, EdD
Assistant Professor, Department of Nursing
California State University, Fresno
Fresno, California
and
Health Ministries/ Parish Nurse Program Coordinator
St. Agnes Medical Center
Fresno, California

Judith Mouch, RSM, MSN, MA, APRN-BC
Assistant Professor of Nursing
University of Detroit Mercy
Detroit, Michigan

Patrice Olin, RNC, MS
Parish Nurse and Parish Nurse Education
Coordinator
Covenant Healthcare and Marquette University
Milwaukee, Wisconsin

Faith Roberts, RN, BSN, CRRN
Coordinator, Community Parish Nurse Program
Carle Foundation Hospital
Urbana, Illinois

Pamela Schroeder, MSN, RN, CHPN
Director, Parish Nurse Ministry
Bon Secours Hampton Roads
Norfolk, Virginia

Marilyn Stember, RN, PhD, FAAN
Professor Emerita
University of Colorado Health Sciences Center
Denver, Colorado

Darla Ura
Clinical Associate Professor
Nell Hodgson Woodruff School of Nursing
Emory University
Atlanta, Georgia

Rosemary Walter, RN, MSN
Parish Nurse Education Program Facilitator
Catholic Charities
Buffalo, New York

Preface

Health care in the United States continues to evolve in chaotic and unplanned ways. It is currently complicated by both a shortage of professional nurses and a shortage of faculty to educate future nurses. Those nurses who are employed in health care settings are expected to do more with fewer resources, at a time when those they care for are more acutely ill than ever.

Despite the challenges and demands of a nursing career, the profession continues to attract more students than there are programs and faculty to teach them. One of the most important aspects of a nursing career, one that has drawn applicants to schools of nursing since their inception, is the desire to serve others. For many in the profession, as well as those aspiring to the profession, the concept of service to others has a basis in one's faith tradition. This spiritual basis motivates and nourishes many nurses to care for others when they are broken or wounded in physical and psychosocial-spiritual ways.

Faith community, parish, or congregational nurses are nurses who minister to faith communities. The heart of their ministry is the caring nurse-client relationship, the caring for fellow children of God. Faith community nursing practice includes service to others, the provision of comfort and relief of pain, healing, education, and support when cure is not possible. Faith community nursing ministries are supported by prayer, by faith community rituals and traditions, and by the belief that spiritual health and wholeness affects all other aspects of health.

Faith Community Nursing was developed and written to meet a specific need identified by graduate level nursing students seeking to develop parish nursing ministries as a part of their community health nursing clinical practicum experiences. It is intended to serve as a primary text for a faith community nursing course, which may be taught as an undergraduate, graduate, or continuing education course; it may also be used as a supplementary text for a community health nursing course. This book may also serve as a reference for practicing faith community nurses. The text integrates the American Nurses Association (ANA)-Health Ministries Association (HMA) *Faith Community Nursing: Scope and Standards of Practice* in each chapter as applicable. It provides the reader with information and resources for beginning and maintaining a faith community nursing ministry. Traditional community health nursing's methods of community assessment, health education, and program planning/evaluation supplement and complement the content about the practice of faith community nursing. Web-based resources and additional resources are provided in each chapter.

Organization of the Text

Italics are used throughout the text to highlight new or key terms, in addition to indicating emphasis and titles of published documents.

Unit I: Faith Community Nursing Practice

In Chapter 1, Philosophical and Theoretical Foundations of Faith Community Nursing, the reader is introduced to the history, philosophy, and descriptions of faith community nursing as well to nursing theory and research. The ANA-HMA *Faith Community Nursing: Scope and Standards of Practice* (2005) are presented as the base for practice. Professional organizations such as the International Resource Center for Parish Nursing and the Health Ministries Association are introduced.

In Chapter 2, Faith Community Nursing Models, Preparation, and Roles, the delivery models of faith community nursing and the educational preparation for faith community nursing practice are presented. The seven roles or functions of a faith community nurse: integrator of faith and health; personal health counselor; health educator; referral agent; coordinator of volunteers; developer of support groups; and advocate are discussed in depth. The research studies and findings related to these roles are presented.

Chapter 3, Holistic Health and the Faith Community, addresses the theology of health, healing, and wholeness, and the faith community nursing role of integrator of faith and health. It looks at health seeking and faith seeking as related processes. The concepts of spirituality, spiritual formation, and faith and healing are presented. Methods of spiritual assessment and spiritual care interventions are discussed.

Unit II: Faith, Health, and the Community

Chapter 4, Working in a Faith Community, presents the elements of beginning a faith community nursing ministry. It includes content on the call to serve, the congregational leader and governance structures, and the expectations of the nurse, the ministry team, and the faith community. The faith community nursing role of working with volunteers is presented. Budgeting, management, and interpersonal challenges are discussed.

Chapter 5, Assessment of the Faith Community and Geopolitical Community, provides direction about how to conduct assessments of both the faith community and the larger community. It discusses the methods to use, as well as how to analyze and utilize the information gathered in the context of faith community nursing practice.

Chapter 6, Diverse Faith Traditions, provides information about the doctrines, branches, and health practices related to the faith traditions of Christianity, Judaism, Buddhism, Hinduism, and Islam.

Chapter 7, Community Connections, addresses the faith community nurse role functions of referral agent and advocate. The concepts of collaboration and advocacy are discussed in depth. Faith community nurse collaborations with colleagues, institutions, and organizations are discussed.

Unit III: Issues in Faith Community Nursing Practice

Chapter 8, Legal Aspects of Faith Community Nursing Practice, discusses nurse practice acts, the scope and standards of practice, living wills and durable power of attorney, accountability, and liability issues. Confidentiality and HIPAA are discussed, as well as the documentation requirements for faith community nursing practice.

Chapter 9, Ethical Issues and Faith Community Nursing Practice, presents ethical theories, frameworks for ethical decision-making, and contemporary ethical issues.

Chapter 10, Complementary and Alternative Modalities, presents information on homeopathy, chiropractic, acupuncture, Reiki, therapeutic touch, guided imagery, herbal medicine, and aromatherapy. For each modality, background information, practice applications, credentialing required of practitioners, and what to look for in a provider are discussed.

Chapter 11, Self-care and the Faith Community Nurse, discusses the personal expectations of the faith community nurse. The chapter includes information about stress and time management and presents strategies for achieving personal peace and nurturing spirituality. Storytelling, journal writing, nature, self reflection and prayer are discussed as self care strategies.

Unit IV: Health Promotion and Disease Prevention

Chapter 12, Planning Health Promotion/Disease Prevention Programs, provides how-to information on program planning, implementation and evaluation. It uses *Healthy People 2010* as a planning guide for program development.

Chapter 13, Health Education, focuses on the health educator and personal health counselor roles of the faith community nurse. This chapter provides a theoretical base for behavioral change and discusses interventions for health behavior change. It also provides a step-by-step guide to the health education process, including assessment of the audience, literacy level, cultural issues, behavioral objectives, and instructional methods. Assessment of educational materials and media is also presented.

Chapter 14, Proposal Writing, gives the reader a detailed description of each of the elements of a grant proposal. Funding sources, proposal writing, and grant management activities are discussed.

Unit V: Faith Community Nursing Practice Concepts

Chapter 15, Faith Community Nursing Practice With Clients With Chronic Illness, discusses using assessment data, making home visits, and using volunteers and support groups in caring for persons with chronic illnesses. The independent nursing interventions of presence, creative arts, humor, and prayer are discussed.

Chapter 16, Faith Community Nursing Practice and Palliative Care, Grief, and Loss discusses the history and challenges of palliative care, grief and loss counseling, and the role of the faith community nurse.

Chapter 17, Vulnerable Populations, presents a discussion of the concept of vulnerability. Each of the vulnerable groups is discussed in terms of an overview of the problem or issue and its effects. Groups presented include persons living in poverty, the homeless, pregnant teens, persons with HIV/AIDS, migrant workers, victims of domestic violence, substance abusers, the mentally ill, and persons with disabilities.

All of the authors who have contributed to this text are Christians and are writing from a Christian faith perspective. However, it is hoped that the content presented will be helpful to nurses of other faith traditions as well.

The author would like to acknowledge and thank those persons who have been most closely involved in the production of this text. The author is grateful for the encouragement of John Friscia and his referral to Margaret Zuccarini who provided editorial direction and assistance. The author wishes to thank Helen Kogut, Dana Irwin, and Betsy Gentzler for their editorial assistance and support and John Owens at Schawk, Inc. for his assistance in the production process.

The author wishes to thank her colleagues who contributed to this book as well as those who reviewed chapter manuscripts. She also wishes to acknowledge the input and support of her graduate nursing students at West Chester University who identified a need for a text of this type.

JANET S. HICKMAN, EdD, RN

Contents

Faith Community Nursing Practice

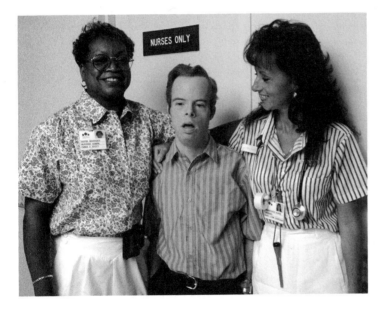

Philosophical and Theoretical Foundations of Faith Community Nursing

Faith community nursing is considered to be one of the newer nursing specialties, yet the concepts underlying this type of nursing practice go back to the very roots of the profession. Faith community nursing practice values the concepts of *holism, caring, health,* and *healing*. A *holistic* perspective views the person as a unified being with complete integration of mind, body, and spirit. *Caring* is watchful attention to and meeting the needs of another person. *Health* is defined as "the experience of wholeness, salvation, shalom. It is the integration of the physical, psychological, social, and aspects of the patient and harmony with self, others, the environment, and God. Health may be experienced in the presence or absence of disease or injury" (American Nurses Association and Health Ministries Association [ANA-HMA], 2005). *Healing* is the process of integrating the mind, body, and spirit to achieve wholeness, health, and a sense of well-being, even when the curing of disease does not occur (ANA-HMA, 2005, p. 37).

What is faith community or parish nursing? *Parish nursing* was the term used by the Rev. Granger Westberg to describe the unique, specialized practice of professional nursing in faith communities to promote holistic health. The principles of holistic health arise from the premise that human beings strive for wholeness in relationship to their God, themselves, their families, and the society in which they live. At first, parish nurse programs were more common in Judeo-Christian faith communities, but, currently, the concept of parish nursing has grown to include many other faith traditions. The term *parish nursing* is not universally acceptable to all faith traditions. As a result, several titles have been created to describe nursing in different faith community settings. They include parish nurse, congregational nurse, health ministry nurse, and wellness nurse. To be inclusive of all faith traditions and to accurately label the location and central focus of practice, the current terminology used in the *Scope and Standards* document is "faith community nursing" (ANA-HMA, 2005, p. 2). The International Parish Nurse Resource Center, however, is retaining the title "parish nurse." These titles will be used interchangeably in the text.

Speaking from a Christian perspective, Nist (2003) describes parish nursing as a sacred calling. She says that she feels blessed to be able to work in a religious-based and mission-driven environment that provides an opportunity and resources to emphasize the vital relationship of spirituality to whole health and the role of each of God's children in creating communities of care. She says that she feels privileged to practice in an area of nursing that demands that nurses ask themselves and others the questions that open the door to spiritual reflection on all that life holds—the everyday sacredness, with its everyday crosses and resurrections.

Faith community nursing can be delivered by several models, and the roles and functions of the faith community nurse (FCN) reflect the needs of the faith community served. Westberg (1999) identified the following seven roles of the parish nurse: health educator, personal health counselor, referral agent, coordinator of volunteers, developer of support groups, integrator of faith and health, and health advocate. Each of these roles will be discussed in Chapter 2.

A Historical Perspective

Ebersole (2000) reports that the roots of parish nursing are as old as ancient civilizations. From the beginning of human records, the cleanliness of the body, the interpretation of natural phenomena—birth, death, cure, and healing—have been considered to be aspects of the spiritual leader's role. In the development of scientific thought, the division of church and state, nature and nurture, body and soul, and medicine and health occurred.

Ebersole (2000) says we have now come full circle because churches, mosques, and temples are recognizing and reclaiming their role in integrating the holy with holistic health.

Ancient Civilizations

Koenig, McCullough, and Larson (2001) report that artifacts from predynastic Egypt (5000–600 BC) indicate that mental illness and physical illness were not distinguished from each other, and both were understood in the context of religious terms.

Egyptian hieroglyphics depict the art of laying on of hands and the use of the pulse as a diagnostic tool (5000–1500 BC). Concurrently, Hinduism emerged in India with the use of herbs, water, incantations, dancing, and amulets to cure ills, and in China disease was treated by acupuncture and medication. In 600–500 BC Buddhism emerged out of northeastern India as Gautama the Buddha began his teachings. He authorized a religious ritual to be used for healing the sick and approved the use of medications. Muhammed the Prophet was born in 570 AD, and the Islamic tradition emerged as the Qur'an was revealed to Muhammed. A body of medical knowledge is universally attributed to the Prophet, and the Qur'an sets a high value on health and the restoration of health.

Judaism and Health

The Jewish belief centers on the revelation of God at Sinai, which is contained in the Torah (the Five Books of Moses), and on the historical relationship of God to the Jewish people from the time of Abraham to the present. Dorff (1986) states that many Jewish attitudes about health and medicine are based on rabbinical responses. The responses indicate that the body is God's masterpiece, and people are to take care of their bodies and seek healing. Jewish people are forbidden to live in places where physicians are not available, and lay people are required to visit the sick.

Nursing and Christianity

Christianity originated in the frame of Palestinian Judaism. Christian charity, or love in action, expanded the role of nursing in society and permitted both sexes to engage in helping endeavors. Following the example of Christ, early nurses ministered to those in need. In the first centuries of the Christian Church, organized visiting of the sick began with the establishment of the order of deaconesses. Phoebe, a Greek woman and friend of St. Paul, was the first deaconess and the first visiting nurse. The order of deaconesses attained a position of importance for many years and then gradually died out (Dolan, Fitzpatrick, & Herrmann, 1983).

Groups of Roman matrons succeeded the deaconesses in providing care to the needy in convents and early hospitals. These women included Helena, Marcella, and Fabiola. They recognized the need to educate nurses and to organize and administer institutions to provide care for the infirm (Dolan et al., 1983).

Toward the close of the 11th century, the Seljuk Turks began their tour of conquest. They captured Palestine and erected mosques in the Holy City of Jerusalem. The capture of the Holy Places caused European Christians to unite to stop the Turks. The Holy Wars, or Crusades, lasted for nearly 200 years (1096–1291). Male military nursing orders, such as the Knights Hospitalers of St. John of Jerusalem and the Knights Templars, were formed to meet the needs of the crusading armies. The orders built and staffed hospitals as well as attended the wounded on the battlefields (Kalisch & Kalisch, 2004).

During the Renaissance (1500–1700), tremendous economical, political, social, and intellectual changes occurred. One of the changes, the Reformation, had a profound impact on the development of nursing. The Reformation resulted in the division of the Western Christian Church and the formation of the Protestant churches. In countries, such as Italy and France, where Roman Catholicism remained the dominant faith tradition, nursing orders continued their healing missions in hospitals and in the community.

The rise of Protestantism in other countries closed monasteries and hospitals and suppressed religious nursing orders. This resulted in a nursing workforce of women who had few other employment options. The image of Dickens' character Sairey Gamp is representative of this dark time of nursing history.

Germany, however, saw a rebirth of nursing through the works of Amalie Sieveking and Theodore Fliedner. In 1823, Sieveking developed a sisterhood similar to the Roman Catholic Sisters of Charity, and 10 years later she established a women's society devoted to the care of the sick and the poor. In 1836, Theodore Fliedner, a Lutheran pastor, revived the deaconess movement. He established the first motherhouse at Kaiserswerth, where he needed an organized corps of nurses to staff his new infirmary. The order of deaconesses of the Rhenish Province of Westphalia comprised three classes of members: The first class devoted itself to care of the sick poor, the second class served as teachers, and the third class was known as visitation deaconesses who assumed the responsibilities of regular parochial work. In 1851, Florence Nightingale spent 3 months at Kaiserswerth, and her experiences there helped to form her ideas about nursing education (Kalisch & Kalisch, 1995).

Development of Nursing in the Western Hemisphere

Nursing in the colonies reflected the delivery of health care in the mother countries. The French colonies imported Roman Catholicism and its nursing orders to the New World, and, as a result, hospitals and nursing services appeared early in New France. Founded in 1608, Quebec City had its first hospital by 1639.

In 1738, Marie-Marguérite d'Youville founded the Sisters of Charity of Montreal, an order also known as the Grey Nuns. Because this was a noncloistered order, the nuns could bring nursing services into the homes of the sick. D'Youville is considered to be the mother of community health nursing in Canada (Dolan et al., 1983).

In the British colonies of the 16th and 17th centuries, colonial hospitals were either almshouses or pesthouses (for contagious diseases). Pennsylvania Hospital, the first American hospital, was founded in 1751 at the suggestion of Benjamin Franklin. The second colonial hospital was New York Hospital, founded in 1770. Two medical schools had been established in America by the end of the colonial period: the Medical College of Philadelphia in 1765 and the medical department of King's College in 1767 (Kalisch & Kalisch, 1995).

In 1809, Elizabeth Seton founded the Sisters of Charity in Emmitsburg, Maryland, and in 1850 this order united with the worldwide community of the Sisters of Charity of St. Vincent. In 1829, the Sisters of Our Lady of Mercy of Charleston, South Carolina, undertook the staffing of the Hospital of Working Men. Also deeply involved in nursing were the Sisters of Mercy, an order founded in Dublin in 1827 by Catherine McAuley. The order was introduced to America in 1843, when seven sisters came from Ireland to establish a convent in Pittsburgh, Pennsylvania. During this period, many American hospitals were established under the direction of Roman Catholic orders. However, except for these few religious orders, nursing remained in the hands of the uneducated (Kalisch & Kalisch, 1995, 2004).

Nelson (1997) presents an excellent argument that "modern professional" nursing should be credited to the religious nursing sisters, who accomplished "professional nursing" before the Crimean War and the American Civil War. She states that the modern professional nurse cannot be seen as the product of secularization but as an extension of a religious form of life. As Nightingale viewed nursing as a spiritual enterprise within the context of a transcendent God, she would, no doubt, agree with Nelson!

Nightingale

Florence Nightingale (1820–1910) is considered to be the founder of modern *professional* nursing. She was born of wealthy, influential English parents and received a thorough classical education. Despite the objections of her family, Nightingale undertook nurse's training at Kaiserswerth in 1851. Later in 1853, she visited France and inspected hospitals and religious institutions, and observed surgery. Shortly after came the opportunity to superintend the military hospital in the Crimea where her expertise in nursing, public health, and administration is well documented. On her return to England, Nightingale opened the first official school of nursing in association with London's St. Thomas Hospital. She emphasized that nursing was concerned with the health, comfort, and welfare of patients, with caring being the central theme (Kalisch & Kalisch, 1995, 2004).

According to Macrae (2001), what is not widely known about Nightingale is that she had a profoundly spiritual, as well as scientific, view of nursing practice. She presented her spiritual views in a three-volume, 829-page manuscript entitled *Suggestions for Thought,* which she had privately printed in 1860. An edited version of this work is now available from the University of Pennsylvania Press (Calabria & Macrae, 1994).

Although Nightingale was raised as a member of the Church of England, her father was a prominent Unitarian member of Parliament who was devoted to social reform. In *Suggestions for Thought* (Calabria & Macrae, 1994), Nightingale wrote, "unless you make a life which shall be manifestation of your religion, it does not much signify what you believe" (p. 116).

Macrae contends that Nightingale's study of statistics was not just an intellectual challenge and a means of effecting public health reform; it was also a sacred science. Nightingale believed that an ordered universe was a reflection of a higher intelligence or divine mind. Because she believed that the universe is regulated by natural laws, or the *thoughts of God,* health promotion should occur through the discovery and proper application of universal principles. She wrote emphatically against the prevalent idea of the time—that illness occurs as a punishment for sins. She wrote that without sanitation, cholera will exist among saints as well as sinners (Macrae, 2001).

Macrae writes that Nightingale was not a pantheist (someone who equates nature with God) because she believed that the divine spirit not only permeates but transcends the created world. However, it is Nightingale's sense of divinity *within* the world that gave her work in nursing a profound sense of meaning. Nightingale wrote in *Notes on Nursing* that "God lays down certain physical laws. Upon his carrying out such laws depends our responsibility" (Macrae, 2001, p. 25). Macrae states that for Nightingale, nursing was a means of harmonizing oneself with the divine source of all existence, and thus a sacred process (2001).

Nursing in America: 1849–1990s

After an 1846 visit to Kaiserswerth, William Passavant, a Lutheran pastor from Pennsylvania, brought the deaconess movement to America in 1849. Passavant is credited with opening hospitals, orphanages, and old-age homes. In America, the deaconesses did not become popular until the mid-1880s when seven deaconesses joined the staff of the German Hospital of Philadelphia (later, Lankenau Hospital) and there established a motherhouse (Lindberg, 1986).

Kalisch and Kalisch (1995) report that over 10,000 women served as nurses during the American Civil War. The nurses consisted of salaried employees of the Northern Army, nuns of various orders, temporary employees, black women employed by the War Department, volunteers, camp followers, and women employed by relief organizations. Very few of the women had actual hospital experience or qualifications other than being willing to serve.

After the war, several women who had been nurses helped lead the way to establish nurse training schools. The first 12-month training program was established at the New England Hospital for Women and Children in 1872. This program graduated Linda Richards, America's first professionally trained nurse in 1873. In that year, the New York Training School (affiliated with the Bellevue Hospital) opened. The school was the first in the United States to be modeled after Nightingale's school of nursing at St. Thomas's Hospital in London. Later that year, other Nightingale-model schools were established—the Connecticut Training School for Nurses at New Haven State Hospital and the Boston Training School for Nurses at Massachusetts General Hospital. However, unlike the Nightingale school model, the American schools of nurse's training were *not* financially independent from the hospitals in which they were based. The consequences of this departure from the Nightingale model have been examined by many contemporary nursing historians. Ashley (1976) and Reverby (1982) have written about the negative effects that this error had on the development of the discipline of nursing in America. It led to both paternalism and the exploitation of nursing students. Student nurses were used as free labor to staff American hospitals for many decades, and their "training" involved more labor than learning.

Buhler-Wilkerson (2001) reports that although the introduction of district nursing in America began as a copy of the English system, it evolved into a specifically American approach to home-based care characterized by individualism and pluralism. Despite Nightingale's resistance to the germ theory, Americans recognized infectious diseases as a greater threat to the public's health than flaws in character. Initially, public health nursing was service directed to the sick poor in their homes and was funded by voluntary agencies—visiting nurse associations, (24%), hospitals (15%), and church groups (11%). The mission emphasized health promotion and disease prevention rather than curative and palliative care. As local and state governments began to take responsibility for the health and welfare of their citizens, public health nursing became a part of health department programs. Service was directed to a wide spectrum of people defined by geographic boundaries (city, county, district, parish), special populations (maternal-child, adult health, school health), and specific health problems, such as tuberculosis, venereal diseases, and communicable diseases. In all settings, the public health team practiced with a high degree of autonomy, in collaboration with the community (Ohlson & Wood, 1999).

In the first 3 decades of the 20th century, nursing school graduates functioned as private duty nurses, instructors, and public health nurses, not as hospital nurses. American hospitals were staffed by student nurses who were supervised by a few graduate nurses. Their patients were individuals who could not afford to be cared for by private duty nurses in their homes (Baer, 1999).

In the 1930s the advances of science and technology, as well as the advent of health insurance, moved the location of health care delivery from the home to the hospital. The need for a lay nursing workforce greatly increased as hospitals grew and expanded their services. The delivery of nursing care became highly regimented and task-oriented, with little attention paid to meeting the psychosocial or spiritual needs of patients. Barnum (2003) states that as nursing matured as an aspiring profession, it adopted the scientific paradigm, and all else was deemed too illusory. As a result, the focus of care moved from the holistic view of the person as mind-body-spirit to that of the person as a biopsychosocial being. Barnum argues that nursing had to model itself after medicine and accept the scientific paradigm to enter the turf of academia, which was a major goal. Donley (1991) writes with concern about the loss of the art of nursing in response to technology and profit making. She states, "As some of the art and most of the mystery of healing were lost, it became clear to nurses, and others who worked in hospitals, that they were part of a technical money-making system, not a 'sacred system' " (p. 178). The focus of nursing became curing not caring.

During the 1950s or "biopsychosocial era," nursing curricula were divested of spiritual content and replaced with content about the major world religions. Religious rituals and dietary practices were discussed in relation to nursing care, but any spiritual needs of the patient were to be referred to the appropriate clergy (Barnum, 2003).

Nursing theorists of the 1950s operated from a biomedical model and focused on nursing's functional roles—what nurses do and patient problems or needs. In the 1960s the focus of nursing theories was on the interpersonal relationship between the patient and the nurse. This nurse–patient relationship focus was a result of Peplau's seminal text, *Interpersonal Relations in Nursing* (1952). Theorists of the 1960s looked at how nurses do what they do, and how the patient perceives his or her situation. In 1967, three Yale University faculty members, Dickoff, James, and Wiedenbach (1968) (two philosophers and a nurse, respectively), presented a definition of nursing theory and goals for theory development in nursing. Their paper was published in *Nursing Research* a year later, and it has become a classic document in the history of theoretical thinking in nursing (Dickoff et al.).

In 1979, Jean Watson published *Nursing: The Philosophy and Science of Caring.* In this work, Watson returned the focus of nursing from curing to caring. Leininger (2001) has contended for many years that "human care and caring are the central, distinct, and dominant foci to explain, interpret, and predict nursing as a discipline and profession . . ." (p. 47). She defines caring as "actions and activities directed toward assisting, supporting, or enabling another individual or group with evident or anticipated needs to ease, heal, or improve a human condition or lifeway or face death or disability" (1991, p. 47).

The 1980s and 1990s brought an intense interest in the caring aspect of the profession. Nursing theories were developed with caring as the central focus, and nursing research was conducted to test these theories. In professional practice, nurses returned to living the value of providing humanized care while still working in a highly technical environment. This became a great challenge in an era of cost containment, nursing shortage, and increasing patient acuity levels.

Addressing the history of nursing outside of the context of the social forces of the 20th century is not possible. Major changes in the status of women, the dramatic growth of university education after World War II, medical and information technology, and the changes in the health care system (that continue to be driven by economics) have all had effects on the development of the nursing profession. One outcome of these forces has been the weakening of the link between nursing and the Christian faith tradition.

Parish Nursing: The Beginning

Granger Westberg (1913–1999) was a Lutheran minister who, over the course of his career, broke new ground about the links of religion, medicine, preventive, and whole person health. Westberg served as a parish pastor, hospital chaplain, professor of theology, and teacher of medical students. While at the University of Illinois College of Medicine, he worked on the W. K. Kellogg Foundation-sponsored project that established medical clinics in churches. Westberg reported that evaluations of these settings over a period of 10 years indicated that the quality of care offered when physicians, nurses, and clergy worked together was measurably more whole-person oriented than in the average doctor's office. He stated that it was clear that nurses were the "glue" that bound these three professions together in a common appreciation of the healing talents of each. He reported that evaluators came to the conclusion that the nurses in these settings could speak both the language of science and the language of religion and thus were acting as translators (Westberg, 1999).

When it became impossible to financially sustain the holistic health clinics, Westberg suggested placing a nurse on the staff of a congregation and seeing what would result. In 1984, he approached the Lutheran General Hospital (LGH) in Park Ridge, Illinois, to help him plan and implement the institutionally based program. Westberg described meeting with hospital administrators and church pastors, and noted that, ultimately, LGH agreed to financially subsidize the initial six pilot parish nursing programs over a 3-year period. The history of the parish nursing program is closely tied to the understanding that churches and synagogues, when they are functioning at their best, are dedicated to keeping people well (Westberg, 1999).

Late in 1986, the International Parish Nurse Resource Center (IPNRC) was developed at the Lutheran General Health System, one of the predecessor organizations of Advocate Health Care. Under the leadership of Ann Solari-Twadell, RN, MSN, MPA, the organization grew to a strong leadership role in parish nurse education, research, and support. In December 2001, Advocate Health Care closed the IPNRC and transferred its programs to Deaconess Parish Nurse Ministries in St. Louis, Missouri, another faith-based organization that had supported parish nursing since the 1980s. The IPNRC serves parish nurses throughout the world by offering the annual Westberg Parish Nurse Symposium as well as other educational and programmatic resources. The IPNRC maintains a Web site (http://www.parishnurses.org) that provides its mission and philosophy statements, strategic vision statement, and other resources. It publishes a quarterly newsletter titled *Parish Nursing Perspectives* and a periodic electronic newsletter titled *IPNRC eNotes.* The IPNRC also provides *Parish Nurse Ministry Survey: An Outcomes Measurement Tool,* developed by Wehling and Rethemeyers. For a nominal fee, the IPNRC will provide the tool, tabulate the data, and prepare a formal report of the findings.

In 1989 the Health Ministries Association (HMA) was formed. HMA is an interfaith, multidisciplinary organization. The parish nurse section of the HMA, with input from parish nurses attending the Westberg Symposium, and in conjunction with the ANA, published the first edition of *Scope and Standards of Parish Nursing Practice* in 1998. The second edition, titled *Faith Community Nursing: Scope and Standards of Practice,* was prepared jointly by the ANA and HMA and published in 2005.

Faith Community Nursing: Scope and Standards of Practice

Faith Community Nursing: Scope and Standards of Practice (ANA-HMA, 2005) addresses the independent practice of professional nursing, as defined by the nurse practice act in health promotion within the context of the patient's values, beliefs, and faith practices. The patient focus of an FCN is the faith community, including its family and individual members and the community it serves. Faith community nursing promotes health and healing by empowering the client system to incorporate health and healing practices from its faith perspective to achieve desired outcomes. *Faith Community Nursing: Scope and Standards of Practice* (ANA-HMA) provides a glossary of terms. Selected terms and definitions are presented in Box 1-1.

BOX 1-1
Terminology

Faith community—An organization of groups, families, and individuals who share common values, beliefs, religious doctrine, and faith practices that influence their lives, such as a church, synagogue, or mosque, and that functions as a patient system, a focus for faith community nursing.

Healing—The process of integrating the body, mind, and spirit to achieve wholeness, health, and a sense of well-being, even when the curing of disease may not occur.

Health ministry—The promotion of health and healing as part of the mission and service of a faith community to its members and the community it serves.

Health promotion—Activities and interventions that patients undertake to achieve desired health outcomes. Health promotion outcomes may be primary, the prevention of disease and injury; secondary, the early detection and appropriate intervention in illness/brokenness; or tertiary, the promotion of wholeness and sense of well-being when curing may not occur.

Illness—The experience of discomfort, brokenness, disintegration of body, mind, and spirit; and disharmony with others, the environment, and God.

Patient—A human system (faith community, group, family, individual) and its environment, viewed as an integrated whole for which the faith community nurse provides professional services.

Self-care—Actions that a patient (faith community, family, individual) would take to attain desired health outcomes, if he or she had knowledge, skills, ability resources, and motivation.

Adapted from American Nurses Association and Health Ministries Association. (2005). *Faith community nursing: Scope and standards of practice*. Silver Springs, MD: ANA, pp. 36–38. Used with permission.

Nursing: Scope and Standards of Practice (ANA, 2004) defines standards as the authoritative statements by which the nursing profession describes the responsibilities for which its practitioners are accountable. Standards reflect the values and priorities of the profession, and they provide both direction for professional practice as well as a framework for evaluation of practice outcomes. A nursing specialty, such as faith community nursing, builds upon the generic scope and standards of practice to further delineate the unique scope and standards of practice for the specialty.

The standards of care for faith community nursing practice describe a competent level of faith community nursing care, as demonstrated by the nursing process: assessment, diagnosis, outcome identification, planning, implementation (including coordination of care; health teaching and health promotion; consultation; and prescriptive authority and treatment), and evaluation. The standards of care describe care that is provided to all patients of faith community nursing services and consider their cultural, racial, ethnic worldview and diversity. The standards of professional performance describe a competent level of behavior in the faith community nursing role; quality of practice, education, professional practice evaluation, collegiality, collaboration, ethics, research, resource usefulness, and leadership. Each standard provides measurement criteria for nursing practice and for advanced nursing practice (ANA-HMA, 2005).

Philosophical Base for Faith Community Nursing Practice

A philosophy is a particular set of beliefs about the nature of something. It identifies the meaning and important elements of phenomena. Philosophies can be personal as well as organizational. The IPNRC has developed a philosophy statement about parish nursing that is presented in Box 1-2.

BOX 1-2
Philosophy of Parish Nursing

Parish nursing is a specialty practice and professional model of health ministry distinguished by the following beliefs:

The parish nurse role reclaims the historical roots of health and healing found in many religious traditions. Parish nurses live out the early work of monks, nuns, and deacons and deaconesses, church nurses, traditional healers, and the nursing profession itself.

The spiritual dimension is central to parish nursing practice. Personal spiritual formation is essential for the parish nurse. The practice holds that all persons are sacred and must be treated with respect and dignity. Compelled by the beliefs the parish nurse serves, advocating with compassion, mercy, and justice. The parish nurse assists and supports individuals, families, and communities in becoming more active partners in the stewardship of personal and communal health resources.

The parish nurse understands health to be a dynamic process, which embodies the spiritual, psychological, physical, and social dimensions of the person. Spiritual health is central to well-being and influences a person's entire being. A sense of well-being can exist in the presence of disease, and healing can exist in the absence of cure.

The focus of practice is the faith community and its ministry. The parish nurse, in collaboration with the pastoral staff and congregants, participates in the ongoing transformation of the faith community into a source of health and healing. Through partnership with other community health resources, parish nursing fosters new and creative responses to health and wellness concerns.

IPNRC, 2005, Used with permission.

The first paragraph of the philosophy statement ties parish nursing practice to its historical roots. The second paragraph begins with two key sentences that state, "The spiritual dimension is central to parish nursing practice. Personal spiritual formation is essential for the parish nurse." These two sentences truly describe what this specialty is all about. The integration of faith and health is at the heart of parish nursing practice. The paragraph goes on to speak about the sacred nature of persons and the concept of the nurse and client being partners in the stewardship of health resources. The third paragraph enlarges the concept of person, which includes dimensions of spiritual, psychological, physical, and social. It also addresses the dichotomies of well-being in the presence of illness and healing in the absence of cure. The final paragraph addresses the focus of practice as the faith community and its ministry. It speaks to the concepts of collaboration and partnership with other resources to foster new and creative responses to health and wellness concerns.

Faith Community Nursing and Nursing Theory and Research

Simply defined, a theory provides a direction in how to view facts and events. A nursing theory would therefore provide direction in how to view the facts and events that occur in nursing practice. Polit and Beck (2004) define a theory as a systematic, abstract explanation of some aspect of reality. They state that, in a theory, concepts are knitted together into a coherent system to describe or explain some aspect of the world.

Meleis (1997) defines nursing theory as "a conceptualization of some aspect of reality (invented or discovered) that pertains to nursing. The concept is articulated for the purpose of describing, explaining, predicting or prescribing nursing care" (p. 16).

Theories are composed of concepts (and their definitions) and propositions that explain the relationships between the concepts. For example, Nightingale *proposed* a beneficial relationship between fresh air and health. Theories are based on stated assumptions that are presented as givens. They must be taken as "truths" because they cannot be empirically tested, such as a value statement or ethic. Theories can be presented as models that provide a diagram or map of the content (Hickman, 2002).

Barnum (1998) states that a complete nursing theory is one that identifies four elements: context, content, process, and goal. Context is the environment in which the nursing act takes place; content is the subject of the theory; process is the method that the nurse uses in applying the theory; and goal is the intended aim of the theory, what the nurse hopes to achieve. The nurse acts on, with or through the content elements of the theory.

The *level* of a theory refers to the scope of phenomena to which the theory applies. The level of abstraction of the concepts in the theory is closely tied to its scope. *Metatheory* refers to theory about theory. In nursing, metatheory considers broad issues, such as the processes for generating knowledge and theory development. *Grand theories* are the most complex theories, and they are the broadest in scope. They are nonspecific and composed of abstract concepts that are not operationally defined. Their propositions are also abstract and not subject to testing (McEwen & Wills, 2002). In the same vein, a *school of thought* has been defined by Parse (1998) as a theoretical point of view held by a community of scholars. Theory is a tradition, including specific assumptions and principles, a specified focus of inquiry, and congruent approaches to research and practice.

Middle range theories are narrower in focus. They are made up of a limited number of concepts and propositions that are written at a fairly concrete level. Fawcett (2000) states that middle range *descriptive* theories are the most basic type. Middle range *explanatory* theories specify relationships between concepts, whereas middle range *predictive* theories predict precise relations between concepts or the effects of one or more concepts on one or more other concepts. Predictive middle range theories address how changes occur in a phenomenon. Most importantly, the propositions of middle range theories are testable by clinical research and thus become the basis for nursing practice.

Although nurses use theories from other disciplines to *inform* nursing practice, *only* nursing theories contribute to the body of knowledge that is nursing science. A very important distinction, it underlies the concept of evidence-based or research-based practice in nursing.

Why is nursing theory important to the faith community nurse? The clear answer to this question is that nursing theory provides the rationale for nursing practice. In applied disciplines, such as nursing, practice is based on theories that are validated through the research process; therefore, theory, research, and practice affect each other in a reciprocal, cyclical, and interactive way (Figure 1-1). Middle range theory can be tested in nursing practice by clinical research. The research process may validate a theory, cause it to be modified, or invalidate it. As the volume of research about a theory increases, its usefulness to nursing practice increases. Research findings are published in the periodical literature and, in books, are presented at professional conferences and are available through abstracts, such as Dissertation Abstracts International (Hickman, 2002).

Nursing research may be based on the positivist or naturalistic paradigms (Box 1-3). Positivistic view research is *quantitative*. In this type of research, statistical data represent empirical or observable facts and events. The methodology of quantitative research is the scientific method. Research data are pieces of information obtained in the course of the study. The researcher identifies the variables of interest, develops operational definitions of those variables, and collects relevant data from subjects. The actual values of the study variables constitute the data for statistical analysis. Quantitative research often looks for relationships between different variables. For example, do individuals who attend religious services lead healthier lives?

In the naturalistic view, research is *qualitative* in nature, based on the thoughts, feelings, and beliefs of the research participants. Positivism reflects the cultural phenomenon of

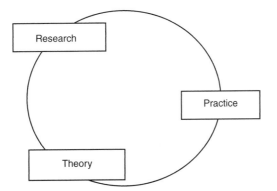

Figure 1-1 Nursing practice is based on theories that are validated through the research process; therefore, theory, research, and practice affect each other in a reciprocal, cyclical, and interactive way.

BOX 1-3
Major Assumptions of the Positivist and Naturalistic Paradigms

ASSUMPTION	POSITIVISTIC PARADIGM	NATURALISTIC PARADIGM
Ontologic (What is the nature of reality?)	Reality exists; there is a real world driven by real natural causes.	Reality is multiple and subjective, mentally constructed by individuals.
Epistemological (How is the inquirer related to those being researched?)	The inquirer is independent from those being researched; findings are not influenced by the researcher.	The inquirer interacts with those being researched; findings are the creation of the interactive process.
Axiologic (What is the role of values in the inquiry?)	Values and biases are to be held in check; objectivity is sought.	Subjectivity and values are inevitable and desirable.
Methodological (How is knowledge obtained?)	Deductive processes. Emphasis on discrete, specific concepts. Verification of researcher's hunches. Fixed design. Tight controls over context. Emphasis on measured, quantitative information, statistical analysis. Seeks generalizations.	Inductive processes. Emphasis on entirety of some phenomenon; holistic. Emerging interpretations grounded in participants' experiences. Flexible design. Context-bound. Emphasis on narrative information, qualitative analysis. Seeks patterns.

Adapted from Polit, D. F., & Beck, C. T. (2004). *Nursing research: Principles and methods* (7th ed., p. 14). Philadelphia: Lippincott Williams & Wilkins. Used with permission.

modernism, whereas naturalism is an outgrowth of the cultural transformation referred to as *postmodernism*. Postmodern thinking emphasizes the value of deconstruction—that is, taking apart old ideas and structures and reconstructing them in new ways. Naturalists take the position of *relativism*, that there are always multiple interpretations of reality that exist in people's minds. They believe that subjective interactions are the primary way to understand phenomena of interest. Therefore, the research findings of this approach will be the product of the interaction between the researcher and participant. Various methods are available to the qualitative researcher (Polit & Beck, 2004) (Box 1-4).

Nursing theories provide a lens for looking at nursing practice. Four concepts have been identified as comprising the metaparadigm or global perspective of nursing: person, health, environment, and nursing. Although there have been endless arguments about whether these concepts could or should be expanded, they do provide a starting point for the novice to look at different theories.

Person refers to a holistic (biopsychosocial-spiritual) being who is more than and different from the sum of the parts. Nursing theorists are often most distinctive in the way they define the concept of person. Some of these definitions are not congruent with the philosophy of parish nursing, and some will not be acceptable to some faith traditions. *Health* is defined in many different ways in the literature, and nursing theorists span the spectrum in their definitions. *Environment* refers to the elements that are external to a person. *Nursing* is the science, art, and practice of the discipline. With the notable exception of Nightingale, the nursing theorists of the last 2 decades most clearly address all four concepts of the metaparadigm.

Berquist and King (1994) presented the first conceptual model of parish nursing. They describe the client as a physiological, emotional, and spiritual person. Health is defined as optimal wellness and wholeness. They identify the faith community to be the environment. They describe parish nursing practice as incorporating roles that include health educator,

---

BOX 1-4
Qualitative Research Methods

RESEARCH TRADITION	AREA OF INQUIRY
Ethnography	Holistic view of a culture
Phenomenology	Lived experiences of individuals
Hermeneutics	Interpretations and meanings of individual's experiences
Grounded theory	Social structural processes within a social setting
History	Descriptions and interpretation of historical events
Case study	In-depth investigations of a single entity or small number of entities
Action	Collaboration between researchers and subjects to define and solve a problem
Narrative analysis	Focuses on *story* in studies, in which the purpose is to determine how individuals make sense of their lives

Adapted from Polit, D. F., & Beck, C. T. (2004). *Nursing research: Principles and methods* (7th ed., p. 249). Philadelphia: Lippincott Williams & Wilkins. Used with permission.

health counselor, leader of individuals and groups, and community liaison. In this model, the goal of parish nursing practice is to enhance the holistic health and well-being of the faith community members. Bunkers (1998, 1999) and Putnam (1995) describes a nursing theory-guided model of health ministry and parish nursing at the First Presbyterian Church in Sioux Falls, South Dakota. The model is a community nursing practice model based on Parse's theory of human becoming paralleled with the Beatitudes. The model was chosen because it focuses on quality of life from the person's/parish's perspective, and it uses the strengths and resources within the church as the foundation for providing care. Parse's theory views health as a process of becoming—a personal commitment to a lived value system (1981, 1987, 1990). He states that quality of life is whatever the person living it says that it is (Parse, 1994).

Bunkers (1995, 1998, 1999) describes the parish nurse practicing with this theory as being open to how others choose to live, without judging their choices. She adds that a nurse living the theory of human becoming in practice is open to a person's uniqueness and possibilities for new ways of evolving.

The Miller Model for Parish Nursing was developed in Miller's doctoral dissertation. The model is based on the theological perspective of evangelical Christianity and contains four components: person/parishioner, health, nurse/parish nurse, and community/parish. The core integrating concept of the Miller Model is the Triune God. Miller (1997) states that the centrality of the concept is what makes her parish nursing model unique. She underscores that health and healing are integral to the Christian church's mission and ministry. Miller diagrams her model in three stained glass windows. The first window details the components and major concepts of the model, which include: Triune God surrounded by health, parish nurse, community and parishioner, ministry, dependence, mission, confession, communion, dignity, shalom-wholeness, and stewardship. The second window presents aspects of the whole person and health-promoting resources. The third window presents the contexts of the parish nurse role.

Wilson (1997) created the Parish Nursing Continuity of Care Model which emphasizes harmony in mind, body, and spirit. It depicts "the nurse as the focal point of the model who connects individuals and families with resources to provide care to a congregation over life's continuum: physical birth, new life—being born again in Christ, suffering—the pains and sorrows of life, surrender—to God's grace and mercy, physical death and resurrection—everlasting life in glory with Christ" (p. 94).

A fourth model of parish nursing, the Circle of Christian Caring, was developed by Maddox (2001). In this model, parish nursing is envisioned as "an opportunity to combine the spiritual and physical dimensions of caregiving and to affirm the church as a place for disease prevention and health promotion" (p. 12). Parish nurse roles are identified as health educator, health counselor, referral resource/client advocate, facilitator/leader, and home visitor.

O'Brien (2003) developed the theory of spiritual well-being in illness. This type is a middle range theory that derives from earlier conceptualizations in the area of spiritual well-being and from the Travelbee Model. The core component of this theory is the concept of finding spiritual meaning in the experience of illness. O'Brien's conceptual model includes personal faith and its components, spiritual contentment and its components, and religious practice and its components—mediated by the severity of illness, social support system, and current stressful life events, which results in spiritual well-being in illness. Empirical testing of this theory has begun, and findings support the following hypotheses: Significant relationships will occur between: (a) the degree of a sick person's personal faith and his or her perceived quality of life in an illness experience, (b) the activity of a sick person's religious practices and his or her perceived quality of life in an illness experience, and (c) the degree of a sick person's spiritual contentment and his or her perceived quality of life. O'Brien recommends that further research about her theory should use methodological triangulation, collecting both quantitative and qualitative data to explore these relationships.

Many nursing theories are appropriate for use in faith community nursing. However, different faith traditions will approach each theory from a different place. For example, some nurse theorists *purposely* choose *not* to explicitly address the concept of God, but their definitions of person and environment encompass the presence of God in a person's life. These theories can be used by persons of diverse faith traditions.

Shelly and Miller (1999) strongly advocate an explicitly Christian theology of nursing. They state that a Christian worldview cannot be superimposed on any other worldview. They define Christian nursing as "a ministry of compassionate care for the whole person, in response to God's grace toward a sinful world, which aims to foster optimum health (shalom) and bring comfort in suffering and death for anyone in need" (p. 18). Stegmeir (2002) and Schoonover-Shoffner (2002) also strongly speak against adjusting nursing theories to Christian beliefs.

Miller (2002) voices concern about nursing theory that is based solely on philosophy. She developed an evaluation tool to assist her students to discover the underlying foundational beliefs of nurse theorists. Her tool includes asking the following questions about a theory/theorist.

"What does the theorist (or you) believe about

- origin and destiny of humankind?
- nature and character of self/other?
- purpose of what exists?
- evidence of plans and patterns regarding what exists?
- problems, such as suffering/disease, death/dying, sin, evil, right/wrong, hope, joy, and peace?
- relatedness?
- time?
- universe/environment?" (Miller, 2002, p. 9)

As a Christian nurse educator, Miller strongly advocates nursing theory to be developed from an explicitly Christian worldview (2002).

Application of Theory to Faith Community Nursing Practice

The case study at the end of the chapter presents a clinical faith community nursing case study. Three nursing theories will be applied to the case study to illustrate the differences of each theoretical approach to practice. Neuman's Systems Model, Watson's Theory of Human Caring, and Parse's Theory of Human Becoming will be used to direct how the nurse would act in the case study situation. Although an overview of each nursing theory will be provided, the reader is referred to nursing theory textbooks for complete presentations of each of the theories.

Application Example: Neuman's Systems Model

Neuman (1995) conceptualizes the client as a unique composite of five interacting variables: physiological, psychological, sociocultural, developmental, and spiritual. These variables function together as the basic structure energy resources of the client and function to attain, maintain, or retain system stability. The client system consists of the flexible lines of defense, the normal line of defense, and lines of resistance. The normal line of defense represents the client's usual level of wellness. The line of defense is considered to be dynamic and can expand or contract over time. The flexible lines of defense act as the client system's first line of defense against invading stressors. When the flexible lines of defense are breached, signs and symptoms occur. The lines of resistance within the client system then respond to these signs and symptoms to support the client's basic structure. When the lines of resistance are effective, signs and symptoms diminish, and the client system returns to a stable state (Neuman). In the case study at the end of the chapter, Mrs. B. is exhibiting signs and symptoms of depression and activities-of-daily-living (ADL) limitations related to rheumatoid arthritis.

Neuman uses the concept of prevention as intervention. She defines primary prevention as intervention that involves the nurse's use of interventions that promote client wellness by stressor prevention and reduction of risk factors. The interventions can begin at any point before a client reaction to a stressor has occurred. The interventions protect the flexible lines of defense and include health promotion activities. Once a reaction to a stressor has occurred, the nurse would use secondary prevention interventions to protect the basic structures by strengthening the lines of resistance. The goal would be to return the client system to a stable state. Reconstitution is the term that represents the return and maintenance of system stability following a nursing intervention for stressor reaction. Tertiary prevention as intervention includes the actions designed to maintain optimum wellness by supporting existing strengths and conserving client system energy (1995). The family in the case study has nursing needs that would be addressed at all three levels of prevention as intervention.

Neuman (1995) designed a three-step nursing process format composed of nursing diagnosis (based on comprehensive data), nursing goals that are mutually set by the nurse and patient, along with mutually agreed-upon prevention as intervention strategies, and nursing outcomes. In this case study, the FCN performs an assessment and arrives at a diagnosis. Together with the patient, plans and goals are discussed and agreed upon, action is taken, and nursing outcomes are evaluated.

Application Example: Parse's Theory of Human Becoming

Parse's theory of human becoming is a human science system of interrelated concepts describing the person's mutual process with the universe in co-creating becoming. It has its roots in the human sciences, which suggests methodologies directed at uncovering the meaning of phenomena as humanly experienced. The methods of inquiry lead to the creation of theories about the lived experiences. A fundamental tenet of Parse's theory is the individual's participation in health (1998). Health is described as a synthesis of values, as a way of living. Health is a continuously changing process that humans co-create in mutual process through the human–universe experience, and it is incarnated as patterns of relating value priorities. From the perspective of this theory, health or quality of life is what the person describes it to be, rather than a standard or norm (Parse, 1981, 1987, 1990).

Parse (1998) describes nursing practice as the art of living human becoming. The art of nursing is described as using the nurse's body of knowledge in service to people with the goal of quality of life from the person's perspective. The assumptions that underlie the nursing process, that the nurse is the authority on health and the person can be "fixed," are not congruent with the theory of human becoming. Parse states that living *true presence* is unique to the art of human becoming. She defines true presence as "an intentional reflective love, an interpersonal art grounded in a strong knowledge base" (p. 71). "True presence . . . is lived in the parish community in a loving, reflective way, bearing witness to others' living health and honoring each person's uniqueness without judging him or her. The nurse, in true presence, respects people as knowing their own way, a chosen personal way of being with the world" (Cody, Bunkers, & Mitchell, 2001, p. 242).

Parse's (1987) practice dimensions are: *illuminating meaning, synchronizing rhythms,* and *moving beyond.* With the true presence of the nurse, Mr. and Mrs. B. *illuminated meanings* concerning their situation of living with both physical and social interaction limitations. They *synchronized rhythms* in developing new patterns of managing chronic disease and relating to each other, to the nurse, and to the faith community. They *moved beyond* their present struggles to engage in new ways of living health.

Choosing to practice nursing using Parse's theory of human becoming requires a major paradigm shift for most practicing nurses.

Application Example: Watson's Theory of Human Caring

In Watson's theory of human caring, love and caring come together to form a new form of deep transpersonal caring. The relationship of love and caring connotes inner healing for self and others that extends to the larger universe. As Watson's theory has evolved over time she has moved from the concept of "carative" to the concept of "caritas," which she states comes from the Greek word meaning to cherish, to appreciate, to give special attention to. Watson says that when we include caring and love in our work we discover and affirm that nursing is more than a job, it is a life-giving and life-receiving career for a lifetime of growth and learning. She advises that such thinking calls for a sense of reverence and sacredness with regard to life and all living things. It also acknowledges a convergence between art, science, and spirituality (Watson, 2001). Watson says that transpersonal caring relationships are foundational to the work of nursing. These relationships seek "to connect with and embrace the spirit or soul of the other, through the processes of caring and healing . . ." (p. 347).

BOX 1-5
Watson's Carative Factors to Clinical Caritas Processes

1. Formation of humanistic-altruistic system of values *becomes* practice of loving kindness and equanimity within the context of caring consciousness.

2. Instillation of faith-hope *becomes* being authentically present and enabling and sustaining the deep belief system and subjective life world of self and one being cared for.

3. Cultivation of sensitivity to one's self and to others *becomes* cultivation of one's own spiritual practices and transpersonal self, going beyond ego self, opening to others with sensitivity and compassion.

4. Development of a helping-trusting human caring relationship *becomes* developing and sustaining a helping-trusting authentic caring relationship.

5. Promotion and acceptance of the expression of positive and negative feelings *becomes* being present to, and supportive of, the expression of positive and negative feelings as a connection with deeper spirit of self and one being cared for.

6. Systematic use of a creative problem-solving caring process *becomes* creative use of self and all ways of knowing as part of the caring process; to engage in artistry of caring-healing practices.

7. Promotion of transpersonal teaching-learning *becomes* engaging in genuine teaching-learning experience that attends to unity of being and meaning, attempting to stay within others' frames of reference.

8. Provision for a supportive, protective, and/or corrective mental, physical, societal, and spiritual environment *becomes* creating environment at all levels (physical as well as nonphysical, subtle environment of energy and consciousness, whereby wholeness, beauty, comfort, dignity, and peace are potentiated).

9. Assistance with gratification of human needs *becomes* assisting with basic needs, with intentional caring consciousness, administering "human care essential," which potentiates alignment of mind-body-spirit, wholeness, and unity of being in all aspects of care, tending both embodied spirit and evolving spiritual emergence.

10. Allowance for existential-phenomenological-spiritual forces *becomes* opening and attending to spiritual forces becomes opening and attending to spiritual mysteries and existential dimensions of one's own life-death; soul care for self and the one being cared for.

Adapted from Watson, J. (2001). Jean Watson theory of human caring. In M. Parker (Ed.), *Nursing theories and nursing practice* (p. 347). Philadelphia: FA Davis. Used with permission.

Nursing theory develops in dynamic ways; therefore, theories may change over time. Watson's theory originally identified 10 carative factors. She has recently revised these 10 carative factors into 10 clinical caritas processes (Box 1-5). Watson says that what differs in the two frameworks is that in the clinical caritas there is a decidedly spiritual dimension and an overt evocation of love and caring merging. Watson states that she views her work more as a philosophical, ethical, intellectual blueprint for nursing's evolving professional matrix, rather than a specific theory per se.

Watson states that a caring occasion occurs whenever the nurse and another come together with their unique human histories. It involves an action and a choice by both the nurse and the other. She says that if the caring moment is transpersonal, each feels a connection with the other at the spirit level. The caring-healing modalities foster harmony, wholeness, and unity.

Because of the high level of abstraction of the theory of human caring, it is less easy to "see" the nursing actions in the case study. The FCN using Watson's theory of human caring views the way in which Mr. and Mrs. B.'s situation is affecting their relationships and the activities that give meaning to their lives. A first step would be for the nurse and one being cared for to reflect on the things that make life meaningful. This process reflects the clinical caritas processes. The FCN learns that Mrs. B. is feeling useless because of her disabilities and embarrassed by her disfigurement and guilty for burdening her husband with her care. The FCN learns from Mr. B that he misses social interaction and that he is concerned about his wife's depression. From the beginning, the FCN engaged the couple in a discussion of ways to promote dignity and harmony of mind, body, and spirit. This entailed a process of mutual reflection on the possibilities for growth and fulfillment in the situation. Ultimately, an antidepressant medication was prescribed with positive results, cleaning help was hired, and the couple were able to increase their social and church participation.

Summary

This chapter has provided the reader with an overview of the history of nursing with attention to its roots in faith traditions. The development of faith community/parish nursing as a nursing specialty was presented from its inception to current practice. Discussion of the philosophy of faith community/parish nursing moved into a broader discussion of the philosophical and theoretical foundations of nursing science, research, and practice. Models and frameworks for parish nursing practice were presented and discussed. Three nursing theories were used as application examples, with a clinical case study.

Reflect and Discuss

1. Reflect on how concepts of caring were addressed in your undergraduate nursing curriculum. Are these concepts evident to you in current nursing practice?
2. Consider the decade in which you graduated from college. What historical events shaped that decade? Did the events have an impact on your nursing education?
3. What is your personal philosophy of nursing? How do you define person, health, environment, and nursing?
4. Compare and contrast the characteristics of qualitative and quantitative research. How might each type of research be conducted in the faith community/parish nursing setting?
5. Reflect on a recent clinical experience and consider what might be different, if you approached it from a different theoretical framework.

Case Study

Mr. B. is a 70-year-old African American man who lives with his wife in a small, single family house in a suburban neighborhood. Mr. B. has a history of hypertension and congestive heart failure, which he manages with medication. Mrs. B. is 68 years old and has severe rheumatoid arthritis, which greatly limits her ability to perform her ADLs. Since his retirement, Mr. B. has gradually assumed most of the household chores and assists his wife with dressing and bathing. The couple were active in their church for many years, but recently they have limited their participation to attending worship services.

Mr. B. calls the faith community nurse (FCN) to share his concern that his wife seems to be depressed and uninterested in doing anything of late. Although he would like to be more active socially and take some day trips, his wife says she would rather stay at home and watch television.

The FCN makes a home visit to Mr. and Mrs. B. to assess their situation. She finds Mrs. B. up and dressed neatly and sitting in a recliner. After some discussion, Mrs. B. shares that she feels that she is useless because of her physical limitations and that she is embarrassed by the disfigurement of her hands. She says she greatly misses cooking for her husband and feeling in control of her life. She admits to feeling guilty for burdening her husband when he should be enjoying his retirement.

In subsequent visits, the FCN explored with Mrs. B. what her hopes for the future were and what changes might improve her situation. A depression screening was performed by the FCN, and Mrs. B. was found to be moderately depressed. Mrs. B.'s physician was consulted by the FCN, and an antidepressant medication was prescribed. Mrs. B. responded well to the medication. Eventually, a biweekly cleaning service was engaged, and the couple began to attend events at church and the local senior center.

References

American Nurses Association. (2004). *Nursing: Scope & standards of practice.* Washington, D.C.: ANA.

Ashley, J. A. (1976). *Hospitals, paternalism, and the role of the nurse.* New York: Teachers College Press.

Baer, E. D. (1999). Commentary: Private duty nursing. In T. M. Schorr & M. S. Kennedy (Eds.), *100 Years of American nursing.* Philadelphia: Lippincott Williams & Wilkins.

Barnum, B. S. (1998). *Nursing theory: Analysis-application-evaluation* (5th ed.). Philadelphia: Lippincott.

Barnum, B. S. (2003). *Spirituality in nursing: From traditional to new age* (2nd ed.). New York: Springer-Verlag.

Berquist, S. & King, J. (1994). Parish nursing: A conceptual framework. *Journal of Holistic Nursing, 12*(2), 155–170.

Buhler-Wilkerson, K. (2001). *No place like home: A history of nursing and home care in the United States.* Baltimore: Johns Hopkins University Press.

Bunkers, S. S. (1998). A nursing theory-guided model of health ministry: Human becoming in parish nursing. *Nursing Science Quarterly, 11*, 7–8.

Bunkers, S. S. (1999). Translating nursing conceptual frameworks and theory for nursing practice. In P. A. Solari-Twadell & M. A. McDermott (Eds.), *Parish nursing: Promoting whole person health within faith communities.* Thousand Oaks, CA: Sage.

Bunkers, S. S. & Putnam, V. (1995). A nursing theory-based model of health ministry: Living Parse's theory of human becoming in the parish community. *Ninth Annual Westberg Parish Nurse Symposium: Parish ministering through the arts.* Northbrook, IL: Advocate Health Care.

Calabria, M. & Macrae, J. (Eds.). (1994). *Suggestions for thought by Florence Nightingale: Selections and commentaries.* Philadelphia: University of Pennsylvania Press. (Original work published in 1860).

Cody, W. K., Bunkers, S. S., & Mitchell, G. J. (2001). The human becoming theory in practice, research, administration, regulation and education. In M. Parker (Ed.), *Nursing theories and nursing practice.* Philadelphia: FA Davis.

Dickoff, J., James, P., & Wiedenbach, E. (1968). Theory in a practice discipline, Part 1: Practice-oriented theory. *Nursing Research, 17,* 197–203.

Dolan, J. A., Fitzpatrick, M. L., & Herrmann, E. K. (1983). *Nursing in society: A historical perspective* (15th ed.). Philadelphia: WB Saunders.

Donley, R. (1991). Spiritual dimensions of health care: Nursing's mission. *Nursing & Health Care, 12,* 178–183.

Dorff, E. N. (1986). In R. L. Members & D. W. Amundsen (Eds.), *Caring and curing: Health and Medicine in Western religious traditions* (pp. 5–39). New York: Macmillan.

Ebersole, P. (2000). Parish nurse leaders. *Geriatric Nursing, 21*(3), 148–149.

Fawcett, J. (2000). *Analysis and evaluation of contemporary nursing knowledge: Nursing models and theories.* Philadelphia: FA Davis.

Health Ministries Association and American Nurses Association. (2005). *Faith community nursing: Scope and standards of practice* (2nd ed.). Washington, DC: American Nurses Publishing.

Health Ministries Association and American Nurses Association. (1998). *Scope and standards of parish nursing practice.* Washington, DC: American Nurses Publishing.

Hickman, J. S. (2002). An introduction to nursing theory. In J. B. George (Ed.), *Nursing theories: The base for professional practice* (5th ed.). Upper Saddle River, NJ: Prentice Hall.

International Parish Nurse Resource Center. (2005, February 8). A word about "parish nurse" ministry (p. 3). *IPNRC eNotes.*

International Parish Nurse Resource Center. (2004). Available at: http://www.ipnrc.parishnurses.org.

Kalisch, P. A. & Kalisch, B. J. (1995). *The advance of American nursing* (3rd ed.). Philadelphia: Lippincott Williams & Wilkins.

Kalisch, P. A. & Kalisch, B. J. (2004). *American nursing: A history* (4th ed.). Philadelphia: Lippincott Williams & Wilkins.

Koenig, H. G., McCullough, M. E., & Larson, D. B. (2001). *Handbook of religion and health.* New York: Oxford University Press.

Leininger, M. (1991). *Culture care diversity and universality: A theory of nursing.* New York: NLN Press.

Leininger, M. & McFarland, M. R. (2001). *Transcultural nursing: Concepts, theories, research, and practice* (3rd ed.). New York: McGraw-Hill.

Lindberg, C. (1986). The Lutheran tradition. In R. L. Members & D. W. Amundsen (Eds.), *Caring and curing: Health and medicine in Western religious traditions* (pp. 5–39). New York: Macmillan.

Macrae, J. A. (2001). *Nursing as a spiritual practice: A contemporary application of Florence Nightingale's views.* New York: Springer-Verlag.

Maddox, M. (2001). Circle of Christian caring: A model for parish nursing practice. *Journal of Christian Nursing, 18*(3), 11–13.

McEwen, M. & Wills, E. M. (2002). *Theoretical basis for nursing.* Philadelphia: Lippincott Williams & Wilkins.

Meleis, A. I. (1997). *Theoretical nursing: Development and progress* (3rd ed.). Philadelphia: J. B. Lippincott.

Miller, B. J. (2002). Who needs theories, anyhow? Critical thinking about faith, reason & nursing theory. *Journal of Christian Nursing, 19*(3), 6–10.

Miller, L. W. (1997). Nursing through a lens of faith: A conceptual model. *Journal of Christian Nursing, 14*(1), 17–21.

Nelson, S. (1997). Pastoral care and moral government: Early nineteenth century nursing and solutions to the Irish question. *Journal of Advanced Nursing, 26,* 6–14.

Neuman, B. (1995). *The Neuman systems model,* 3rd ed. Norwalk, CT: Appleton & Lange.

Nist, J. A. (2003, January–February). Parish nursing programs: Through them, faith communities are reclaiming a role in healing. *Health Progress, 84*(1), 50–54.

O'Brien, M. A. (2003). *Parish nursing: Healthcare ministry within the church.* Subury, MA: Jones and Bartlett.

Ohlson, V. & Wood, V. (1999). Commentary: Public health and community health nursing. In T. M. Schorr & M. S. Kennedy (Eds.), *100 Years of American nursing.* Philadelphia: Lippincott Williams & Wilkins.

Parse, R. R. (1990). Health: A personal commitment. *Nursing Science Quarterly, 3,* 136–140.

Parse, R. R. (1998). *The human becoming school of thought.* Thousand Oaks, CA: Sage.

Parse, R. R. (1981). *Man-living-health: A theory of nursing.* New York: Delmar.

Parse, R. R. (1987). *Nursing science: Major paradigms, theories, and critiques.* Philadelphia: WB Saunders.

Parse, R. R. (1994). Quality of life: Sciencing and living the art of human becoming. *Nursing Science Quarterly, 7,* 16–20.

Peplau, H. E. (1952). *Interpersonal relations in nursing.* New York: GP Putnam's Sons.

Polit, D. F. & Beck, C. T. (2004). *Nursing research: Principles and methods* (7th ed.). Philadelphia: Lippincott Williams & Wilkins.

Reverby, S. M. (1982). Ordered to care: The dilemma of American nursing 1850–1945. London: Cambridge University Press.

Schoonover-Shoffner, K. (2002). Does "adjusting" go far enough? *Journal of Christian Nursing, 19*(3), 12–13.

Shelly, J. A. & Miller, A. B. (1999). *Called to care: A Christian theology of nursing.* Downers Grove, IL: InterVarsity Press.

Stegmeir, D. (2002). Faith & nursing: Adjusting nursing theories to Christian beliefs. *Journal of Christian Nursing, 19*(3), 11–15.

Watson, J. (2001). Jean Watson theory of human caring. In M. Parker (Ed.), *Nursing theories and nursing practice.* Philadelphia: FA Davis.

Watson, J. (1979). *Nursing: The philosophy and science of caring.* Boston: Little, Brown and Company.

Wehling, B. & Rethemeyer A. (2002). Perish nurse ministry survey: An outcomes measurement tool. [On-line]. Available http://www.ipnrc.parishnurses.org/westsymp2002survey.phtml

Westberg, G. (1990). *The parish nurse: Providing a minister of health for your congregation.* Minneapolis: Augsburg.

Westberg, G. (1999). A personal historical perspective of whole person health and the congregation. In P. A. Solari-Twadell & M. A. McDermott (Eds.), *Parish nursing: Promoting whole person health within faith communities.* Thousand Oaks, CA: Sage.

Wilson, R. P. (1997). What does the parish nurse do? *Journal of Christian Nursing, 14*(1), 13–16.

Additional Resources

Alligood, M. R. & McGuire, S. L. (2000). Perceptions of time, sleep patterns and activity in senior citizens: A test of a Rogerian theory of aging. *Visions: The Journal of Rogerian Nursing Science, 8*(1), 6–14.

Berry, A. B. (1999). Mexican-American women's expressions of the meaning of culturally congruent prenatal care. *Journal of Transcultural Nursing, 10*(3), 203–212.

Cortis, J. D. (2000). Caring as experienced by minority ethnic patients. *International Nursing Review, 47*(1), 53–62.

Gigliotti, E. (2001). Empirical tests of the Neuman systems model: Relational statement analysis. *Nursing Science Quarterly, 14*(2), 149–157.

Gigliotti, E. (1999). Women's multiple role stress: Testing Neuman's flexible line of defense. *Nursing Science Quarterly, 12,* 36–44.

Goodwin, Z., Kiehl, E. M., & Peterson, J. Z. (2002). King's theory as foundation for an advance directive decision-making model. *Nursing Science Quarterly, 15*(3), 237–241.

Miller, L. W. (1996). A nursing conceptual model grounded in Christian faith. (PhD dissertation, University of Victoria.)

Parse, R. R. (2003). The lived experience of feeling very tired: A study using the Parse research method. *Nursing Science Quarterly, 16,* 319–325.

Raeside, L. (2000). Clinical. Perceptions of environmental stressors in the neonatal unit. *Journal of Neonatal Nursing, 6*(3), 93–99.

Schaefer, K. M. (2002). Reflections on caring narratives: Enhancing patterns of knowing. *Nursing Education Perspectives, 23*(6), 286–293.

Stepans, M. B. F. & Knight, J. R. (2002). Application of Neuman's framework: Infant exposure to environmental tobacco smoke. *Nursing Science Quarterly, 15*(4), 327–334.

Swanson, K. M. (1999). What is known about caring in nursing science: A literary meta-analysis. In A. S. Hinshaw, S. L. Feetham & J. L. F. Shaver (Eds.), *Handbook of clinical nursing research* (pp. 31–60). Thousand Oaks, CA: Sage.

Taylor, S. G., Geden, E., Isaramalai, S., & Wongvatunyu, S. (2000). Orem's self-care deficit nursing theory: Its philosophic foundation and the state of the science. *Nursing Science Quarterly, 13,* 104–110.

Wall, L. M. (2000). Changes in hope and power in lung cancer patients who exercise. *Nursing Science Quarterly, 13*(3), 234–242.

Watson, J. (2002). *Assessing and measuring caring in nursing and health science.* New York: Springer-Verlag.

Winsted-Fry, P. (2000). Rogers' conceptual system and family nursing. *Nursing Science Quarterly, 13,* 278–280.

Yamashita, M. (1999). Neuman's theory of health applied in family caregiving in Canada. *Nursing Science Quarterly, 12*(1), 73–79.

Yeh, C. (2001). Adaptation in children with cancer: Research with Roy's model. *Nursing Science Quarterly, 14*(2), 141–148.

Zhan, L. (2000). Cognitive adaptation and self-consistency in hearing-impaired older persons: Testing Roy's adaptation model. *Nursing Science Quarterly, 13*(2), 158–165.

→ Web Resources

http://www.ualberta.ca/~jrnorris/nttheory.html   Nursing theories home page

http://www.nursing.oakland.edu/king   Imogene King

http://www.neumann.edu   Click on UG programs, nursing, then Neuman's Systems Model

http://www.lemmus.demon.co.uk/neuman1.html   Neuman's Systems Model

http://www.muhealth.org/~nursing   Orem's Self Care   Click on scdnt

http://www.uwcm.ac.uk/uwcm/ns/martha   Society of Rogerian Scholars

http://www.forums.nyu.edu   Martha Rogers Listserv

http://www2.bc.edu/~royca   Roy Adaptation Model

http://www.tcns.org   Transcultural Nursing Society

http://www.tc.umn.edu/~hoym003/   Margaret Newman

http://www.utoronto.ca/icps   International Consortium of Parse Scholars

http://www.uwo.ca/nursing/homepg/peplau.html41   Hildegarde Peplau

http://www.uchsc.edu/ctrsinst/chc   Center for Human Caring

http://www.fau.edu   Choose "Colleges" then "Nursing"   Link to Lynn Center for Caring

http://www.kumc.edu/service/clendening/florence/florence.html   Kansas University Medical Center—Nightingale

http://www.ahna.org   American Holistic Nurses Association

http://www.healthministriesassociation.org   Health Ministries Association

http://www.parishnurses.org   International Parish Nurse Resource Center

http://www.ivcf.org/ncf   Nurses' Christian Fellowship

http://www.stephenministry.org   Stephen Ministries Foundation

http://www.deaconess.org   Deaconess Foundation

http://www.florence-nightingale-foundation.org.uk   Florence Nightingale Foundation

http://www.dcfl.org/eliz.htm   Elizabeth Ministries

http://www.vincenter.org/tree/svdp/index.html   Society of St. Vincent de Paul

2

Faith Community Nursing Models, Preparation, and Roles

This chapter will present the various models through which faith community nursing is delivered. The advantages and disadvantages of each of the models will be discussed. A profile of faith community nursing in the United States will be presented. Actual and ideal educational preparation for parish/faith community nursing will be discussed. A review of the research literature about faith community nursing roles will be presented, and the findings will be analyzed.

Models of Faith Community Nursing Practice

Essentially, four models exist through which faith community nursing services are delivered: the congregational volunteer model, the congregational paid model, the paid consortium model, and the institutional model, in which faith community nurses (FCNs) are employed and paid by a health care organization that provides care to congregations through a contractual agreement.

The original parish nurse pilot project, coordinated by Granger Westberg with the Lutheran General Hospital, was an institutional model where the parish nurses were employed by the hospital. The congregations shared a portion of the costs of providing the parish nursing services according to a contractual agreement. In the 25-year history of parish nursing, different kinds of structures have been formed to meet the needs of faith communities and the communities in which they reside.

Regardless of the faith community nursing model chosen, the most important element for success of a faith community nursing program is the support and endorsement of the faith community leader and the ministry team. The literature is rife with personal stories of well-intentioned nurses who have attempted to launch faith community nursing programs with the *permission* of the congregational leader, as opposed to that individual's endorsement and support. The stories describe disillusionment, frustration, and program failures. A second element for the success of a faith community nursing program is the ability of the structure to provide the financial support for resources over the long term. Many faith community nursing programs that were launched on "soft" or grant monies were discontinued or downsized when the funding period ended. And a third important element for success is that the faith community embraces health and healing within their mission and organizational strategic planning. This element includes program and personnel evaluation and identifying program outcomes and their measurement. A fourth element for success is the educational preparation of the FCN. As discussed in Chapter 1, *Faith Community Nursing: Scope and Standards of Practice* (ANA-HMA, 2005) defines FCN practice and recommends a baccalaureate or higher degree in nursing with academic preparation in community health nursing (p. 5).

Institutional Model

Many faith community nursing programs (previously called *parish nurse programs*) were started in the 1990s when hospitals and health care systems were looking for community outreach partnerships. This happened in response to extreme competition for clients in health care. Community outreach provided "positive" community service and served as a marketing tool for health care providers. It also provided a safety net for uninsured populations. The institutional model can be offered in a variety of ways. In some cases the institution employs a faith community nurse manager or coordinator who is paid by the institution. This coordinator assists congregations in establishing faith community nurse programs using paid or unpaid nurses. The coordinator provides resources and consultation. In other cases, the institutionally paid FCN provides direct services to one or several congregations.

Institutional models are most often hospital-directed, but long-term care facilities and community health agencies have also provided faith community nurse programs. When institutional models are driven purely by economic values, faith community programs are discontinued when the costs outweigh the benefits. Unfortunately, this was the trend in the late 1990s in the Northeast. Institutions in other regions of the country have been more supportive of faith community nursing programs, recognizing that although these programs are not revenue-producing, they provide needed and cost-effective services to vulnerable populations.

In the institutional model, the FCN is a paid employee of the health care institution and may or may not be a member of the faith community served. The mission, goals, and expected program outcomes are determined by the employing institution and therefore take priority over those of the faith community. For some faith communities, incompatible missions between the health care institution and the faith community will be unacceptable.

Important advantages of the institutional model are the resources of the employing institution. For the nurse, this will mean paid benefits, institutional liability coverage, a position description, a network of peers within the system, access to staff development, and travel reimbursement. For the program, it will mean availability of health supplies and literature, referral opportunities, uniform documentation of client service, and access to interdisciplinary professional consultation.

Smith (2000, 2003) labels the institutional model the "marketplace model." She states that the term "parish nurse" is inappropriate in the marketplace model because the efforts of these programs are not on behalf of the congregation, and the church setting is simply the venue. Smith argues that secular nursing and secular health care in churches are not the same as Christian nurses doing ministry as insider-experts in their own congregations.

Schumann (2000) responds to Smith's argument by stating that there are many secular institutions that advocate for holistic health—including spiritual health. In promoting spiritual wellness, institutions contribute to the overall well-being of the community by helping the churches to "do church" and care for the Christian family in a godly way. Clearly, this is an ecumenical viewpoint that allows for a diversity of faith traditions to benefit from faith community nursing.

Paid Congregational Model

In this model, members of the congregation are served by a paid FCN who is a member of the faith community. The FCN discerns a spiritual call to serve in this ministry role. The focus is not on the nurse but on the persons served. Authority for the position comes from being called by God to the ministry and by being endorsed or installed by the congregation. As an employee of the faith community, the FCN is usually accountable to the faith community leader and a board or other faith community organizational structure. The objectives of the faith community nursing program and the position description of the FCN are directed by the ministry goals of the congregation. Benefits, travel reimbursement, liability insurance coverage, and staff development are negotiated as a part of the hiring process.

Smith (2000, 2003) labels this model (as well as the volunteer congregation-based one) as the mission/ministry model. The congregationally based models are the only models that she believes are deserving of the title *faith community nurse*, as in these, the Christian ministry aspect of faith community nursing is paramount.

Paid FCNs serve their faith communities as full-time or part-time employees. Goals and expectations need to be congruent with the hours worked, and this concept is easier stated than accomplished! Many FCNs serve in part-time capacities and need to be realistic in both goal setting and outcome expectations. Programs and services are planned and implemented based on the assessed needs of the faith community and the personnel, financial, and time resources available.

Paid Consortium Model

In the consortium model of faith community nursing, the FCN is paid by a consortium of faith communities. The FCN may divide her time equally between the congregations in the consortium, or the FCN may develop health programming that rotates the delivery setting between the congregations in the consortium, to share resources. Many consortium arrangements were originally funded with grant monies. As the funding terms ended, the only way some faith communities could afford to retain their faith community nursing program was to share costs with others.

Congregational Model: Volunteer

In the voluntary model, the FCN is considered to be a part of the ministry team of the congregation but provides services without compensation. The job description and selection of the FCN is determined by the organizational structure of the congregation. Documentation requirements are established with the pastor/board of the congregation, with consideration of the nurse's professional accountability.

The part-time, volunteer model of faith community nursing is the one most frequently found. Part-time, as well as retired nurses are functioning effectively as voluntary FCNs, while maintaining all aspects of professional nursing standards. Many FCNs see advantages and flexibility in the voluntary model of parish nursing. Voluntary models do allow the FCN flexibility in terms of role focus, program implementation, and scheduling.

Smith (2003) lists three areas of concern related to the volunteer model: (a) church volunteers versus ministry staff, (b) pastoral and administrative support, and (c) professional accountability (p. 20). She states that the term "ministry staff" denotes mutual expectations of both the church and the nurse, whereas responsibilities are negotiable when the term "volunteer" is used. She voices concern that the pastoral administrative leadership needs to give visible support for the faith community nursing program and clearly tie it to the mission of the faith community. Even though the volunteer FCN feels a call to serve, that does not negate professional responsibilities to public regulations and nurse practice acts. Smith believes that the volunteer model leaves much to be desired. She questions whether working nurses can do justice to a faith community nursing program while operating on a volunteer basis and whether volunteer retired nurses want to do all that is required for professional accountability.

Summary of Models

In terms of creating a vibrant and comprehensive faith community nursing program, the literature recommends the full-time compensated model. However, in reality, the majority of FCNs function effectively as part-time volunteers, while maintaining all aspects of professional nursing standards.

Because of the financial constraints of faith communities and health care providers, more and more models are evolving and blending the four traditional models in new ways to meet local needs. As the number of persons over age 65 continues to grow, faith community nursing needs will grow accordingly. It may be unrealistic to expect that nurses will be able to expand the functions of faith community nursing when they are working in unpaid capacities.

In addition to various health care providers forming collaborative partnerships with faith communities, university schools of nursing are using faith communities as community health nursing clinical settings for student practicum experiences (Maddox, 2003; Patillo, Chesley, Castles, & Sutter, 2002). These creative collaborations help to extend and expand services to congregants as well as to meet the learning needs of students. Collaborations and partnership models will be addressed in greater detail in Chapter 7.

Faith Community Nurse Profile

In 1993, McDermott and Burke reported that 69% of the 109 parish nurses surveyed were between ages 35 and 54, and all but one were female. Over half of these nurses were salaried, either by a faith community or an institution. They found that satisfactions with the parish nurse role were personal and spiritual growth, the ability to practice holistically and the opportunity to establish long-term relationships with clients. Frustrations cited were unrealistic expectations for the time allotted, ambiguity of the role and its boundaries, and lack of resources, including financial compensation and support systems.

Solari-Twadell (1999) reports the findings of three national parish nurse surveys conducted by the International Parish Nurse Resource Center (IPNRC) in 1992, 1994, and 1996. The number of respondents were: 1992−N = 293, 1994−N = 509, and 1996−N = 536. The data reflect that when institutions invest in a parish nurse partnership, it will usually be a paid model. In contrast, congregational models were likely to be volunteer models because congregations were not as frequently offering paid positions. The congregational unpaid model was the most frequently reported by the respondents. The responses indicate that parish nursing is ecumenical, representing both Christian and non-Christian faith traditions. The data reflect that most parish nurses consistently provide health education, personal health counseling, and referrals. The education levels of the respondents in 1996 were LPN, 1%; diploma, 11%; ADN, 27%; BSN, 29%; non-Nursing BS, 9%; MSN, 11%; non-Nursing MS, 11%; and doctorate, 1%. This was a concern because almost half of the respondents had no formal course and clinical practicum in community health nursing.

Kuhn (1997) surveyed a convenience sample of parish nurses in Pennsylvania in 1995; 128 questionnaires were mailed with a 59% response rate. Many of the respondents (36%) were not active parish nurses, so only 48 questionnaires were analyzed. Interviews using the same questionnaire were conducted with five active parish nurses to obtain more in-depth responses and to validate mailed survey findings.

Kuhn found that the vast majority of her subjects (N = 47) were women (97.9%), women age 50 and older (73%), and women who were educated in diploma schools of nursing (62%). Twenty-seven percent were educated in ADN programs, and only 12% in BSN programs. Once again, the lack of formal education in community health nursing is a concern. Seventy-five percent of the respondents were congregation-based volunteer parish nurses. Congregation-based paid parish nurses and institutionally based paid parish nurses comprised 12.5%, respectively. When the nurses were paid, they received a salary ranging from $10–$18 per hour. Part-time employment was the norm (85%).

Kuhn (1997) asked her subjects to indicate their titles. Fifty-eight percent were called *parish nurses,* but other titles included *health ministries coordinators, health and whole team coordinators, health promoters, parish nurse educators,* and *nurses in the congregation.* Professional liability insurance was maintained by only 46% of the active parish nurses. Of the 46%, 40% indicated that their liability coverage was employer-paid.

Kuhn (1997) also assessed the methods by which parish nurses were evaluated. Twenty-five percent of the subjects did not answer the question, and 25% indicated there was no formal evaluation process in place. The remaining 50% were formally evaluated quarterly or annually. The basis for evaluation of the nurses included whether goals were met, number of programs offered, and the number of clients visited. All respondents answered open-ended questions about the frustrations and satisfactions of the parish nurse role. Satisfactions in the role were reported as the freedom to speak about God and the role of spirituality in health and illness, the opportunity to provide holistic care, to develop and maintain relationships with clients, to act as an advocate, and to be a health educator. The subjects were asked to describe the ways that they incorporate spirituality into their role. Selected comments included: "praying with clients when it seems right," "take Communion to clients," "by promoting wellness of body, mind, and soul," "show compassion and caring for all," and "frequent discussions as to client's spiritual concerns" (Kuhn, 1997, p. 28). Additional education for this role was considered important by 62% of the respondents. Subject areas for additional education included physical assessment (especially with the elderly), counseling in general and in relation to grief and loss in particular, spiritual assessment, interviewing skills, small group facilitation, home safety assessment, listening skills, and updates on diagnostic procedures and the treatment of chronic diseases.

Patterson (2003) reports that in the United States there are approximately 4,000 nurses who have completed the IPNRC Basic Preparation course, and probably several thousand other parish nurses who have attended other parish nurse preparation, as well as registered nurses working as parish nurses without training. She estimates that there are close to 10,000 parish nurses in the United States. Coluccio, Porter, and Robbins (2005) report that there are 7,500 trained faith community nurses in America. However, they do not cite a source for this figure.

Educational Preparation for Parish/Faith Community Nursing

The IPNRC offered the first continuing education program on parish nursing in 1987. This evolved into the Annual Westberg Symposium on Parish Nursing, which is held in St. Louis, Missouri. Each symposium has an annual theme—"Parish Nursing: At the Crossroads" is the theme for 2005. A nurse keynote speaker is selected as well as a clergy presenter, and workshops and poster presentations are part of the event.

In 1996, the IPNRC conducted an educational programming needs assessment, using a convenience sample of 50 parish nurse coordinators. They were queried regarding the content of their own basic parish nurse educational preparation and any additional education that they had experienced to help prepare for the role. The findings from the needs assessment served as the basis for a 3-year collaborative effort between Marquette University (Milwaukee, WI), Loyola University (Chicago, IL), and the IPNRC. The outcome of this effort was the development of curricula for basic parish nurse preparation and for the coordinator role (McDermott, Solari-Twadell, & Matheus, 1999). These curricula, a statement of philosophy for parish nurse education, and a vision statement for parish nurse education are available on the IPNRC Web site http://www.parishnurses.org.

BOX 2-1
Learning Modules for the IPNRC Basic Preparation Course

1. Health, Healing, and Wholeness in the Faith Community (3)
2. History and Philosophy of Parish Nursing (1)
3. Ethics in Parish Nursing (1.5)
4. Legal Issues and Accountability in Parish Nursing (2)
5. Self-Care for Parish Nurses (2)
6. Assessment: Individual, Family, Faith Community (1.5)
7. Function of the Parish Nurse: Integrator of Faith and Health (3)
8. Function of the Parish Nurse: Personal Health Counselor (1)
9. Function of the Parish Nurse: Health Educator (1.5)
10. Health Advocate (1)
11. Function of the Parish Nurse: Referral Agent (1)
12. Function of the Parish Nurse: Coordinator of Volunteers (1)
13. Function of the Parish Nurse: Accessing and Developing Support Groups (1)
14. Getting Started (2)
15. Functioning within a Ministerial Team (1.5)
16. Health Promotion and Wellness (2)
17. Prayer and Worship Leader (2)
18. Grief and Loss (2)
19. Family Violence (2)
20. Documentation (2)

International Parish Nurse Resource Center. (2004). Information for educators. Available at: http://www.ipnrc.parishnurses.org/basic.phtml. Used with permission.

The 2004 curriculum revision was directed by the IPNRC in collaboration with Eden Theological Seminary and Webster University (all of St. Louis, MO). A Curriculum Advisory Committee composed of parish nurse educators in the United States and Canada met in November 2003 to begin the development of a curriculum revision plan. Twenty modules were identified as being the core content of the Basic Parish Nurse Preparation Curriculum. In addition, 11 modules were identified for an Advanced Parish Nurse Preparation curriculum to be developed in 2005. Every effort was made to involve a diverse group in every aspect of the curriculum revision process (IPNRC, 2004).

The assumptions regarding the Basic Parish Nurse Curriculum are as follows.

The curriculum:

- Focuses on core concepts of spiritual formation: professionalism and shalom as health wholeness and community, incorporating culture and diversity.
- Encourages individual spiritual growth.
- Is developed from a Judeo-Christian theological framework of care and is applicable to and respective of other faith traditions.
- Is inclusive of sociocultural and geographical diversity, including ethnicity, gender, lifestyle, sexual orientation, and faith traditions.
- Includes various ways of thinking and knowing, such as the application of nursing process that involves assessment, planning, implementation, and evaluation; a theological perspective is also emphasized.
- Develops the nurse for a leadership role in collaborative health ministry.
- Supplies the content to develop and sustain a parish nursing practice.
- Fosters interdisciplinary collaboration among educators. (IPNRC, 2004; used with permission)

The IPNRC Basic Preparation Curriculum for Parish Nursing is written at the baccalaureate level. It can be offered for college credit or as continuing education. Box 2-1 presents the 20 modules with recommended clock hours of instruction in parentheses.

The IPNRC (2004) also addresses the process component of parish nurse education. Process dynamics allow for a deeper personal engagement of the learner and provide opportunities to form meaningful networks with others. Hospitality is a process dynamic that is defined as the creation of a safe, sacred space where others are welcomed, offering an open heart and allowing for a stance of availability and acceptance. The character of the space, the religious nature, and the contemplative demeanor of the learners draw attention to the spirituality that is the core of parish nursing practice. Each curricular module provides a reflective activity intended to draw the learners into the sacred space and to share as a community of learners.

Process dynamics also include active learning experiences through retreat experiences, round table discussions, interactive online learning, and mentoring. Inclusion of worship experiences as a component of the educational process is a distinctive element of parish nursing education. Prayer, devotions, a healing service, and music are vehicles for spiritual learning and personal growth. A service of dedication to the ministry of the parish is recommended for the completion of the educational preparation (IPNRC, 2004).

The IPNRC Web site lists over 100 educational partners who provide the basic preparation course in the United States and four international affiliates representing Australia, Canada, Korea, and Switzerland. There are also parish nurse educational programs in other universities and institutions who have chosen not to partner with the IPNRC but who offer comparable courses and/or certificate programs. Educational formats vary, with online, traditional, and a mix of online/on-site courses available. The author offers an online format that concludes with a weekend on-site retreat.

Faith Community Nursing: Scope and Standards of Practice Professional Performance Standard 8: Education states, "The faith community nurse attains knowledge and competency that reflects current nursing practice" (ANA-HMA, 2005, p. 25). The measurement criteria for this standard are as follows. The FCN:

- Participates in ongoing educational activities related to spiritual care, professional nursing practice, and related professional issues.
- Demonstrates a commitment to lifelong learning through self-reflection and inquiry to identify learning needs.
- Seeks learning experiences that reflect current practice in order to maintain knowledge, skills, and competence in all dimensions of faith community nursing.
- Acquires knowledge and skills appropriate to faith community nursing practice.
- Maintains professional records that provide evidence of competency and lifelong learning in the speciality.
- Seeks experiences and formal and independent learning activities to maintain and develop the necessary professional skills and knowledge to provide spiritual care.
- Uses current research findings and other evidence to expand knowledge and enhance role performance.

Faith Community Nursing Roles

Granger Westberg identified seven roles for the parish nurse: integrator of faith and health, personal health counselor, health educator, health advocate, referral agent, coordinator of volunteers, and developer of support groups (1990, 1999). The language of the 2004 Basic Parish Nurse Preparation Curriculum uses the term "function" of the parish nurse instead of the term "role" (IPNRC, 2004).

Faith Community Nursing: Scope and Standards of Practice (ANA-HMA, 2005, pp. 17–21) Standard 5: Implementation (5a–5d) details the roles or functions. Standard 10: Collegiality states that the faith community nurse interacts with and contributes to the professional development of peers and colleagues (p. 27).

The roles or functions that an FCN actually assumes in the job setting will be dependent on many things. Clearly, time will be a factor that can limit the number of roles any FCN can actualize. Obviously, a full-time FCN nurse will have more time to develop more fully any or all of the roles. The needs of the congregation, the presence or absence of a health ministry team, and the personal preferences and priorities of the FCN will affect which roles are actualized.

BOX 2-2
Role Comparison of the FCN and Home Care Nurse

TYPE OF NURSING SERVICES	PARISH NURSE NO HANDS-ON SERVICES	HOME CARE NURSE HANDS-ON SERVICES
Focus of care	Health promotion/disease prevention; emphasis on spiritual care	Treatment of disease
Physician's orders	Not needed	Mandatory
Functions	Counselor, referral source, educator, advocate	Case manager, direct caregiver
Payment method	No payment from any source	Client or third-party payment
Nurse's compensation	Voluntary or paid by faith community or health care institution	Salary from home care agency
Nurse/client relationship	Continuing	Episodic
Location of visit	Home, nursing home, hospital, church or temple	Home visit
Visit limit	Variable, one visit to ongoing	Restricted by third-party payers

Adapted from Cassidy, K. (2002). Partners in healing: Home care, hospice, and parish nurses. *Home Healthcare Nurse, 20*(3), 179–183. Used with permission.

Cassidy (2002) looks at faith community nursing roles more broadly. She compares the roles of the FCN with the roles of home care nurses (See Box 2-2). Before discussing each of the FCN roles, the research findings related to these roles will be discussed.

Review of the Research Literature about Faith Community Nursing Roles/Functions

Tables 2-1 and 2-2 provide a summary of the research about faith community nursing. Table 2-1 presents studies in which parish nurses were the respondents. Table 2-2 presents studies in which congregants were the respondents.

The research findings presented provide support for the FCN roles of integrator of faith and health, health educator, health counselor, advocate, and referral agent. No research findings support the roles of coordinator of volunteers and facilitator of support groups; however, the study by Weis, Schank, Coenen, and Matheus (2002) does support aggregate activities of the FCN. The activities were described as health education-related as opposed to support groups. This study also adds the FCN role of ministry team member.

TABLE 2-1

Research on Faith Community Nursing Roles

AUTHOR/DATE	PURPOSE	SAMPLE	DATA GENERATION	FINDINGS
Rydholm (1997)	To describe the content of parish nurse practice	1,800 elders	Analysis of field notes and reduction of content to assessment, intervention, and outcome components as they pertained to functional, physiological, psychosocial, psychospiritual, and safety/environmental domains	Advocacy, referral, assistance finding, active listening, and supportive education efforts served to increase access to care. Facilitating access meant earlier, simpler, more cost-effective treatment. Half of the cases were related to psychosocial-spiritual concerns, half to physical concerns.
Weis, Schank, Coenen, & Matheus (1999)	To describe parish nursing practice, using the Nursing Minimum Data Set	19 parish nurses practicing in 22 faith communities	1,557 encounters for services provided to 1,730 nursing diagnoses and 3,451 nursing interventions	Most frequent nursing interventions were active listening and spiritual support. The parish nurse roles of educator, counselor, referral agent, integrator of faith, and health advocate and facilitator were identified.
Weis & Schank (2000)	To describe parish nursing practice, using the Nursing Minimum Data Set	408 older adults	Survey	Health-seeking behaviors, active listening, emotional support, and spiritual support were the most frequently used nursing diagnoses.
Tuck & Wallace (2000)			Ethnography	A taxonomy of parish nursing roles, which included health educator, group leaders, visitor, coordinator, program developer, liaison, health screener, healer, and advocate. A taxonomy of parish nurse offerings emerged, which included educational classes, skill building classes, health screenings, and focused meetings, such as Bible study and prayer meetings.

(continued)

TABLE 2-1

Research on Faith Community Nursing Roles *(continued)*

AUTHOR/DATE	PURPOSE	SAMPLE	DATA GENERATION	FINDINGS
Mayhugh & Martens (2001)	To describe parish nursing practice	67 church members, 6 parish nurses, and 1 pastor; 54% of respondents were > age 65, 79% were women, and 73% were married	Survey	Parish nursing practice should focus on helping people to stay well and to manage physical or emotional disease. Half reported that the parish nurse should offer education about spiritual health; less than 25% thought the parish nurse should consult about spiritual problems. Health education programs were the preferred services (80%).
Tuck, Wallace, & Pullen (2001)	To explore spirituality in parish nurses and the variables related to their practice	119 parish nurses; mean age, 50.8 years; 97% women; 35% diploma; 15% ADN; 34% BSN; 25% MSN; 76% Protestant; 23% Roman Catholic; mean hours/wk = 16.5.	Survey	Parish nurses scored high on spirituality scales; the most frequent foci of care were: holistic care health promotion and education. Most frequent nursing activities were screening, educating, and visiting. The most frequently reported spiritual intervention was praying, offering communion, and offering spiritual guidance. Professional activities included assessment, referral, and education.
Chase-Ziolek & Iris (2002)	To study parish nurses' perspectives on the distinctive aspects of providing care in a faith community setting	17 parish nurses	Content analysis of focus group and interview transcripts	Parish nurses reported they had the greatest impact through health promotion and prevention, advocacy, health education, and health counseling, including spiritual care.
Weis, Schank, Coenen, & Matheus (2002)	To describe parish nursing practice	10 parish nurses in 22 faith communities	Surveys using NANDA and NIC	The most frequent nursing diagnoses and intervention emphasized health promotion and disease prevention. Roles of educator, counselor, referral agent, and advocate were described. Being a member of the ministerial team was an additional role described.

TABLE 2-2

Research of Client Perceptions of Parish Nursing Practice

AUTHOR/DATE	PURPOSE	SAMPLE	DATA GENERATION	FINDINGS
Scott & Sumner (1993)	To investigate client experiences with parish nurses	47 clients (75% women > age 61)	20-minute telephone interviews	Three of the top four concerns of clients were related to health and illness. Half of the clients said that they discussed spiritual topics with the parish nurse. Responses were overwhelmingly positive.
Chase-Ziolek & Gruca (2000)	To investigate client perceptions of distinctive aspects of congregational nursing	11 clients in 2 urban Catholic churches	Content analysis of interviews	Distinctive attributes revealed included the manner of care, the focus of care, and the outcomes achieved. The ambiance, convenience, time for interaction, and reflection of the connection between faith and health were seen as distinctive characteristics of the congregational setting
Wallace, Tuck, Boland,& Witucki (2002)	To study client perceptions of parish nursing	—	Face-to-face interviews and Spradley's ethnographic approach	Five themes emerged: (a) being available; (b) integrating spirituality and health; (c) helping is to help ourselves; (d) exploring parish nursing; and (e) evaluating parish nursing. Client viewed parish nursing as useful, meaningful, and effective.

The research findings about faith community nursing roles indicate that faith community nursing practice is unique to each faith community served, with some congregations preferring the more traditional nursing services of health education and health promotion and less spiritual care, and others preferring the opposite. FCN roles also are negotiated with other members of the ministry team and health ministry goals. It can be hypothesized that FCN roles and programs will look different in particular denominations and in different geographical regions. Further research is needed to test these hypotheses.

Integrator of Faith and Health

Integrator of faith and health is the central, overarching role of faith community nursing practice. It extends like an umbrella over all of the other roles. Every contact made by an FCN assists people to strengthen their spiritual lives to become and stay more whole and healthier. To actualize this role, the FCN needs to be knowledgeable about the human spirit, spirituality, and how spirituality and religion differ and overlap—in the context of the faith tradition of the congregation. Practice in this area requires both spiritual maturity and openness to spiritual growth on the part of the nurse. Spiritual assessment skills are required, and spiritual resources need to be in place for referral. Spiritual interventions are developed collaboratively with other members of the ministry team. Spiritual resources include prayer, music, worship, sacraments, and healing services, again, within the context of the faith tradition.

Many of the individuals who seek faith community nursing services are in some form of life crisis, transition, or loss situation. These individuals need introspection and reflection to make sense of what is happening to them. At these times, individuals may express doubt or question their faith. The FCN, through active listening and reflection, can assist individuals and families to use the crisis, transition, or loss to further grow in one's faith and thus in overall health. For congregants who are not experiencing any form of life crisis, the FCN may provide a stimulus for congregants to open themselves to more fully incorporate the holy into their lives through reflection, prayer, or meditation.

Tuck, Pullen, and Wallace (2001) compared spiritual interventions of mental health nurses and parish nurses. They found that parish nurses identified ideal spiritual interventions: praying, listening, touching, being present, and being available. The parish nurses reported that praying, listening, and supporting were their most frequent spiritual interventions in the 2 weeks prior to completing the questionnaire. The mental health nurses believed that listening, referring, and encouraging were the interventions that best supported patients' spirituality.

The integrator of faith and health role is highly supported by current research findings related to faith community nursing roles. Chapter 3 will further develop this central FCN role. It will discuss the theology of health, healing and wholeness, spiritual formation, and models of spiritual care.

Health Educator

Health education is appropriate within a faith community because people view their health through the lens of their faith tradition. Many people try to be good stewards of what they have been given and wish to attain or maintain good health. Acting in the health educator role, the FCN provides the faith community with the opportunity to participate in well-organized seminars, workshops, forums, classes, and discussion groups covering a wide range of wellness and health topics. The FCN may conduct some of the health education events or coordinate and facilitate the use of the expertise and talents of congregational and community members. In doing this, the FCN increases the community's awareness of how health and faith issues relate.

Often, the FCN identifies a need for a specific type of health programming, based on ongoing assessment of the faith community. Assessment data will also assist the FCN in planning events at days and times that are convenient to the target audience. Organizational skills are needed to plan the health education event and to market it to the congregation.

Health education events can serve as a means for case-finding for the FCN. Attendees at events may arrange to speak privately with the FCN about their particular concerns related to the topic presented. This type of contact sets the stage for follow-up by telephone or home visiting.

Knowledge of the principles of teaching and learning, and knowing what facilitates learning and what blocks learning, will add to the success of health education programs. Attention should be paid to the literacy level of the materials provided to participants as well as to age-appropriateness. All health education programs should include measurable learning objectives that can later be used in the evaluation process.

The health educator role of the FCN covers the spectrum—from teaching an individual at a teachable moment to sharing health literature with the whole congregation. It includes making sure that information provided is current, accurate, and available. Sermons, children's stories, and health fairs are other ways to provide health education in faith communities. Information may be shared through use of bulletin boards, pamphlets or poster displays, articles in newsletters, and bulletin inserts.

Information on the health educator role of the FCN will be expanded in Chapters 12 and 13. Also, the "how-to's" of health education programming and evaluation will be discussed in-depth, and health education resources will be provided.

Personal Health Counselor

According to the research findings presented earlier in this chapter, FCNs spend much of their time in health counseling activities. As a personal health counselor, the FCN assesses the health needs of individuals, families, and groups. The FCN may schedule appointments for counseling or may post "walk-in" hours. Personal health counseling needs may arise at health screening or health education events.

As all nurses know, much personal health counseling is sought and given in casual and unplanned interactions. The unplanned counseling can then lead to more formal discussion and problem solving. Availability and flexibility are important aspects of this role.

Although some personal health counseling will occur in the worship setting, FCNs also visit congregants in homes, hospitals, and nursing homes. The counseling role assists people to express their feelings, identify health issues of concern, identify possible ways to deal with health issues, and evaluate the effectiveness of newly learned skills.

Depending upon the size of the ministry team and the size and needs of the congregation, the FCN may be asked to co-counsel with faith group leaders. Olson (2000) reports that an advantage to co-counseling is that the perspectives and expertise of two disciplines are combined for a richer counseling experience. Because most FCNs are women and many faith leaders are men, the potential benefit of different gender perspectives exists. Olson states that enriched marital and family counseling experiences have resulted in combining the expertise of a male clergyperson and a female FCN.

Westberg (1990) identified three representative groups that sought out parish nurses for health counseling: the elderly, parents of preadolescents and teenagers with substance abuse or sexual issues, and men over age 40. Research findings certainly support that the elderly seek out personal health counseling services from parish nurses (Scott & Sumner, 1993; Rydholm, 1997; Weis & Schank, 2000; Mayhugh & Martens, 2001). Research findings about teens and men over age 40 seeking parish nurse services were not found in the published research literature.

Referral Agent and Liaison with Community Health Organizations

To be an effective referral agent and liaison with community health organizations, the FCN must be aware of the resources within the faith community and the resources external to the faith community. The FCN must also have an awareness of which community resources are and are not acceptable to the members of the faith community. If the FCN has a community health nursing background in the local community and is a member of the faith community, much of this information will be known. However, complete information can be gathered by conducting a comprehensive community assessment. The community assessment process identifies internal and external resources available to the faith community. The assessment process is presented in-depth in Chapter 5.

Operating in the referral agent role, the FCN matches the needs of congregants with appropriate and available resources. The FCN needs to know when, where, and how to refer people. The FCN assists congregants in understanding and negotiating the health care system and recognizes the factors that promote or deter people from using services. Follow-up with congregants about the effectiveness and satisfaction with services used is important as well. The role of referral agent and liaison with community health organizations is highly supported by current research findings. All of the studies addressing FCN roles support this role as central to practice. Chapter 7 presents expanded content about community connections.

Coordinator of Volunteers

The coordinator of volunteers role refers to the training and coordinating of lay people to extend the helping ministries of the faith community. Olson states that facilitating volunteer activities is one way to ensure that the health ministry belongs to the broader congregation (2000). Examples of volunteer health ministries include a Stephen Ministry Program, which trains people to be one-to-one caregivers, transportation services, foster grandparents, friendly visitor programs, or outreach ministries. The FCN collaborates with congregational volunteer structures, assesses needs of the congregation, and serves as a clinical resource to volunteers.

Current research findings about faith community nursing roles do not identify this role as central to FCN practice. Whether this is a reflection of the kinds of data collected or whether it is a role that is not being actualized (at least not by FCNs) in faith community settings is unclear. Solari-Twadell (1999) reports that in IPNRC National Surveys of 1992, 1994, and 1996, the trainer of volunteers role was the least developed. She states that because the largest organizational model reported was the unpaid, part-time congregational model, it is understandable that parish nurses would not have the time to develop this role. Professional Performance Standard 10: Collegiality, in the *Faith Community Nursing: Scope and Standards of Practice,* states that the FCN interacts and contributes to the professional development of peers and colleagues (ANA-HMA, 2005, p. 27). Further descriptive research is needed to affirm this FCN role.

Developer of Support Groups

Faith communities share beliefs and values, and they come together to worship and to support each other in those beliefs. The FCN may formalize support group structures to meet various needs within the congregation. Examples would include a caregivers group, smoking cessation groups, weight management groups, loss, and grieving groups.

This role is not identified in the research literature and not specifically addressed by the *Faith Community Nursing: Scope and Standards of Practice* (ANA-HMA, 2005). Solari-Twadell reports that the data from the IPNRC National Surveys of 1992, 1994, and 1996 indicate that this role was not well developed (1999). In the research literature, group counseling and group classes were subsumed under the more global category of health promotion activities of the parish nurse (Weis et al., 2002). Support groups can also be a part of the social ministry activities of the faith community and are not as clearly defined as a nursing role.

Hurley and Mohnkern (2004) report that FCNs have the opportunities and background to organize and facilitate psycho-educational support groups that promote wholeness and healing. They define psycho-education as preventive or growth-focused education that supports skill attainment and coping. A church-based psycho-educational support group focuses on the whole person and the connection between mind, body, and spirit. The biblical perspective for understanding life events and one's responses to God's provisions form the foundation and context for group activities and discussions. The authors contend that support groups are cost-effective. Their article provides step-by-step instructions on guiding the group process.

Health Advocate

An important role of the FCN is health advocacy. *Advocacy* is derived from the Latin *advocatus*, which means one who summons to give evidence (Webster, 1991). *Advocate* is a noun and a verb: to act for, speak for, plead for, or defend. *Advocacy* is the function of these verbs and has been described as advising, informing, or counseling (Mitchell & Bournes, 2000). Rydholm defines advocacy as the gift of translating needs into attention-getting language (1997, p. 48). While not having the centrality of the integrator of faith and health role, advocacy is a part of each of the roles of the FCN and is based on the belief that all persons are sacred and should be treated with respect and dignity. In this role the FCN works with the client, the faith community, and all available resources to provide whatever is in the best interests of holistic health. Reinhard, Grossman, and Piren (2004) state that the nurse's ethical responsibility is to transfer as much knowledge as possible to the client and to support the client in making informed choices. Advocacy becomes teaching, nonjudgmental support of the person's decisions, and assistance in acting on those choices. The FCN listens and learns the needs of the client, assists the client in decision making and acting, and speaks for the client when the client is unable to.

Advocacy occurs at the client level and at the system level. Client-focused definitions of advocacy emphasize client autonomy and assist clients in voicing their values (Connolly, 1999). Systems-level or community-level advocacy refers to influencing systems or communities to improve or change services (Stuart & Laraia, 2001).

Advocacy by nurses is far from a new concept. Advocacy has been prevalent since Nightingale advocated for a clean hospital environment in Scutari. Foley, Minick, and Kee (2002) state that advocacy as a central role for nurses was formalized during the 1970s when terms such as "loyal obedience" and "obeying physicians' orders" disappeared from the professional literature. In 1976, the ANA published its *Code of Ethics* with a definition of patient advocacy. This statement is the first to mention that nurses are *required* to protect patients from the "incompetent, unethical, or illegal practice of any person" (ANA, 1976, p. 8).

Empirical research about the advocacy role is meager. The studies are qualitative in nature, and sample sizes are small. Segesten's (1993) study, conducted in Sweden, found that advocacy situations arose for nurses when patients were perceived as powerless or when health care workers or family members viewed patients' wishes as contrary to what they believed were the patients' best interests. Millette (1993) explored nurses' preferences for bureaucratic advocacy (institutional loyalty), physician advocacy (loyalty to the physician), and client advocacy (loyalty to the patient). Her findings show that the client advocacy model was the most preferred by the nurse respondents; however, when nurses were given hypothetical situations, the nurses more frequently chose to use the bureaucratic advocacy model or the physician advocacy model. Snowball (1996) interviewed nurses regarding advocacy in their practice. She found that the important factors leading to advocacy included nurses and clients sharing a common humanity and the cultural environment, being one of care. Snowball concluded that a therapeutic relationship was central to advocacy. Foley, Minick, and Kee (2000) interviewed military nurses about their advocacy practices during a military operation. One pattern, safeguarding or keeping patients safe from harm, was identified. Related themes included advocating as protecting, advocating as attending the whole person, advocating as being the person's voice, and advocating as preserving personhood. Foley et al. (2002) studied how nurses develop the skill of advocating for patients. Their findings indicate that for the nurses in their study, developing advocacy skills was more haphazard and situation-dependent than it was methodically taught in their nursing education programs.

As the health care system continues to become increasingly complex, the FCN, in the advocate role, educates and assists clients to navigate within the system. This can include activities such as facilitating welfare applications, teaching clients about food banks, assisting families in finding domestic violence shelters, accessing legal aid, and negotiating with health insurers.

The advocacy role is well supported in the research findings related to faith community nursing roles and clearly identified in the *Faith Community Nursing: Scope and Standards of Practice* (ANA-HMA, 2005) and in the IPNRC's Philosophy of Parish Nursing. Advocacy interventions have both ethical and legal aspects, which will be discussed in-depth in Chapters 8 and 9.

Summary of Faith Community Nursing Roles/Functions

As discussed, the literature is supportive of the traditional FCN roles of integrator of faith and health, health advocate, health educator, personal health counselor, and referral agent. The literature is less supportive of the traditional FCN roles of coordinator of volunteers and developer of support groups. Ward (personal communication, 2003) suggests that the traditional FCN roles are too narrow in scope. She suggests broadening the roles in the following way:

- Integrator of faith and health—*Integrating faith and health*
- Health advocate—*Advocating for health*
- Health educator—*Educating about holistic health*
- Personal health counselor—*Counseling about personal health*
- Referral agent—*Linking to the community*
- Coordinator of volunteers—*Sharing assets*
- Developer of support groups—*Supporting others*

The author believes that the roles of coordinator of volunteers and developer of support groups should be folded into a role label of "ministry team member." This role was identified by Weis et al. (2002). They state that the role may involve weekly ministerial meetings, participation in worship services, faith community meetings, such as the human concerns group, Elizabeth Ministry (focused on the needs of pregnant women), Stephen Ministry (caregiver preparation), health and homeless ministry board, interfaith meetings, and serving as the faith community representative to various community groups. An important piece of the ministry team member role is that it is negotiated between the faith community leader and the rest of the ministry team. As the team sets goals, roles and expectations will be divided among the staff members to meet the needs of the specific faith community. Depending on the size of the team and the needs of the faith community, social ministries may or may not be under the purview of the FCN.

Nist (2003) affirms the pastoral partner or health ministry member role and adds yet another faith community nursing role—initiating caring relationships with the elderly, the chronically ill, and the "worried well." Although it can be argued that the initiation of caring relationships with all clients is a part of all of the traditional FCN roles, nurses are very familiar with the concept of working with "worried well" clients.

Sellers and Orfanelli (2003) identify four faith community nursing roles: educator, counselor, liaison, and advocate. They fold the functions of trainer of volunteers and developer of support groups into the advocate role.

Derrickson (2001) participated in planning a clinical pastoral education (CPE) course for FCNs. He identified three important themes described by FCNs. The first theme was identity issues and the need to "fix it"—no matter what "it" was. For some FCNs, the identity issues arose because of the newness of the role; for others there was a desire to change the role as it had grown beyond any reasonable ability to fulfill it. Derrickson states that struggling with the desire to "fix it" provoked discussions of personal limits and boundary setting. A second theme identified related to gaining credibility within the congregation, and the third theme was the importance of the FCN negotiating his or her role with the clergy. Derrickson also identifies the importance of the FCNs navigating transitions in their roles as programs develop and grow.

Hahn, Radde, and Fellers (2001) state that all members of the health ministry team, assuming that they have the requisite skills and training, collaborate in providing pastoral care and counseling. They state that clear role descriptions are vital. How health ministry teams will provide such services will depend on the setting, which of them is available, and which of them has the necessary training. Role functions unique to one member of the pastoral care team, such as sacramental functions, are not difficult to identify and differentiate. In such cases, team members need to know when to refer.

Case Study

Linda is the FCN at an African American church that has an active women's group called the Angels of Peace. The Angels asked Linda to provide a guest speaker for their monthly luncheon. At the time of the request, Linda was precepting a graduate student, Anne Marie, for a community health nursing practicum experience. Because the graduate student had a strong background in emergency department nursing, Linda asked her to be the speaker at the Angels monthly meeting. Together they decided that the graduate student's topic would be "When to go to the emergency room."

On the appointed day, Linda and Anne Marie attended the luncheon worship service. After the meal, Anne Marie spoke to the group about when to go to the emergency room, and she discussed what kinds of information would be important to share with health professionals. The question-and-answer period gave Anne Marie and Linda additional opportunities to provide health promotion information.

The case study illustrates the FCN roles of health educator, personal health counselor, referral agent, integrator of faith and health, and advocate. Health information was provided in a group setting, the FCNs participated in the worship service with the clients, individual questions were answered, and the group was referred to community resources and was assisted in navigating the health care system in an informed way.

Summary

This chapter presented and discussed the advantages and disadvantages of each of the models through which faith community nursing programs are delivered. A profile of faith community nursing in the United States was presented. The educational preparation for faith community nursing was discussed.

A review of the research literature regarding faith community nursing roles was provided. These findings support the traditional parish roles of integrator of faith and health, health educator, personal health counselor, advocate, and referral agent. The roles of trainer of volunteers and developer of support group groups were not supported by research findings. An additional role, that of health ministry team member, was identified and supported by research findings.

Reflect and Discuss

1. Discuss four specific nursing interventions that you could use to integrate faith and health in a client situation.
2. Compare and contrast the FCN role with that of the public health nurse.
3. Review Standard of Care 5: Implementation in *Faith Community Nursing: Scope and Standards of Practice* (ANA-HMA, 2005). Compare this standard to the traditional FCN roles described in the chapter.
4. Review Professional Performance Standard 8: Education in *Faith Community Nursing: Scope and Standards of Practice* (ANA-HMA, 2005). Reflect on the content required for faith community nursing, and consider this content in relation to your own nursing education. Are there content areas that you need more preparation in?
5. Reflect on your personal experiences in nursing when you acted in the role of client advocate. Consider your comfort level and success (or lack of success) in carrying out this role.

References

American Nurses Association. (1976). *Code for nurses with interpretative statements.* Kansas City, MO: Author.

American Nurses Association & Health Ministries Association. (2005) *Faith community nursing: Scope and standards of practice.* Silver Springs, MD: ANA.

Cassidy, K. (2002). Partners in healing: Home care, hospice, and parish nurses. *Home Healthcare Nurse, 20*(3), 179–183.

Chase-Ziolek, M. & Gruca, J. A. (2000). Client's perceptions of distinctive aspects in nursing care received within a congregational setting. *Journal of Community Health Nursing, 17*(3), 171–183.

Chase-Ziolek, M. & Iris, M. (2002). Nurse's perspectives on the distinctive aspects of providing nursing care in a congregational setting. *Journal of Community Health Nursing, 19*(3), 173–186.

Coenen, A., Weis, D. M., Schank, M. J., & Matheus, R. (1999). Describing parish nursing practice using the nursing minimum data set. *Public Health Nursing, 16*(6), 412–416.

Coluccio, M., Porter, R. R., & Robbins, K. A. (2005). Healing ministries in health care. In M. de Chesnay (Ed.), *Caring for vulnerable populations* (pp. 271–275). Sudbury, MA: Jones and Bartlett.

Connelley, P. M. (1999). Consumer advocacy. In C. A. Shea, L. R. Pellitier, E. C. Poster, G. W. Stuart, & M. P. Verhey (Eds.), *Advanced practice nursing in psychiatric and mental health care* (p. 387). St. Louis: Mosby–Year Book.

Derrickson, P. (2001). Parish nursing and clinical pastoral education. *Journal of Health Care Chaplaincy, 11*(2), 15–25.

Foley, B. J., Minick, M. P., & Kee, C. C. (2002). How nurses learn advocacy. *Journal of Nursing Scholarship, 35*(2), 181–186.

Foley, B. J., Minick, M. P., & Kee, C. C. (2000). Nursing advocacy during a military operation. *Western Journal of Nursing Research, 22*(4), 492–507.

Hahn, K., Radde, J. M., & Fellers, J. E. (2001). Spiritual care: Bridging the disciplines in congregational health ministries. *Journal of Health Care Chaplaincy, 11*(2), 49–61.

Hurley, J. E. & Mohnkern, S. (2004). Mobilize support groups to meet congregational needs. *Journal of Christian Nursing, 21*(4), 34–40.

International Parish Nurse Resource Center. (2004). Information for coordinators. Available at: http://www.ipnrc.parishnurses.org/coordbrochure.phtml.

International Parish Nurse Resource Center. (2004). Information for educators. Available at: http://www.ipnrc.parishnurses.org/basic.phtml.

International Parish Nurse Resource Center. (2004). Information for parish nurses. Available at: http://www.ipnrc.parishnurses.org/forpn.phtml.

Kuhn, J. K. (1997). A profile of parish nurses. *Journal of Christian Nursing, 14*(1), 26–28.

Maddox, M. (2003). Clinical experience in parish nursing. *Journal of Christian Nursing, 20*(2), 18–20.

Mayhugh, L. J. & Martens, K. H. (2001). What's a parish nurse to do? Congregational expectations. *Journal of Christian Nursing, 18*(3), 14–16.

McDermott, M. A. & Burke, J. (1993). When the population is a congregation: The emerging role of the parish nurse. *Journal of Community Health Nursing, 10*(3), 179–190.

McDermott, M. A., Solari-Twadell, P. A., & Matheus, R. (1999). Educational preparation. In P. A. Solari-Twadell & M. A. McDermott (Eds.), *Parish nursing: Promoting whole person health within faith communities* (pp. 269–276). Thousand Oaks, CA: Sage.

Millette, B. (1993). Client advocacy and the moral orientation of nurses. *Western Journal of Nursing Research, 15,* 607–618.

Nist, J. A. (2003, January–February). Parish nursing programs: Through them, faith communities are reclaiming a role in healing. *Health Progress, 84*(1)50–53.

Olson, J. K. (2000). Functions of the nurse as health promoter in a faith community. In M. B. Clark & J. K. Olson (Eds.), *Nursing within a faith community: Promoting health in times of transition* (pp. 141–155). Thousand Oaks, CA: Sage.

Patterson, D. L. (2003). *The essential parish nurse: ABCs for congregational health ministry.* Cleveland, OH: Pilgrim Press.

Reinhard, S. C., Grossman, J., & Piren, K. (2004). Advocacy and the advanced practice nurse. In L. A. Joel (Ed.), *Advanced nursing practice: Essentials for role development.* Philadelphia: FA Davis.

Rydholm, L. (1997). Patient-focused care in parish nursing. *Holistic Nursing Practice, 11*(3), 47–60.

Schumann, R. (2000). Collaborating for mission. *Journal of Christian Nursing, 17*(1), 22–23.

Scott, L. & Sumner, J. (1993). How do parish nurses help people? A research perspective. *Journal of Christian Nursing, 10*(1), 16–18.

Segesten, K. (1993). Patient advocacy: An important part of the daily work of the expert nurse. *Scholarly Inquiry for Nursing Practice, 7,* 129–135.

Sellers, T. M. & Orfanelli, K. A. (2003, April 14). Parish health ministries. *Advance for Nurses, 5*(9), 31, 32.

Smith, S. D. (2000). Parish nursing: A call to integrity. *Journal of Christian Nursing, 17*(1), 18–20.

Smith, S. D. (Ed.) (2003). *Parish nursing: A handbook for the new millennium.* New York: Haworth Pastoral Press.

Snowball, J. (1996). Asking nurses about advocating for patients: "Reactive" and "proactive" accounts. *Journal of Advanced Nursing, 24,* 67–75.

Solari-Twadell, P. A. (1999). Nurses in churches: Differentiation of practice. In P. A. Solari-Twadell & M. A. McDermott (Eds.), *Parish nursing: Promoting whole person health within faith communities* (pp. 249–256). Thousand Oaks, CA: Sage.

Stuart, G. W. & Laraia, M. T. (2001). *Principles and practice of psychiatric nursing* (7th ed.). St. Louis: Mosby–Year Book.

Tuck, I., Pullen, L., & Wallace, D. (2001). A comparative study of the spiritual perspectives and interventions of mental health and parish nurses. *Issues in Mental Health Nursing, 22,* 593–605.

Tuck, I., & Wallace, D. C. (2000). Exploring parish nursing from an ethnographic perspective. *Journal of Transcultural Nursing, 11*(4), 290–299.

Tuck, I., Wallace, D., & Pullen, L. (2001). Spirituality and spiritual care provided by parish nurses. *Western Journal of Nursing Research, 23*(1), 441–453.

Wallace, D. C., Tuck, I., Boland, C. S., & Witucki, J. M. (2002). Client perceptions of parish nursing. *Public Health Nursing, 19*(2), 128–135.

Webster's Ninth New Collegiate Dictionary. (1991). Springfield, MA: Merriam Webster Inc. Publishers.

Weis, D. & Schank, M. J. (2000). Use of a taxonomy to describe parish nurse practice with older adults. *Geriatric Nursing, 21*(3), 125–130.

Weis, D. M., Schank, M. J., Coenen, A., & Matheus, R. (2002). Parish nurse practice with client aggregates. *Journal of Community Health Nursing, 19*(2), 105–113.

Westberg, G. (1990). *The parish nurse.* Minneapolis: Augsburg Fortress.

Additional Resources

American Nurses Association. (2004). *Nursing: Scope and standards of practice.* Washington, DC: Author.

Boultinghouse, P. (2003). *Hugs for nurse: Stories, sayings and scriptures to encourage and inspire.* West Monroe, LA: Howard Publishing.

Brueggemann, W. (1976). *Living toward a vision: Biblical reflections on shalom.* Philadelphia: United Church Press.

Carson, V. B. & Koenig, H. G. (2004). *Spiritual caregiving: Healthcare as a ministry.* Philadelphia: Templeton Foundation Press.

Cusveller, B., Sutton, A., & O'Mathuna, D. (2003). *Commitment and responsibility in nursing: A faith-based approach.* Sioux City, IA: Dordt College Press.

DeMaria, D. A. (2003). A parish nurse practitioner. *Journal of Christian Nursing, 21*(3), 32.

Hewitt, J. A. (2002). Critical review of the arguments debating the role of the nurse advocate. *Journal of Advanced Nursing, 37*(5), 439–445.

Homan, D. & Pratt, L. C. (2002). *Radical hospitality: Benedict's way of love.* Brewster, MA: Paraclete Press.

Kumar, K. (2004). Spiritual care: What's worldview got to do with it? *Journal of Christian Nursing, 21*(1), 24–28.

Mallik, M. (1997). Advocacy in nursing: A review of the literature. *Journal of Advanced Nursing, 25,* 130–138.

Mallik, M. & Rafferty, A. M. (2000). Diffusion of the concept of advocacy. *Journal of Nursing Scholarship, 32*(4), 399–404.

Menz, R. (2003). *A pastoral counselor's model for wellness in the workplace: Psychergonomics.* Binghamton, NY: Haworth Pastoral Press.

Millette, B. (1993). Client advocacy and the moral orientation of nurses. *Western Journal of Nursing Research, 15,* 607–616.

Mitchell, G. & Bournes, D. (2000). Nurse as patient advocate? In search of straight thinking. *Nursing Science Quarterly, 13*(3), 204–209.

O'Brien, M. E. (2003). *Prayer in nursing: The spirituality of compassionate caregiving.* Sudbury, MA: Jones and Bartlett.

O'Brien, M. E. (2003). *Spirituality in nursing: Standing on holy ground.* Sudbury, MA: Jones and Bartlett.

Quenstedt-Moe, G. (2003). Parish nursing and home care. *Journal of Christian Nursing, 20,* 26–30.

Rowe, L. (2003). *On call: Daily encouragement for all nurses.* Grand Rapids, MI: Baker Book House.

Schweitzer, R., Norberg, M., & Larson, L. (2002). The parish nurse coordinator: A bridge to spiritual health care leadership for the future. *Journal of Holistic Nursing, 20*(3), 212–231.

Stephenson, C. & Wilson, K. (2004). Does spiritual care really help? *Journal of Christian Nursing, 21*(2), 26–29.

Young, C. & Koopson, C. (2005). *Spirituality, health, and healing.* Thorofare, NJ: Slack.

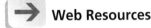 **Web Resources**

http://www.marquette.edu/dept/nursing/parish.htm
  Marquette University
http://www.carroll.edu/parishnurse/
  GettingStarted.htm   Carroll University

http://www.nursingworld.org   American Nurses
  Association
http://www.via-christi.org/cchmweb.nsf/mainview
  Center for Congregational Health Ministry
http://www.ihpnet.org   Interfaith Health Programs
http://www.augie.edu/dept/nurs/marya.htm
  Augustana College
http://www.capital.edu/nursing/nursmsnparish.html
  Capital University
http://www.synodofcovenant.org/HMPN.html   Parish
  Nursing
http://www.lcms.org/bhcm/hm/pn.htm
  Congregational Health Ministry
http://www.elca.org/dcs/healthmin/html   Division for
  Church in Society
http://www.patientadvocacy.org   Center for Patient
  Advocacy
http://www.florenceproject.org/   Florence Project: The
  Heartbeat of Health Advocacy
http://www.hopkinsmedicine.org/   Johns Hopkins
  Medical Institutions: Patient Advocacy Numbers
  (Clearinghouse)

3

Holistic Health and the Faith Community

The connections between faith, healing, wholeness, and faith communities are long-standing. Every faith tradition explores the meaning of major life events, such as birth, illness, suffering, and death. The focus of this chapter is to provide an overview of holistic health and the faith community and to demonstrate how the parish nurse promotes whole person health.

Health

Traditional dictionary definitions of health include the condition of being sound in body, mind, and spirit; especially freedom from physical disease or pain; the general condition of the body (in poor health or in good health); and well-being (Merriam-Webster, 1991). Definitions of health are culturally bound and have evolved over time.

The Greek goddess Hygeia represented the idea that people could remain healthy, if they lived rationally. Health was defined holistically and thought to be influenced by one's lifestyle and personal habits. Historically, however, physical wholeness and mental soundness were a major importance for acceptance in social groups. Persons with disfiguring diseases, congenital anomalies, or inappropriate behaviors were ostracized from society because of fear that they were either contagious or that they harbored evil spirits (or both).

With the advent of germ theory, the causes of illnesses were understood in scientific terms, and the curing of illness became a scientific and medical challenge. Because diseases could be attributed to specific microbial causes, being free from the causative agent became synonymous with health. Health and illness were viewed on a continuum as polar opposites. The medical community's mindset was to "rule out" specific conditions to diagnose health. This mindset was the prevalent medical worldview for the first half of the 20th century.

The World Health Organization (WHO) Constitution (2004) defines health as "a state of complete physical, mental, and social well-being, and not merely the absence of disease and infirmity" (http://www.who.int./about/en). Pender, Murdaugh, and Parsons (2002) state that the WHO definition was revolutionary because it:

- increased the number of components to consider in assessing health.
- called attention to the multidimensionality of health.
- reflected concern for the individual as a total person.
- placed health in the context of the social environment.
- equated health with productive and creative living.

Using the WHO definition as a base, Ware, Kosinski, Gaandek, Aaronson, Apolone, and, Bech (1998) propose five dimensions as a minimum standard for a comprehensive health measure: physical health (functional and structural integrity), mental health (emotional and intellectual functioning), social functioning, role functioning, and general perceptions of well-being. These dimensions are reflected in *Healthy People 2010,* the 10-year plan for improving the nation's health.

Faith Community Nursing: Scope and Standards of Practice (ANA-HMA, 2005) states that health is "the experience of wholeness, salvation, or shalom. It is the integration of the spiritual, physical, psychological, and social aspects of the patient to create a sense of harmony with self, others, the environment, and a higher power". It further states that "health may be experienced in the presence or absence of disease or injury" (p. 37).

Theoretical Perspectives on the Health of Individuals

The concept of health can be approached from different theoretical perspectives. The following sections will look at the concept of health as stability, actualization, a combination of stability and actualization, and holism.

HEALTH AS STABILITY

For individuals, stability-based definitions of health are derived from the physiologic concept of adaptation to environmental stressors, which, ultimately, result in homeostasis, steady state, balance, harmony, or stability. Health exists when one is able to function successfully in the environment. Theorists representative of this approach include Dubos (1965) and Parsons (1958). Nurse theorists who use this approach include Levine [Schaefer & Pond, 1991 (Eds.)], Johnson (1990), Neuman (1995), and Roy (1999).

HEALTH AS ACTUALIZATION

Dunn (1959) was an early advocate for a definition of health emphasizing actualization. He coined the term *high level wellness,* which he defined as integrated human functioning that maximizes individual potential. Pender et al. (2002) state that actualization models have been criticized because of the difficulty in measuring subjective perceptions, because perceptions vary according to age and culture, and because actualization is not clearly distinguished from other global concepts, such as happiness or quality of life. Nurse theorists who use this approach include Orem (1995), Newman (1999), and Parse (1998).

HEALTH AS BOTH STABILITY AND ACTUALIZATION

Some conceptual models combine the idea of maximizing one's potential with flexibility to adapt to the environment. King (1990), Smith (1983), and Pender (2002) are nurses who have each developed definitions of health based on a combination of actualization and adaptation.

Pender defines health as "the actualization of inherent and acquired human potential through goal-directed behavior, competent self-care, and satisfying relationships with others, while adjustments are made as needed to maintain structural integrity and harmony with relevant environments" (p. 22). Her definition has led to a classification system that describes affective and behavioral expressions of health by individuals, which include five culture-free dimensions: affect, attitudes, activity, aspirations, and accomplishments. The dimensions are further divided into 15 subcategories that may be culture-specific. Her system is based on the assumption that health is a manifestation of person and environment interactional patterns that become increasingly complex throughout the life span.

HEALTH AND HOLISM

Narayanasamy (1999) states that *holism* relates to the study of whole organisms or whole systems, and that its spelling is derived from the Greek word "holos," meaning "whole." Holism refers to a perspective that an individual is a whole person—an integration of mind, body, and spirit, which are inseparable. She states that, in regard to spirituality, holism emphasizes that a continuous harmonious interaction between the spirit, mind, and body is required to maintain an individual's health.

Although the WHO definition initiated the concept of health as having many dimensions, until recently, the traditional views in nursing, medicine, and public health divided the dimensions of persons into discrete parts: bio-psycho-social-spiritual. Although the professional disciplines "officially" stated the whole person was an entity more than and different from the sum of the parts, students were taught that content related each component separately. Beginning with Rogers' (1970) concept of unitary man and continuing with nurse theorists Roy (1999), Parse (1998), and Newman (1999), a strong argument has been made that persons can be understood as *only* holistic beings. The American Holistic Nurses Association (AHNA) stresses the interconnectedness of the bio-psycho-social-spiritual dimensions and recognizes two views of holism. The AHNA has publicly stated that "holistic nursing responds to both views, believing that the goals of nursing can be achieved within either framework" (Dossey, Keegan, & Guzzetta, 2005, p. 86).

Judeo-Christian Definitions of Health

Shelly and Miller (1999) state that the goal of nursing is health, but that definitions of health vary in our society and from culture to culture. How health is defined impacts how nursing is practiced and how nursing outcomes are evaluated. In biblical theism, wellness or health is being able to live as God created us, to be as integrated, whole living beings in loving relationship with God, self, and others (Ps 16). Shelly and Miller state that health is central to the Old Testament concept of *Shalom* (Ps 38:3, Jer 33:6) and the New Testament understanding of salvation—to be made whole (Lk 18:42). They further state shalom incorporates all the elements that go into making a God-centered community—peace, prosperity, rest, safety, security, justice, happiness, health, welfare, and wholeness. A God-centered wholeness enables the person to live in harmony with self, God, others, and to be responsible stewards of the environment. Shelly and Miller provide these biblical definitions of health as a basis for the practice of nursing in Judeo-Christian settings.

Westberg (1999), the founder of parish nursing, further elaborates that Jesus, in his healing ministry always dealt with people as whole persons. Parish nurses are positioned to deliver "whole-health care." He states that the parish nurse movement is closely tied to the understanding that when churches are functioning at their best, they are dedicated to keeping the whole person well. Westberg reminds us that the whole person movement takes a person's belief system seriously. "If one's belief system is faulty, it affects the way the body functions. If whole-person concepts can be integrated with one's religious beliefs, then each will provide motivation for the other" (p. 40).

The Eastern Perspective of Health

Eastern medical traditions are based on the assumption that human beings are made up of energy systems and a vital life force. The flow and balance of the energy provide the underlying principle of traditional Chinese medicine (TCM), Ayurvedic medicine, and other traditions. To maintain health, the energy connecting mind and body must be moving, flowing freely, and balanced, because its stagnation causes disease.

Saylor (2004a) presents a representation of health that she calls the circle of health. The design of her model is based on the TCM symbol that represents the balance and harmony between the fundamental principles of yin and yang. The model is intended for teaching clients and health providers about health improvement. Saylor defines health as optimal function, well-being, and quality of life, and she places these concepts at the center of the circular model. The center core circle is surrounded by a ring that is part light in color and part dark, a symbol that both activity/performance and renewal/recovery are necessary for health and are a part of well-being and quality of life. The activity and performance (lighter side) of the model encompasses the concepts of energy, strength, fitness, stamina, happiness, enjoyment, satisfaction, growth and development, and occupational and social role performance. The darker side of the figure represents the passive, inner qualities similar to the yin dimension of the TCM symbol and is labeled renewal and recovery. Included in this side of the model are: rest, relaxation, peacefulness, nourishment, social support, sense of purpose and meaning, balance, adaptation, and resiliency. Saylor's model may be helpful to parish nurses who practice in various settings.

The Research Base for Faith and Health

Dr. David B. Larson (1947–2002), an epidemiologist and psychiatrist, was a pioneer in the field of health and spirituality. He developed an award-winning, objective, quantitative research methodology called the "Systematic Review." This method of review of research brought to light the potential relevance of religion/spirituality research, medical education, and clinical health care. In 1991, Larson founded the National Institute for Healthcare Research, which became the International Center for the Integration of Health and Spirituality (ICIHS). Larson authored more than 270 professional publications and coauthored the *Handbook of Religion and Health* (2001). To honor Dr. Larson's work, the Library of Congress announced the endowed David B. Larson Fellowship in Health and Spirituality in 2004. To further honor Dr. Larson's memory, colleagues Drs. Harold Koenig and Jeff Levin have coedited *Faith, Medicine and Science* (2004), a collection of Larson's scientific papers and tributes written by his peers (Saylor, 2004a).

In 1998, a landmark article appeared in the *Archives of Family Medicine* (Matthews, McCullough, Larson, Koenig, Swyers, & Milano), which reviewed the research literature about religious commitment and health status. The article reported that empirical data suggest that a religious commitment may play a beneficial role in preventing mental and physical illness, improving how people cope with mental and physical illness, and facilitating recovery from illness. The authors suggested that practitioners who make several small changes in how patients' religious commitments are broached in clinical practice may enhance health outcomes, which was a landmark in that the positive link between health and religion was presented in a prestigious, mainstream medical periodical.

In his book, *God, Faith, and Health,* Jeff Levin presents the strong research base for the positive link between health and religion. Levin is an epidemiologist who is credited with identifying and presenting the epidemiology of religion. From the base of health and religion research, Levin has derived the seven principles of theosomatic medicine (2001). He states that "theosomatic medicine" is literally a model or view of the determinants of health based on the apparent connections between God, or spirit, and the body. The principles are based on the findings of hundreds of studies about God, faith, and health. Levin's seven principles of theosomatic medicine are as follows:

1. Religious affiliation and membership benefit health by promoting healthy behavior and lifestyles.
2. Regular religious fellowship benefits health by offering support that buffers the effects of stress and isolation.
3. Participation in worship and prayer benefits health through the physiologic effects of positive emotions.
4. Religious beliefs benefit health by their similarity to health-promoting beliefs and personality styles.

5. Simple faith benefits health by leading to thoughts of hope, optimism, and positive expectation.
6. Mystical experiences benefit health by activating a healing bioenergy or life force or altered state of consciousness.
7. Absent prayer for others is capable of healing by paranormal means or by divine intervention. (pp. 13, 14)

Chamberlain and Hall (2000), in their book, *Realized Religion* (2000), present research findings about the relationship between religion and health as related to mental health, life satisfaction, marital satisfaction, suicide, and alcohol use and abuse. They conclude that religion (with the possible exception of extreme fundamentalism) is generally good for human health because it promotes a healthy lifestyle, opposes self-indulgent and self-destructive behavior, encourages moral behavior, provides vital social support and an ethical value system, establishes an interpretative framework to understand the complexities of life, and promotes spiritual growth. Furthermore, religion provides access to a divine force (God), who has the perceived power or sovereignty to influence human events (transcendence) and who hears prayers that are health promotive, if not healing.

Coyle (2002) suggests that people are better able to cope with, or recover from, illness when they feel they are not completely in control of their own destiny. She states that a spirituality based on transcendence or religious commitment may provide the opportunity for a shared sense of responsibility through a connectedness with a higher power.

Theology of Faith, Healing, and Wholeness

"Not a single faith fails to address the issues of illness and wellness, of disease and healing, of caring and curing. People turn to their faiths to interpret their misfortunes, to summon the strength to fight illness, to rally their communities and a larger public to promote well-being" (Marty, 1990, p. 14). The HMA-ANA (2005) defines healing as, "the process of integrating the body, mind, and spirit to bring about wholeness, health, and a sense of spiritual well-being, although the patient's disease may not be cured" (p. 37).

Through lifestyle choices we can facilitate health and healing, but God, or the Almighty, is the true source of health and healing. "In Hebrew scriptures, health is portrayed as one of God's great gifts and responsibility is placed on people to lead lives that cherish and protect this gift" (Wylie & Solari-Twadell, 1999, p. 25). Historically, faith communities were considered to be places of healing. Stories of health and healing are interspersed throughout the Bible. Two examples are Mark 10:46–52, "Blind Bartimaeus Receives His Sight," and Luke 17:11–19, "Ten Healed of Leprosy." Both gospel stories stress the importance of faith in healing. In Mark 10, Jesus tells Bartimaeus to "Go; your faith has healed you," and in Luke 17, Jesus tells the tenth leper who returned to give praise to God to "Rise and go; your faith has made you well." (See www.ncf-jcn.org/jcn/archive/04sp/04sp_jsp3.html for a full overview of the healing accounts in Scripture.)

A theoretical framework for nursing in early Christianity to the present is discussed in Chapter 1. Several historical events influenced the relationship between the church and conventional medicine that warrant mentioning at this time. First, Emperor Constantine gave Christians complete freedom of worship and equality with other religions. Until that time, Christians endured tremendous persecution. The Nicaean Council established a special, privileged status for the bishops of Jerusalem; they now had full authority over the churches (the Emperor Constantine and Jerusalem, http://www.jeru.huji.ac.il/ed31.htm). This move was intended to strengthen the Christian churches, and, in part, it did by adding an organizational component. Yet some believe that this resulted in a change of the delivery of humanitarian services from a faith community base to a community or institutional base.

The second event was the reintroduction of dualism. Dualism is an ancient notion deeply rooted in Greek thought. The Greeks believed that a man's soul and body were two different and distinct entities. In the 1600s Descartes expanded on the concept of dualism and held that the body, including the brain, was purely mechanistic or machinelike in operation, and disease occurred when the machine broke down. The mind, soul, and body are autonomous and do not interact, thus study of the mind was the domain of religion and philosophy, and study of the body was the domain of medicine. This dualistic view of man had a profound impact on Western civilization and was the beginning of the biomedical model of health (the Internet Encyclopedia of Philosophy, http://www.utm.edu/research/iep/d/descarte.htm).

Starr's (1982) riveting account of the history of American medicine, from its infancy to the early 1980s, follows the evolution of the medical health establishment. It details the industrial rise in power, both economically and culturally, and reveals how medicine supports the concept of dualism by the development of specializations. This action, by the medical establishment, further delineated exclusively the church's position in caring for matters of the spirit and the medical community in caring for matters of the body.

Post-World War II ushered in the beginnings of a renewed emphasis and acceptance of whole person health. Reconciliation between clergy and physicians and the two worlds of spirit and body began to occur (Wylie & Solari-Twadell, 1999).

Faith

Faith is a belief and trust in God and doctrines of a religion. A belief in something cannot be proven but is accepted anyway. Thomas Merton (1972) defines faith as being an "intellectual assent. It perfects the mind, it does not destroy it. It puts the intellect in possession of Truth which reason cannot grasp by itself" (p. 127). Faith is a way of communicating with God. Fowler (1995) notes that "Faith is a person's way of seeing him or herself in relation to others against a background of shared meaning and purpose" (p. 4). "Faith . . . is an endless pilgrimage of the heart. We know that our awareness of God's Truth is always beyond our secure apprehension; yet we are committed to seeking after it diligently and then living faithfully according to the measure of Truth given to us" (Seeger, 2001, p. 112).

Individuals develop in a holistic way: body, mind, and spirit. Many theologians and psychologists have identified stages and progression of spiritual development. Peck (1993), a physician and counselor, recognizes four stages: chaotic antisocial, formal/institutional fundamental, skeptic/individual, and mystic/communal. Barnum (2003) notes that "Peck breaks down traditional boundaries . . . between psychiatry and religion remaining within a traditional religious perspective" (p. 65). Fowler's (1995) Stages of Faith explore people's lifelong development of faith in totality. The stages are loosely associated with age. Transition to the next stage is dependent on many factors, and people can be in more than one stage at one time. Fowler's Stages of Faith are frequently cited, therefore, further explanation is warranted at this time.

Fowler's Stages of Faith Development

Primal Faith (Infancy)

Fowler (1995) defines the time period from birth to age 2 years as a prestage known as *infancy and undifferentiated faith*. Conceptual thought and language are not yet possible, and the foundation for trust versus mistrust is being built. The infant is forming "pre-images of God" and of the kind of world in which they live. Fowler believes that this basic foundation of trust or mistrust is what faith is built upon. Religious experiences in the future will have to confirm that basic trust. Primal faith developmental tasks include separation without anxiety and consistent, loving, respectful responses from parent/caregivers/nurturers.

INTUITIVE–PROJECTIVE FAITH (EARLY CHILDHOOD)

This stage of faith development ranges from ages 2 to 7 years. It is dynamic, filled with change and growth. Imagination is developing, and the child does not possess the kind of logic to question his or her perceptions or fantasies. During this stage, the child's mind is religiously fertile. Experiences that take place during this period often have powerful and lasting effects on the child's faith life. Developmental tasks of this stage include reacting and listening to stories and fantasies.

MYTHIC–LITERAL FAITH (CHILDHOOD AND BEYOND)

During this stage, the child is able to develop order and meaning to his or her world. "Capable of inductive and deductive reasoning, . . . this child works hard and effectively at sorting out the real from the make-believe" (Fowler, 1995, p. 135). Narrative is the gift of this stage. The child can share meaningful experiences with others in the form of stories. Because of the literalness of this stage, the child has difficulty reflecting on the meaning of stories, symbols, and myths and accepts things at face value. *Mythic–Literal Faith* developmental tasks include: acceptance of the inerrancy of the book of faith, adherence to behavior codes that can be traced to a specific Scripture verse or verses, and possession of concrete mythical images of God, heaven, and hell.

SYNTHETIC–CONVENTIONAL FAITH (ADOLESCENCE AND BEYOND)

This stage usually begins around age 12 or 13. This stage is marked by what Piaget calls *formal operational thinking.* The adolescent is capable of reflecting on his or her own thoughts. Establishing an identity and feeling accepted by significant other people is a major concern. A sense of self or identity is an outcome of this stage. A distinguishing characteristic of this stage is the tendency to compose images of God as a friend who deeply values the relationship. Adolescents want to feel accepted and valued by God, and this perceived relationship can facilitate that feeling. Developmental tasks of this stage include: talking with friends about the meaning of faith or spirituality, believing that God is the only one who really knows them, yet, at the same time, questioning the existence of God.

Fowler's stages are loosely associated with specific ages, but this stage could be an adult stage. Many members of faith communities are best described by their faith that was formed during their adolescence.

INDIVIDUATIVE–REFLECTIVE FAITH (YOUNG ADULTHOOD AND BEYOND)

During this stage, the individual is forced out of or decides to leave his or her comfort zone. The challenge of this stage is that the person must now reflect upon self as separate from the groups and the shared world that defines his or her life. This transition usually begins between ages 17 and 20 and is completed between the mid-20s and 30s. The later transition occurs, the more difficult it is to personally manage, and the relationship needs to be reworked. Many people are unable to complete transition to this stage. Fowler (1995) notes that "for a genuine move to occur there must be an interruption of reliance on external sources of authority" (p. 179).

In this stage, boundaries are of utmost importance, discerning self from others and identifying with groups that can be compellingly embraced as opposed to other groups. This stage is very concerned with being true to self and creating a fit between whom we perceive ourselves to be in a group and any beliefs or commitments to which we are attached. Development tasks include struggling with faith and developing an intimacy with or a withdrawal from faith.

CONJUNCTIVE FAITH (EARLY MIDLIFE AND BEYOND)

In the mid-30s to age 40, some people transition to the stage of *Conjunctive Faith*. Conjunctive faith is a type of awakening to the knowledge that everything that you thought was clear and concise, in terms of boundaries and identity, is not. This stage helps one to recognize that self is both conscious and unconscious.

While dealing in the unconscious, to realize how our social conscious has affected us is important. Cultural mores, standards, and beliefs that were learned all along shape our behavior and are the cause of our reactions. Looking at those reactions and recognizing their roles in our lives lets us know we are able to accept other persons who may be of different faiths and have different goals or schools of thought. This stage is a time when one is open to the truth, not a truth that is black-and-white, but one that has many shades of gray. These different shades of the truth need to be understood and embraced. Conjunctive faith developmental tasks include: discussions of early midlife in relation to faith, discussions of ecumenism and religious diversity/pluralism, and prayers of contemplation and meditation.

UNIVERSALIZING FAITH (MIDLIFE AND BEYOND)

Persons in this stage begin to live as though what Christians and Jews call the kingdom of God were already a fact. These are persons who, in a sense, have gone beyond self for the sake of affirming God. Fowler (1995) states, "The rare persons who may be described by this stage have a special grace that makes them seem more lucid, more simple, and yet somehow more fully human than the rest of us. . . . Such persons are ready for fellowship with persons at any of the other stages and from any other faith tradition" (p. 201). Some examples of people who are representative of this stage are Dorothy Day, Mother Teresa of Calcutta, Martin Luther King, Jr., Thomas Merton, and Gandhi. Universalizing faith developmental tasks include: serving in social ministries and living a lifestyle that places faith as the basis and framework for living.

Faith and Healing

Interesting to think about is how faith, healing, and wholeness are so closely intertwined. Levin (2001) notes that "For religious believers or the spiritually committed, hope provides a substantial link between active *faith* and psychological factors in disease prevention and healing. Being hopeful represents a cognitive state or process that mobilizes beliefs and emotions that . . . may reduce the risk of illness as well as hasten recovery. Faith, through its provision of hope and positive expectations, is epidemiologically significant" (p. 138).

Healing and wholeness are even further enmeshed. Healing is the precursor to wholeness. Frequently, the terms *healing* and *cure* are interchanged, which is an error. You can experience one or the other, even both, but they are mutually exclusive. Koenig (1999) notes that "Healing can include dramatic, sudden physical cures, but . . . for most people, the healing power of faith involves a healing of the mind and emotions, of the intangible spirit, and of relationships with others" (p. 298). This type of healing often leads to inner peace, which may very likely lessen the physical burden of illness. Wholeness is what we all desire to achieve and is an attempt at balance between body, mind, and spirit.

Religion

Religion is defined as an organized system of beliefs, rituals, practices, and worship with which an individual identifies and wishes to be associated. It usually involves worshipping a deity or supreme being and gathering to worship with persons of like beliefs. Levin (2001) states that religion has denoted three things: particular churches or organized religious institutions; a scholarly field of study; and the domain of life that deals with things of the spirit and matters of "ultimate concern." Clark describes the concept of religion as "a community within which to share reflection and celebration around experiences of being in relationship with" (2000, p. 25). This final concept stresses the dimension of *sharing* within a *community*. Thich Nhat Hanh in *Living Buddha, Living Christ* (1995) notes:

> The faith community is a vehicle that allows people the opportunity to learn and emulate the teachings of Jesus or Buddha. Faith communities, "with all their shortcomings, are the best way to make the teachings available to people. The Father, Son and the Holy Spirit need the church in order to be manifested. . . . People can touch the Father and the Son through the church. That is why we say that the church is the mystical body of Christ. Jesus was very clear about the need to practice the teaching and to do so in community. He told His disciples to be the light of the world. For a Buddhist, that means mindfulness. The Buddha said that we must each be our own torch. Jesus also told His disciples to be the salt of the world, to be real salt. His teaching was clear and strong. If the church practices well the teachings of Jesus, the Trinity will always be present and have a healing power to transform all that it touches" (p. 70).

The importance of faith communities is stressed in the writings of Dietrich Bonhoeffer. He was a minister, spiritual writer, musician, social activist, and a prisoner of the Nazi concentration camps and was later executed in the camp at Flossenbürg. Bonhoeffer's (1954) *Life Together* grew out of personal experience of the deep meaning of Christian community found in the concentration camp. He writes that "The physical presence of other Christians is a source of incomparable joy and strength to the believer" (p. 19) and "The Christian needs another Christian who speaks God's Word to him. He needs him again and again when he becomes uncertain and discouraged" (p. 23). Clearly, the strength of all faith communities lies in the unlimited opportunities for sharing with God and others.

It can be a daunting undertaking for the new parish nurse to try to understand the concepts of faith, spirituality, theology, and religion. It requires a commitment to continual learning, drawing from nursing science, theology—both scholarly and narrative—philosophy, sacred writings, and the behavioral sciences.

Callister, Bond, Matsumura, and Mangum (2004) state that it is critical that spirituality be addressed in nursing education and practice. They believe that the struggle to discover, understand, and more fully embrace the spirituality of the human community, in the midst of a world preoccupied by its more scientifically observable materiality, may be the key to affirming positive health behavior and reducing negative health risks.

Spirituality

"Spirituality is the core of a person's being and is usually conceptualized as a 'higher' experience or a transcendence of oneself. Often, such an experience involves a perception of a personal relationship with a supreme being (such as God)" (Mauk & Schmidt, 2004, p. 2). Spirituality also encompasses feelings and thoughts that bring meaning and purpose to life. *Ruah*, the Hebrew word for *spirit*, translates as wind, breath, and exhalation. Thus, spirit is the life force that motivates people and actively commits them to living (Goldberg, 1998).

Levin (2001) states that, traditionally, the term *spirituality* refers to a state of being that is acquired through religious devotion, piety, and observance. Attaining spirituality, or union with God or the divine, is the ultimate goal of religion and is a state that not everyone reaches. According to this usage, spirituality is a subset of a larger phenomenon, religion, and any definition is sought through religious participation. Levin states that in the past 20 years, the term *spirituality* has taken on a new meaning. Popular writing by New Age authors and the media, often hostile to organized religion, defines spirituality as the larger phenomenon, with the term *religion* reserved for that subset of spiritual activity that involves organized religious activities.

Goldsmith (1997), a pastor and qualified Myers-Briggs practitioner, stresses the importance of knowing yourself and understanding your personality and how it affects your spiritual life. He notes that "There is a great need for each of us to discover a pathway of spirituality which is appropriate for us individually" (p. 19). Parish nurses need to be open to, and to understand, what spirituality means to those they minister to and to themselves. A starting place for inquiry into spirituality is the nursing literature. Macrae (2001) notes that for "Nightingale, spirituality is not an intellectual belief, but an actual experience. Saying 'I believe in God' is different from saying 'I feel the divine presence in my life.' She felt that experience, rather than belief by itself, is the transformative element" (p. 21). Ellis (1980) identifies spirituality as the "quality of having a dynamic and personal relationship with God" (p. 42), whereas O'Brien (1982) defines spirituality as "that which inspires in one the desire to transcend the realm of the material" (p. 88). Barnum (2003) defines spirituality as "a person's search for, or expression of, his connection to a greater and meaningful context. For some people, that will be seen as a connection with God; for others, it may be finding their place in the universe, and that may involve in-depth searching for a greater sense of self" (p. 1). Additional definitions for spirituality are presented in Box 3-1.

Moberg (1984) compares studying spirituality to walking a "tightrope of trying to avoid a misleading reductionism while being sufficiently effective to fulfill scientific and practical needs" (p. 359). McSherry and Draper (1998) believe that "The challenge to the nursing profession is to develop a definition of spirituality which is broad enough to accommodate the uniqueness of all individuals, patients and nurses, and indeed the whole of humanity irrespective of beliefs, values, or religious orientation" (p. 690). Spirituality is the essence of our being and has a distinct meaning to each of us. Whom we become spiritually is all part of life's journey. Is it important for parish nurses to have a definitive definition of spirituality? Probably not, but all nurses would benefit from a broad understanding of this human phenomenon, while knowing that it manifests in each of us in a unique way. A good starting place for understanding spirituality is within us.

Common Spiritual Needs

We all have needs in life: physical, emotional, and spiritual. Some are more obvious than others, such as the need for food, air, water, safety, and belonging. Some are more difficult to ascertain, such as the need to feel God's love and presence. Frequently, spiritual needs are more difficult to identify. Clark (2000) defines spirituality as an "experience of being in relationship with . . ." (p. 21). The distinction between faith and spirituality is an awareness of the "experience *of* being." Spiritual needs, problems, and concerns come into play when this engaging relationship is threatened. Stallwood and Stoll (1975) identify spiritual need as "any factors necessary to establish and maintain a person's dynamic personal relationship with God" (p. 1086). O'Brien (1982) notes that spiritual needs "are seen as involving any essential variables required for the support and viability of that element which inspires in man the desire to transcend the realm of the material" (p. 85).

Spiritual needs can be related to self, others, groups, and God. They range from a need for purpose and meaning, to forgiving others, to staying active in community groups, and to experiencing God's presence (Taylor, 2002). Spiritual needs can result from positive or negative stressful experiences.

BOX 3-1
Definitions of Spirituality

Nightingale (1860)	Spirituality "is not an intellectual belief, but an actual experience." (Macrae, 2001, p. 21).
Vailot (1970)	Spirituality is "the quality of those forces which activate us, or are the essential principle influencing us. Spiritual, although it might, does not necessarily mean religious; it also includes the psychological. The spiritual is opposed to the biological and mechanical, whose laws it may modify" (p. 30).
Ellis (1980)	Spirituality is a "quality of having a dynamic and personal relationship with God" (p. 42).
Colliton (1981)	Spirituality is "the life principle that pervades a person's entire being, including volitional, emotional, moral-ethical, intellectual, and physical dimensions, and generates a capacity for transcendent values" (p. 492).
O'Brien (1982)	Spirituality is "that which inspires in one the desire to transcend the realm of the material" (p. 88).
Amenta (1986)	"The spiritual is the self, or I, the essence of personhood, the God within, that part which communes with the transcendent. It is that part of each individual which longs for ultimate awareness, meaning, value, purpose, beauty, dignity, relatedness, and integrity" (p. 117).
Stoll (1989)	Spirituality involves a vertical dimension (i.e., a person's relationship with God, the transcendent, supreme values) and a horizontal dimension (i.e., which "reflects and 'fleshes out' the supreme experiences of one's relationship with God through one's beliefs, values, life-style, quality of life, and interactions with self, others, and nature") (p. 7).
Reed (1992)	"Spirituality refers to the propensity to make meaning through a sense of relatedness to dimensions that transcend the self in such a way that empowers and does not devalue the individual. This relatedness may be experienced intrapersonally (as a connectedness within oneself), interpersonally (in the context of others and the natural environment), and transpersonally (referring to a sense of relatedness to the unseen, God, or power greater than the self and ordinary resources)" (p. 350).
Fowler (Fowler & Peterson, 1997)	"Spirituality is the way in which a person understands and lives life in view of her or his ultimate meaning, beliefs, and values. It is the unifying and integrative aspect of the person's life and, when lived intentionally, is experienced as a process of growth and maturity. It integrates, unifies, and vivifies the whole of a person's narrative or story, embeds his or her core identity, establishes the fundamental basis for the individual's relationship with others and with society, includes a sense of the transcendent, and is the interpretive lens through which the person sees the world. It is the basis for community for it is in spirituality that we experience our co-participation in the shared human condition. It may or may not be expressed or experienced in religious categories" (p. 47).
Narayanasamy (1999)	"Spirituality is rooted in an awareness which is part of the biological makeup of the human species. Spirituality is therefore present in all individuals and it may manifest as inner peace and strength derived from perceived relationship with a Transcendent God/an Ultimate Reality, or whatever an individual values as supreme. The spiritual dimension evokes feelings which demonstrate the existence of love, faith, hope, trust, awe, and inspirations; therein providing meaning and a reason for existence" (pp. 274, 275).
Barnum (2003)	Spirituality is "a person's search for, or expression of, his connection to a greater and meaningful context. For some people, that will be seen as a connection with God; for others it may be finding their place in the universe, and that may involve in-depth searching for a greater sense of self" (p. 1).
Dossey, Keegan; & Guzzetta (2004)	"Spirituality is a unifying force of a person; the essence of being that permeates all of life and is manifested in one's being, knowing, and doing; the interconnectedness with self, others, nature, and God/Life/Force/Absolute/Transcendent" (p. 7).

BOX 3-2
Manifestations of Spirituality: Common Spiritual Needs

CATEGORY OF SPIRITUAL NEED	EXAMPLES OF SPIRITUAL NEEDS	ILLUSTRATIVE STATEMENTS OR BEHAVIORS
Needs related to self	Need for meaning and purpose	"Sometimes I wonder what the purpose of my life is."
	Need to feel useful	"No one needs me anymore, it seems."
	Need for vision	"It's hard to think that there is anything more I can contribute to this world."
	Need for hope	"I feel desperate—nothing can help me overcome my problem."
	Need for support in coping with life transitions	"I realize how important it is now for me to have my friends and loved ones helping me."
	Need to adapt to increasing dependency	"I don't want my family to have to take care of me when I'm old."
	Need to transcend life challenges	"I wish I could find a silver lining in all my problems."
	Need for personal dignity	"I wish the staff would respect my privacy more."
	Need to express feelings	"Ha! Who wants to listen to me?"
	Need to be thankful	"Feeling grateful makes me feel better."
	Need to accept and prepare for death	"I'm afraid to die."
	Need of fellowship with others	"I miss being able to go to my support group every week."
	Need to love and serve others	"I try to help others who, like me, are coping with breast cancer."
	Need to confess and be forgiven	"I wish I could tell my dad how sorry I am about what I did to him."
	Need for continuity with the past	"Praying to my grandma makes me feel better." (Or making a scrapbook, studying personal genealogy, or reminiscing).
Needs related to others	Need to forgive others	"I feel so betrayed; and I know my anger is eating me inside."
	Need to cope with loss of loved ones	"I miss my loved one so much; I can't live without him/her."
Needs related to the Transcendent	Need to be certain there is a God or ultimate power in the Universe	"How can anyone be absolutely sure there is some guiding force running this world?"
	Need to believe that God is loving	"Because of all the bad stuff that has happened to me, I wonder if God is loving or if He loves me."
	Need to experience God as present	"I wish I could feel God more personally–like a friend."
	Need to serve and worship God	"Going to synagogue and keeping mitzvah allow me to return love to God."
	Need to learn Scripture or other sources considered inspired by God	"I like to read my Bible every day; it helps me to understand the world."

BOX 3-2
Manifestations of Spirituality: Common Spiritual Needs *(continued)*

CATEGORY OF SPIRITUAL NEED	EXAMPLES OF SPIRITUAL NEEDS	ILLUSTRATIVE STATEMENTS OR BEHAVIORS
Needs among and within groups	Need to contribute to the improvement of one's community	A business club that raises funds for a school.
	Need to recognize the power for positive change that groups of individuals can make	"Individually, I can do a little to better the world; collectively, we can do a lot to change the world."
	Need to understand duties and responsibilities	A service organization that modifies its vision and mission to meet the needs of a community.
	Need to be respected and valued	A sociocultural group of persons (e.g., impoverished, disabled, Latinos, Haitians) who unify to demand better treatment from those who oppress them.
	Achievement of personal growth of members of group.	A religious organization that fosters spiritual growth of its members.
	Knowing what and when to give and take.	A nature club that strives to preserve natural habitat or a prayer group that prays for its community and leaders.

Adapted from: Taylor, E. J. (2002). *Spiritual care: Nursing theory, research, and practice* (pp. 17–20). Upper Saddle River, NJ: Prentice Hall; Koenig, H. & Pritchett, J. (1998). *Religion and psychotherapy*. In H. Koenig (Ed.), *Handbook of religion and mental health* (Chapter 22). San Diego, CA: Academic Press; and Nolan, P. & Crawford, P. (1997). Towards a rhetoric of spirituality in mental health care. *Journal of Advanced Nursing, 26,* 289–294. Used with permission.

Examples of spiritual needs vary but may include the need to feel purpose and a sense of belonging, to be able to forgive, to be grateful, or to believe that God loves. Nurses need to be sensitive to how spiritual needs manifest as a first step in determining the need for spiritual care. Box 3-2 offers examples of spiritual needs.

Spiritual Care

If you ask a parish nurse what a typical workday is like, you may have to wait some time before getting an answer. It would probably be easier to explain an atypical day. One thing for sure, this nurse is working or standing on holy ground. What exactly does it mean to stand on holy ground? O'Brien (2003) believes that when parish nurses stand before their parishioners they are truly standing on holy ground; they are present for their "parishioners' pain and loneliness and fear" (p. 152). This intimacy of their troubles is the gift that people give to the parish nurse. This does not suggest that only parish nurses receive this gift or blessing; all nurses are in a position to stand on holy ground, in the hospital, in the clinic, in a doctor's office, or in the community. The first part of the prayer *Holy Ground* (by Columban Father Pat Sayles) states "Loving God, we believe you live among us and the place where you are is Holy Ground" (The Columban Fathers mission net, http://www.st.columban.org/prayer/hg.html). Holy ground is not so much a physical place but a spiritual place where we can meet and minister to the needs of those in our care. One advantage of being a parish nurse is the emphasis on providing spiritual care. Providing spiritual care is a way of caring for another holistically while integrating faith and health.

Sawatzky and Pesut (2005) present a brief historical review of spiritual care in nursing practice. They state that three eras characterized by particular approaches have shaped spiritual care in nursing. The first era was the religious approach in which nursing was considered a calling and individuals cared for others out of a sense of duty and the glory of God. The second era was the scientific approach that occurred through the middle part of the 20th century. During this period, spiritual care was primarily enacted using the nursing process. Spiritual assessments, diagnoses, and interventions were the components of spiritual care, with the assumptions that a person's spirituality could be assessed and modified via specific interventions.

Recent authors have proposed an existential approach to spiritual care, which emphasizes the importance of dialogue. Hall (1997) describes the goals of spiritual care to be "self-in-relation," with the role of the nurse to be caring and present during the patient's search for meaning. Sawatzky and Pesut (2005) suggest that all of the approaches contribute important understandings about spiritual care. They state that the religious perspectives are important for those whose faith-based historical traditions are essential to their spiritual well-being. The scientific perspectives encourage systematic thinking about spirituality in the larger context of knowledge development. The existential perspectives have redefined spirituality as a broader, universal human dimension. These authors propose that "Spiritual care nursing is an intuitive, interpretive, altruistic, and integrative expression that is contingent on the nurse's awareness of the transcendent dimension of life but that reflect the patient's reality" (p. 23).

Spiritual Assessment

Nurses assess routinely and in-depth physical or emotional needs for patients, but how many nurses assess spiritual needs comfortably? Assessing spiritual needs makes many nurses uncomfortable, even parish nurses; especially new parish nurses may have some difficulty with this type of assessment. Spiritual assessment is very intimate, and according to Maugens (1996) and Peterson (1987), spiritual assessment should be an ongoing process. Building trusting relationships with faith community members lays down a foundation for approaching spiritual assessment.

Several models for spiritual assessment come from the disciplines of nursing, pastoral care, psychology, psychiatry, and even medicine. No one "preferred" model for spiritual assessment exists; all have value because they help the parish nurse formulate ideas and questions for an inclusive spiritual assessment. Unknown is how many parish nurses actually use specific spiritual assessment tools per se, but they do assess spirituality through observation within the faith community, relationship building, and listening to people's stories or narrative theology. However, it is important to look at many assessment tools and decide on those you are most comfortable with, and to understand that as you grow in experience you may use different assessment tools or you may develop your own assessment tool.

Pruyser's (1976) book, *The Minister as Diagnostician,* is one of the most influential works about spiritual assessment. Pruyser was a psychologist who had a strong interest in spiritual care and counseling. In Chapter 5 of his book, Pruyser identifies seven guidelines in the form of seven theological themes. These guidelines for pastoral diagnosis have become the foundation of more specific models of spiritual assessment. They include:

1. Awareness of the holy
2. Providence
3. Faith
4. Grace or gratefulness
5. Repentance
6. Communion
7. Sense of vocation

An interesting way to approach spiritual assessment is by using Maugens' (1996) SPIRIT mnemonic; it keys the parish nurse to remember the important areas to be covered while doing an assessment. The SPIRIT mnemonic stands for **S**piritual belief system, **P**ersonal spirituality, **I**ntegration and involvement with a spiritual community, **R**itualized practices and restrictions, and **I**mplication and **T**erminal events planning. Maugens offers some sample questions for each of the areas in the model.

S—Spiritual belief system

- What is your formal religious affiliation?
- Name and describe your spiritual belief system.

P—Personal spirituality

- Describe the beliefs and practices of your religion or personal belief system.
- Describe the beliefs or practices you do not accept.
- What does your spirituality mean to you?
- What is the importance of spirituality/religion in daily life?

I—Integration with a spiritual community

- Do you belong to a spiritual/religious group or community? What is your role or position?
- What importance does this group have to you? Is it a source of support? In what ways?
- Does or could this group provide help in dealing with health issues?

R—Ritualized practices and restrictions

- Are there specific practices that you carry out as part of your religion/spirituality?
- Are there certain lifestyle activities or practices that your religion/spirituality encourages or forbids? Do you comply? What significance do these practices have for you?
- Are there specific elements of medical care that are forbidden on the basis of religious grounds?

I—Implications for care

- What aspects of your religion/spirituality would you like me to keep in mind as I care for you?
- Would you like to discuss religious or spiritual implications of health care?
- What knowledge or understanding would strengthen our relationship as caregiver and client?
- Are there any barriers to our relationship based on religious or spiritual issues?

T—Terminal events planning

- As we plan for end-of-life care, how does your faith affect your decisions?
- Are there particular aspects of care that you wish to forgo or have withheld because of your faith?

Parish nurses often minister to their faith community members in various settings: in a church, temple or mosque, in someone's home, in a restaurant, or while sitting on a fence in a parking lot. Timing is everything when doing spiritual assessment; the SPIRIT mnemonic is easy to remember and can be used easily in any setting.

Puchalski and Romer (2000) developed the FICA Model, which assists in gathering data about a client's spiritual and religious background. The FICA Model is user-friendly and flexible enough to use with diverse populations. Questions that the nurse can use for each element are as follows:

F—Faith and belief

- What is your faith or belief?
- Do you consider yourself to be spiritual or religious?
- What things do you believe in that give meaning to your life?

I—Importance

- Is your faith important in your life?
- Have your beliefs influenced how you take care of yourself?
- What role do your beliefs play during this illness?
- Will your beliefs affect your recovery?

C—Community

- Are you a part of a spiritual or religious community?
- Is this of support to you and how?
- Is there a group of people you really love or who are important to you?

A—Address

- How would you like me, your health care provider, to address these issues in your health care?

Anandarajah and Hight (2001) offer another spiritual assessment model, based on the acronym HOPE:

H—Sources of **h**ope, meaning, comfort, strength, peace, love, and connection
O—Organized religion
P—Personal spirituality and practice
E—Effects on medical care and end-of-life issues

Two additional examples of spiritual assessment tools are the JAREL Spiritual Well-Being Scale (Box 3-3) and Stoll's Guidelines for Spiritual Assessment (Box 3-4). The JAREL Scale uses a Likert scale, is quick and easy to administer, and is an effective tool for an initial spiritual assessment. Stoll's model is considered a classic model; it requires more time to administer, is contemplative in nature, but it renders more in-depth data.

Regardless of the type of spiritual assessment used, the goal is to identify spiritual needs and to determine appropriate spiritual care, remembering that there are many approaches.

Diagnosis

The North American Nursing Diagnosis Association (NANDA, 2003) has approved three nursing diagnoses specifically related to spirituality: spiritual distress, risk for spiritual distress, and readiness for enhanced spiritual well-being. See Box 3-5 for definitions of these terms.

Spiritual Care Interventions

Providing spiritual care is the essence of parish nursing. Although this specialty focuses on holistic health and wellness and prevention, the spiritual component is what makes it so unique. Many ways provide spiritual care, but what is important to remember is that it is not

BOX 3-3
Jarel Spiritual Well-Being Scale

Directions: Please circle the choice that best describes how much you agree with each statement. Circle only one answer for each statement. There is no wrong answer.

	Strongly Agree	Moderately Agree	Agree	Disagree	Moderately Disagree	Strongly Disagree
1. Prayer is an important part of my life.	SA	MA	A	D	MD	SD
2. I believe I have spiritual well-being.	SA	MA	A	D	MD	SD
3. As I grow older, I find myself more tolerant of others' beliefs.	SA	MA	A	D	MD	SD
4. I find meaning and purpose in my life.	SA	MA	A	D	MD	SD
5. I feel there is a close relationship between my spiritual beliefs and what I do.	SA	MA	A	D	MD	SD
6. I believe in an afterlife.	SA	MA	A	D	MD	SD
7. When I am sick I have less spiritual well-being.	SA	MA	A	D	MD	SD
8. I believe in a supreme power.	SA	MA	A	D	MD	SD
9. I am able to receive and give love to others.	SA	MA	A	D	MD	SD
10. I am satisfied with my life.	SA	MA	A	D	MD	SD
11. I set goals for myself.	SA	MA	A	D	MD	SD
12. God has little meaning in my life.	SA	MA	A	D	MD	SD
13. I am satisfied with the way I am using my abilities.	SA	MA	A	D	MD	SD
14. Prayer does not help me in making decisions.	SA	MA	A	D	MD	SD
15. I am able to appreciate differences in others.	SA	MA	A	D	MD	SD
16. I am pretty well put together.	SA	MA	A	D	MD	SD
17. I prefer that others make decisions for me.	SA	MA	A	D	MD	SD
18. I find it hard to forgive others.	SA	MA	A	D	MD	SD
19. I accept life situations.	SA	MA	A	D	MD	SD

Hageman, J., Kneel-Rossi, E., Klasson, L., & Stollenwerk, R. (1987). Marquette University School of Nursing, Milwaukee, WI 53201. Used with permission.

BOX 3-4
Stoll's Guidelines for Spiritual Assessment

CONCEPT OF GOD OR DEITY

1. Is religion or God significant to you? If yes, can you describe how?
2. Is prayer helpful to you? What happens when you pray?
3. Does a God or deity function in your personal life? If yes, can you describe how?
4. How would you describe your God or what you worship?

SOURCES OF HOPE AND STRENGTH

1. Who is the most important person to you?
2. To whom do you turn when you need help? Are they available?
3. In what ways do they help?
4. What is your source of strength and hope?
5. What helps you the most when you feel afraid or need special help?

RELIGIOUS PRACTICES

1. Do you feel that your faith (or religion) is helpful to you? If yes, would you tell how?
2. Are there any religious practices that are important to you?
3. Has being sick made any difference in your practice of praying? In your religious practices?
4. What religious books or symbols are helpful to you?

RELATIONS BETWEEN SPIRITUAL BELIEFS AND HEALTH

1. What has bothered you the most about being sick (or in what is happening to you)?
2. What do you think is going to happen to you?
3. Has being sick (or what has happened to you) made any difference in your feelings about God or the practice of your faith?
4. Is there anything that is especially frightening or meaningful to you now?

Excerpted from Stoll, R. I. (1979). Guidelines for Spiritual Assessment. *American Journal of Nursing, 79*, 1574–1577. Used with permission.

so much about delivering care but more about facilitating the process of achieving spiritual well-being. A few examples of spiritual care are presented in Box 3-6.

Van Dover and Bacon (2001) state that "Spiritual care addresses the core of the human being, the human spirit; therefore, nurses who give spiritual care are engaging the core of who they are in caring for others. This level of interaction creates meanings and memories that are life- and health-giving for the nurse as well as the patient" (p. 28). They cite Wendell Berry's (1998) poetry "To give words to the awesome, humbling experience it is to give and receive spiritual care" (p. 28):

> And we are here
> as we have never been before,
> sighted as not before, our place
> holy, although we knew it not. (p. 94)

BOX 3-5
NANDA Definitions

Spiritual distress	Impaired ability to experience and integrate meaning and purpose in life through the individual's connectedness with self, others, art, music, literature, nature, or a power greater than oneself.
Risk for spiritual distress	At risk for altered sense of harmonious connectedness with all of life and the universe in which dimensions that transcend and empower the self may be disrupted.
Readiness for enhanced spiritual well-being	Ability to experience and integrate meaning and purpose in life through connectedness with self, others, art, music, literature, nature, or a power greater than oneself.

Carpenito-Moyet, L. J. (2004). *Nursing diagnosis: Application to clinical practice* (10th ed.). Philadelphia: Lippincott Williams & Wilkins. Used with permission.

Grant (2004) surveyed 299 nurses in a large university hospital in the Southwest. This institution had recently taken several significant steps to recognize the importance of the sacred in medical care. He found that five spiritual interventions were used by the majority of the respondents. These interventions were holding a client's hand (92%), listening (92%), laughter (84%), prayer (71%), and being present with a client (62%). Nurse respondents (30% to 40%) have offered massages, therapeutic touch, music therapy, guided imagery, and meditation. Virtually all of the nurses thought that spiritual care resources should be made available to clients. Grant's findings are congruent with those of Tuck, Wallace, and Pullen (2001), who studied spiritual care interventions provided by parish nurses. They found that praying was the primary spiritual intervention used by parish nurses. Other interventions included being with, caring, listening, and providing spiritual services.

The *Nursing Interventions Classification* (NIC, 2004) defines a nursing intervention as "*Any treatment, based upon clinical judgment and knowledge, that a nurse performs to enhance patient client outcomes*" (p. xxiii). The NIC lists priority interventions, suggested interventions and additional optional interventions related to each NANDA nursing diagnosis. Priority interventions for the diagnoses of spiritual distress and risk for spiritual distress include spiritual growth facilitation and spiritual support. The priority intervention for the diagnosis of readiness for enhanced spiritual well-being is spiritual growth facilitation.

Taylor (2002) notes that "The complexity and variety of spiritual needs of diverse clients certainly require numerous approaches to spiritual care" (p. 150). A few examples of spiritual care will be discussed in detail; this does not imply that they are preferred methods but rather demonstrates a few approaches. One example of spiritual care that is limitless in expression is

---

BOX 3-6
Examples of Spiritual Care

- Being present (physically, psychologically, or spiritually)
- Active listening
- Prayer
- Reading religious texts
- Reminiscence
- Touch
- Creative arts
- Religious practices or customs
- Social support
- Guided imagery
- Journaling
- Meditation
- Presencing
- Kything
- Labyrinths

prayer. Ameling (2000) states that prayer is an ancient healing practice, which is the simple act of turning our mind to the sacred. Although there are as many types of prayer as there are ways of praying, the traditional categories of prayer include:

1. *Petition*: asking something for one's self
2. *Intercession*: asking something for others
3. *Confession*: expressing repentance of wrongdoing and asking forgiveness
4. *Lamentation:* crying out in distress and asking for vindication
5. *Adoration:* giving honor and praise
6. *Invocation:* summoning the presence of the Almighty
7. *Thanksgiving:* offering gratitude (Ameling, 2000, p. 43)

Prayer is a way of connecting and becoming aware of God's presence. DelBene, Montgomery, and Montgomery (1988) speak of the importance of prayer when ministering to the seriously ill. Breath prayer is a simple form of prayer that "arises from the heart and becomes as natural as breathing" (p. 31). Breath prayer is individualized and personal but can be shared with others. Prayer will not always change the situation, but prayer brings about change in us. Prayer is a vehicle to discovering sources of "hope, strength and courage that we didn't know we had" (p. 82). It brings people together, crosses theologies, and is not hindered by distance. The following case study illustrates the use of prayer.

Case Study

Mallory, a parish nurse, was scanning messages on an online group for parish nurses. One message was a prayer request for a nurse named Mary Lou who wanted to start a parish nurse ministry in her church and was preparing to do a final presentation before the faith community board. Mallory responded to the e-mail and prayed for this request. A few days later, Mary Lou posted that she had received approval to start the parish nurse ministry, but now she was faced with a personal health challenge. She wanted prayers for herself. A few months ago her ophthalmologist noted a lesion in her eye, possibly a melanoma. She was scheduled to return for a follow-up visit and requested prayers for healing. Mallory read the e-mail and responded by sending Mary Lou a favorite prayer she used for request of healing. The next afternoon Mary Lou posted an e-mail noting that just before she left for her doctor's appointment she read the prayer. She went to the appointment and the physician was amazed. The lesion in her eye had so significantly decreased that the physician commented that he must have made a mistake last visit. Mary Lou could not contain herself. Later that day she e-mailed the group and thanked Mallory for the special prayer and the group for all of their prayers. Her comment was that the doctor thought he had made a mistake, but we know what really happened.

Another unique way of ministering to another person spiritually is through Kything, which is described as "a conscious act of spiritual presence" (Savary & Berne, 1988). Kything can be established by "physical presence and touching, . . . psychological presence and communication, . . . and spiritual presence and communion" (pp. 9, 10). Three steps comprise the process of Kything: becoming centered, focusing on the person with whom you want to Kythe, and establishing a connection with that person. Rupp (1989) speaks of Kything with a friend who was critically ill. She explained to her friend that every day she would Kythe or be spiritually present with her. Rupp describes it as a way of sending God's loving energy to fill one's spirit and being.

Labyrinths also serve as an excellent tool in facilitating spiritual care. Labyrinths have been around for over 3,500 years and are used by people of many different religions. Labyrinths are not mazes but have one path that leads to the center and back out again. Walking a labyrinth or using a finger labyrinth is symbolic of a journey to the divine; it is a form of walking prayer. "At its most basic level the labyrinth is a metaphor for the journey to the center of your deepest self and back out into the world with a broadened understanding of who you are" (*The Labyrinth: Walking Your Spiritual Journey,* http://www.lessons4living.com/labyrinth.htm). When a person walks the labyrinth over time, he or she forms a "deeper connection with the sacred," experiences more "creative surges," develops a "growing acceptance of others," and "experiences joy and transformation" (Geoffrion, 2000, p. xv).

The use of creative arts is an innovative way of providing spiritual care. Many people are moved by listening to music or favorite hymns, or looking at beautiful pieces of art, even creating art. One technique that taps into our creativity is drawing a mandala. "The word 'mandala' is from the classical Indian language of Sanskrit. Loosely translated to mean 'circle,' a mandala is far more than a simple shape. It represents wholeness and can be seen as a model for the organizational structure of life itself—a cosmic diagram that reminds us of our relation to the infinite, the world that extends both beyond and within our bodies and minds" (http://www.mandalaproject.org/Mandalas/index_new.htm). Anyone can draw a mandala— from children to the elderly. It is not about how artistic someone is, but rather a form of drawing prayer. Gerding (2001) notes: "There is something about creating a circular design which seems to draw us inward. . . . It fits well into our explorations as we open our inner selves to God" (p. 46).

Remembering that the possibilities for spiritual care are endless is important. The case study on pp. 66–67 presents a parish nurse/parishioner situation in which the importance of *relationship* is demonstrated.

Evaluation of Spiritual Care

The Iowa Outcomes Project, *Nursing Outcomes Classification* (Moorhead, Johnson, & Maas, 2004), defines spiritual health as "connectedness with self, others, higher power, all life, nature, and the universe that transcends and empowers the self" (p. 519). This outcome can be measured using the NOC spiritual health overall rating scale, which has 21 indicators of spiritual health that are measured on a five-point Likert scale ranging from "severely compromised" to "uncompromised."

The NOC also provides a list of suggested outcomes for each NANDA diagnosis. These measures will be helpful to all parish nurses to assess the outcomes of spiritual care interventions with individuals.

Rethemeyers and Wehling (2004) designed a tool to measure the practice of parish nursing in faith communities. Specific questions that the tool addressed were:

- Do parish nurses effect change in the health behaviors of those served?
- Are parish nurses easily accessible to members of the congregation?
- What are the benefits of using the parish nurse for health needs?
- What are the disadvantages, if any, of using a parish nurse for health needs?
- Do parish nurses provide services that are commensurate with their roles?

In January 2003, they surveyed 760 people, representing five denominations: Lutheran; Catholic; United Church of Christ; Christian Church, Disciples of Christ; and Presbyterian. Results showed that those participating in the survey felt that the congregation benefited from the services offered by the parish nurse. Participants indicated that they had no problems contacting the parish nurse; they received answers to their questions and were comfortable praying with the parish nurse. They also indicated that the parish nurse encouraged self-development and self-reflection and had a positive impact on their health. The most frequently reported health practices that were impacted by the parish nurse included: regular blood pressure checks (49.3%), participating in worship (41.1%), eating healthier foods (38.7%), learning the warning signs of a heart attack (39.6%) or stroke (35.4%), attending church-sponsored programs (35.1%), and getting regular exercise (31.8%). This survey is available to parish nurses on the International Parish Nurse Resource Center Web site, http://www.ipnrc.parishnurses.org.

Characteristics of Faith Communities

What encompasses a faith community? The answers are faith, spirituality, theology, religion, and its members. All of these, and more, are true. A faith community is a place where "we can sense the relationship between God and God's creation" (Gunderson, 1997, p. 21). A faith community is also a place where we can feel love and give love, comfort others and be comforted, where we can "grow with God" in the midst of all of life's stressors and sufferings (O'Brien, 2003). When a nurse is blessed with the opportunity of becoming a parish nurse, the faith community becomes her or his client. Because most schools of nursing do not prepare nurses for this role, it is advantageous for the new parish nurse to seek basic preparation educational programs early on in their ministries.

Working within a faith community, the nurse must be grounded somewhere between nursing science and theology. For new parish nurses understanding the characteristics of faith communities is important when finding one's way in this specialty. It should be noted that "nurses have already made significant contributions in this area by reflecting on the terms *spirit, spiritual,* and *spirituality.* The concepts of religion, religious, and religiosity have received considerably less attention, with other related ideas, like faith and theology, receiving only passing mention or referred to theological literature" (Barnum, 1996; Carson, 1989; Stuart, Deckro, & Mandle, 1989).

Many ways exist of viewing faith communities. One interesting way of looking at the members is generationally. Poling-Goldenne (1998) suggests that each of the present generations in the United States offers "generational gifts" particular to their subset. Although nothing is absolute, this approach offers a unique overview of members of faith communities. Five current generations are defined: the GI generation, the builder or booster generation, baby boomers, the first postmodern generation, and the millennial kids' generation. A few highlights of each generation are as follows:

The GI generation "born prior to 1930 is . . . fiercely reliable and values honor." The builder or booster generation "born between 1930 and 1945 . . . is rooted in tradition and values hard work." The baby boomers "born between 1946 and 1964 . . . are creative and want to be involved and make a difference." The postmodern generation "born between 1965 and 1981 . . . value personal experiences and feelings . . . are accepting of ethnic diversity and balanced power between genders." The millennial kids born between 1982 and the current time are "the first generation to accept nontraditional families. . . . They are more ethnically diverse than the generations born before them" (pp. 30, 31). These generational characteristics may be helpful to the parish nurse in planning activities for different age groups.

In contrast, Clark (2000) looks at faith communities through the concepts of "faith, spirituality, theology, and religion as constitutive elements undergirding the practice of nursing in a faith community" (p. 18). She describes, rather than defines, each concept and demonstrates how each concept is connected to the original concept. The first concept, faith, is described as "being in relationship with" the key word, being *relationship* (p. 19). Many relationships exist within faith communities, how people relate to each other, religious customs, and services to the community at large and to the environment. Through observation, assessment, and inquiry the parish nurse can better understand people in the faith community and how they "view health, life, suffering, self-care, and social responsibility" (p. 21). The second concept, spirituality, is described as "an experience of being in relationship with" (p. 21). Perceiving the subtle distinction between *experience* and *being* is the difference between faith and spirituality. *Being* is more of an abstract state, whereas to *experience* is more involved, more connected. Spirituality is more involved and answers the questions of how members relate with their God, with each other, and with their environment. The third concept, theology, is described as "reflection and celebration around experiences of being in relationship with" (p. 24).

Many nurses today view theology as a scholarly discipline, but theology did not start out this way. Initially, it was a way of sharing stories about "the god, goddesses, heroes, and heroines of ancient civilization" (Bowker, 1997, p. 970). This form of narrative theology brings people closer together by sharing beliefs, experiences, and traditions of the faith community. "The sharing of stories, music and the arts in general provide the natural means to help us engage with people of all backgrounds and interest" (The Northumbria Community, 2002, p. 9). The importance of narrative theology or hearing the story is made evident in this prayer:

> Teach me to hear that story, through each person, to cradle a sense of wonder in their life, to honor the hard-earned wisdom of their sufferings, to waken their joy that the King of all kings stoops down to wash their feet, and looking up into their face says, I know—I understand. (p. 199)

Narrative theology is a wonderful way for faith community members and the parish nurse to develop a personal theology; it is a way to *reflect on experiences of being in relationship with.* Celebration and worship can also be facilitated through art, dance, song, instrumentation, and the use of symbols.

Faith Seeking and Health Seeking as Interrelated Processes

Many of us, knowingly or unknowingly, seek faith and health in an interrelated fashion. This may mean connecting with a faith community, or a meditation group, or a group that focuses on spirituality and spiritual connection, but not necessarily associated with a particular religion. Wherever we feel spiritually connected is our ideal place for combining faith and health. In such surroundings is where the concept of holism flourishes.

Parish nurses are situated within faith communities, and one of their ministerial roles is to help people discover how to integrate faith with health. Koenig (1999) notes many ways "to enhance the health benefits of faith, based on scientific research" (p. 277). This topic is covered in more detail in his book *The Healing Power of Faith: Science Explores Medicine's Last Great Frontier.* A brief overview of Koenig's suggestions for people who are already religious is described:

- Attend services more often and become involved in the faith community.
- Identify your gifts and use them to benefit the faith community or the community-at-large.
- Join prayer groups or religious text study groups.
- Carve out time early in the morning for prayer or quiet time; this time is a wonderful time to listen to God.
- Pray with family members.
- Pray before you make important decisions.
- Pray, pray, pray! Praying is a wonderful way to communicate with God.

Koenig suggests "stepping-out in your faith on a regular basis. . . . If you're white . . . attend an African-American service" or a Latino-American service (p. 280). Ways to "step-out" are endless.

People who are *not* religious benefit from:

- Not denying the existence of God.
- Attempting to reconcile any previous bad experiences with religion.
- Attending services with friends.
- Reading about inspiring people of faith and or religious texts.
- Trying to adopt any of the suggestions given for people who are religious (Koenig, 1999).

Sometimes, people are not ready to consider religion, and they should be encouraged to:

- Find ways to help others in the community.
- Enroll in activities, such as meditation or yoga—something that will have a calming effect.
- Be more introspective about feelings regarding past negative religious experiences and discuss them with close friends. (Koenig, 1999)

Summary

This chapter provides the parish nurse with the basic theology of faith, health, and wholeness. Tools for assessment of spiritual needs and suggestions for providing spiritual care are given. An overview of definitions of spirituality, stages of spiritual development, and suggestions for seeking faith and health interrelatedly is presented.

Reflect and Discuss

1. Discuss the relationship between faith, healing, and wholeness.
2. Identify examples of healing in spiritual texts.
3. How can parish nurses help faith community members integrate faith and health?
4. Identify and discuss the characteristics of your practicing faith community.
5. Why is it important to have an understanding of spiritual development?

Case Study

Betsy, a 59-year-old obese African American woman, would stop by the parish nurse's office after noon-day prayer every Wednesday. She just wanted to check in to see how things were going. After 2 months of visits, she agreed to have her blood pressure (BP) checked. It was high, 180/90. Diane, the parish nurse, did all of the interventions any nurse would do after detecting an elevated blood pressure. She inquired if Betsy had a family doctor, was on medication for her elevated blood pressure, was she taking it, could she afford it? Did she exercise regularly? They discussed diet, salt intake, and stress levels. Diane asked Betsy if she would like her to call her family doctor to report the BP elevation or would she like for Diane to call. Betsy commented that she preferred to make the call and would do so as soon as she got home. Diane informed Betsy that she would call the next day to check on her.

Diane tried the next day and the next to contact Betsy, but there was no answer. The next Wednesday rolled around and Betsy came back for a BP check. Betsy and Diane started this visit with a prayer and then started to talk about Betsy's family and daily routine. Betsy's BP was still elevated. Betsy said she was trying to get a little exercise and to watch her diet. They again discussed medication, diet, reduced salt intake, exercise, stress management, follow-up with a physician, and the serious potential health problems that could occur, if the BP was not adequately treated. These weekly visits achieved many things. They provided a great opportunity to reinforce the importance of lifestyle changes and to observe actual change, time to build a helping–trusting caring relationship, and a chance to focus on spiritual health.

Finally, one day Betsy came to the office for her weekly BP check. She told Diane that she wasn't being completely truthful about her medication and going to the doctor. Betsy had some financial problems, lost her health insurance and was too embarrassed to tell anyone in the church about what was happening. Diane was able to refer her to a local clinic that would see her free of charge. Appointments were arranged, and Diane hoped that Betsy would follow through with the clinic appointment. She did not.

This weekly appointment went on for about 8 or 9 months. Then a month lapsed when Betsy didn't come to the office. Finally, one day Betsy stopped by the office for a visit. She and Diane prayed, and then Betsy announced: "You will be happy to know that my BP is down." After months and months of praying, being present with, educating, caring, and encouraging, Betsy finally decided to do something. She told Diane that she really believed that she cared about her and was truly concerned, and that is why she decided to get some treatment.

References

Ameling, A. (2000). Prayer: An ancient healing practice becomes new again. *Holistic Nursing Practice, 14*(3), 40–48.

Amenta, M. O. (1986). Spiritual concerns. In M. O. Amenta & N. Bohnet (Eds.), N*ursing care of the terminally ill* (pp. 115–161). Boston: Little, Brown and Company.

Anandarajah, G. & Hight, E. (2001). Spirituality and medical practice: Using the HOPE questions as a practical tool for spiritual assessment. *American Family Physician, 63,* 81–89.

Barnum, B. S. (2003). *Spirituality in nursing: From traditional to new age* (2nd ed.). New York: Springer-Verlag.

Barnum, B. S. (1996). *Spirituality in nursing: From traditional to new age.* New York: Springer-Verlag.

Berry, W. (1998). *A timbered choir: The Sabbath poems 1979–1997.* Washington, DC: Counterpoint.

Bonhoeffer, D. (1954). *Life together.* New York: Harper & Row.

Bowker, J. (Ed.) (1997). *The Oxford dictionary of world religions.* New York: Oxford University Press.

Callister, L. C., Bond, A. E., Matsumura, G., & Mangum, S. (2004). Threading spirituality throughout nursing education. *Holistic Nursing Practice, 18*(3), 160–166.

Carpenito-Moyet, L. J. (2004). *Nursing diagnosis: Application to clinical practice* (10th ed.). Philadelphia: Lippincott Williams & Wilkins.

Carson, V. B. (1989). *Spiritual dimensions of nursing practice.* Philadelphia: WB Saunders.

Chamberlain, T. J. & Hall, C. A. (2000). *Realized religion: Research based on the relationship between religion and health.* Philadelphia: Templeton Foundation Press.

Clark, M. B. (2000). Characteristics of faith communities. In M. B. Clark & J. K. Olson (Eds.), *Nursing within a faith community: Promoting health in times of transition* (pp. 17–29). Thousand Oaks, CA: Sage Publications.

Colliton, M. (1981). The spiritual dimension of nursing. In I. Beland & J. Y. Passons (Eds.), *Clinical nursing* (4th ed.). New York: Macmillan.

Columban Fathers Mission. (2003). Available at: http://www.st.columban.org/prayer/hg.html.

Coyle, J. (2002). Spirituality and health: Towards a framework for exploring the relationship between spirituality and health. *Journal of Advanced Nursing, 37*(6), 589–597.

DelBene, R., Montgomery, H., & Montgomery, M. (1988). *Into the light: A simple way to pray with the sick and the dying.* Nashville, TN: The Upper Room.

Dossey, B. M. & Guzzetta, C. E. (2005). Holistic nursing practice. In B. M. Dossey, L. Keegan, & C. E. Guzzetta, *Holistic nursing: A handbook for practice* (4th ed.) (pp. 5–37). Sudbury, MA: Jones and Bartlett.

Dubos, R. (1965). *Man adapting.* New Haven, CT: Yale University Press.

Dunn, H. L. (1959). What high level wellness means. *Canadian Journal of Public Health 50*(11), 447–457.

Ellis, D. (1980). Whatever happened to the spiritual dimension? *The Canadian Nurse, 76*, 42–43.

Fowler, J. W. (1995). *Stages of faith: The psychology of human development and the quest for meaning.* San Francisco: HarperCollins.

Fowler, M. & Peterson, B. S. (1997). Spiritual themes in clinical pastoral education. *Journal of Training and Supervision in Ministry, 18,* 46–54.

Geoffrion, J. (2000). *Living the labyrinth: 101 Paths to a deeper connection with the sacred.* Cleveland, OH: The Pilgrim Press.

Gerding, J. (2001). *Drawing to God: Art as prayer, prayer as art.* South Bend, IN: Sorin Books.

Goldberg, B. (1998). Connection: An exploration of spirituality in nursing care. *Journal of Advanced Nursing, 27*(4), 836–846.

Goldsmith, M. (1997). *Knowing me, knowing God: Exploring your spirituality with Myers-Briggs.* Nashville, TN: Abingdon Press.

Grant, D. (2004). Spiritual intervention: How, when, and why nurses use them. *Holistic Nursing Practice, 18*(1), 36–41.

Gunderson, G. (1997). *Deeply woven roots: Improving the quality of life in your community.* Minneapolis: Fortress Press.

Hageman, J., Kneel-Rossi, E., Klasson, L., & Stollenwerk, R. (1987). Marquette University School of Nursing, Milwaukee, WI 53201. Used with permission.

Hall, B. A. (1997). Spirituality in terminal illness: An alternative view of theory. *Journal of Holistic Nursing, 15,* 82–96.

Health Ministries Association/American Nurses Association. (2005). *Scope and standards of faith community nursing* (2nd ed.). Washington, DC: Author.

Internet Encyclopedia of Philosophy. (2004). Available at: http://www.utm.edu/research/iep/d/descarte.htm.

Johnson, D. E. (1990). The behavioral systems models for nursing. In M. E. Parker (Ed.), *Nursing theories in practice* (pp. 23–32). New York: NLN Press.

Johnson, M., Maas, M., & Moorhead, S. (Eds.). (2000). *Nursing outcomes classification (NOC)* (2nd ed.). St. Louis: Mosby–Year Book.

King, I. M. (1990). Health as the goal for nursing. *Nursing Science Quarterly, 3*(3), 123–128.

Koenig, H. G. (1999). *The healing power of faith: Science explores medicine's last great frontier.* New York: Simon & Schuster.

Koenig, H. & Pritchett, J. (1998). Religion and psychotherapy. In H. Koenig (Ed.), *Handbook of religion and mental health* (Chapter 21). San Diego, CA: Academic Press.

The Labyrinth: Walking your spiritual journey. (2004). Available at: http://www.lessons4living.com/labyrinth.htm.

Levin, J. S. (2001). *God, faith, and health: Exploring the spirituality-healing connection.* New York: John Wiley and Sons.

Levin, J. S. & Vanderpool, H. Y. (1991). Religious factors in physical health and the prevention of illness. *Prevention in Human Services, 9,* 41–64.

Levine, M. E. (1991). The conservation principles: A model for health. In M. Schaefer & J. B. Pond (Eds.), *Levine's conservation model: A framework for nursing practice* (pp. 1–11). Philadelphia: FA Davis.

Macrae, J. A. (2001). *Nursing as a spiritual practice: A contemporary application of Florence Nightingale's views.* New York: Springer-Verlag.

Marty, M. (1990). Health, medicine, and the faith traditions. In M. Marty, M. Solberg, & S. Pittman (Eds.), *Healthy people 2000: A role for America's religious communities.* Chicago & Atlanta: Carter Center of Emory University & Park Ridge Center of the Study of Health, Faith, and Ethics.

Matthews, D. A., McCullough, M. E., Larson, D. B., Koenig, H. G., Swyers, J. P., & Milano, M. G. (1998). Religious commitment and health status. *Archives of Family Medicine, 7,* 118–124.

Maugens, T. A. (1996). The SPIRITual history. *Archives of Family Medicine, 5,* 11–16.

Mauk, K. L. & Schmidt, N. A. (2004). *Spiritual care in nursing practice.* Philadelphia: Lippincott Williams & Wilkins.

McCloskey, J. C. & Bulechek, G. M. (Eds.). (2000). *Nursing interventions classification (NIC).* St. Louis: Mosby–Year Book.

McCloskey, J.C. & Bulechek, G. M. (Eds.). (2004). *Nursing intervention classification (NIC),* 4th ed. St. Louis: Mosby.

McSherry, W. & Draper, P. (1998). The debates emerging from the literature surrounding the concept of spirituality as applied to nursing. *Journal of Advanced Nursing, 27,* 683–691.

Merriam-Webster. (1991) *Webster's Ninth New Collegiate Dictionary.* Springfield, MA: Merriam-Webster Inc., Publishers.

Merton, T. (1972). *New seeds of contemplation* (26th ed.). New York: New Directions Publishing Corp.

Moberg, D. O. (1984). Subjective measures of spiritual well-being. *Review of Religious Research, 25,* 351–364.

Moorhead, S., Johnson, M., & Maas, M. (Eds.). (2004). *The Iowa outcomes project: Nursing Outcomes Classification (NOC).* St. Louis: Mosby–Year Book.

Narayanasamy, A. (1999). ASSET: A model for actioning spirituality and spiritual care education and training in nursing. *Nurse Education Today, 19,* 274–285.

Narayanasamy, A. (1999). A review of spirituality as applied to nursing. *International Journal of Nursing Studies, 36,* 117–125.

Neuman, B. (1995). *The Neuman systems model* (3rd ed.). Stamford, CT: Appleton & Lange.

Newman, M. A. (1999). *Nursing as expanding consciousness* (2nd ed.). New York: NLN Press.

Nhat Hanh, T. (1995). *Living Buddha, living Christ.* New York: Berkley Publishing Group.

Nightingale, F. (1860, 1992). *Notes on Nursing.* Philadelphia: J.B. Lippincott Company.

Nolan, P., & Crawford, P. (1997). Towards a rhetoric of spirituality in mental health care. *Journal of Advanced Nursing, 26*, 285–294.

North American Nursing Diagnosis Association (NANDA). (2003). *Nursing diagnosis: Definitions and classification 2003–2004*. Philadelphia: Author.

Northumbria Community Trust, Ltd., The. (2002). *Celtic daily prayer*. New York: HarperCollins.

O'Brien, M. E. (1982). The need for spiritual integrity. In H. Yura & M. B. Walsh (Eds.), *Human needs and the nursing process* (pp. 85–115). Norwalk, CT: Appleton-Century-Crofts.

O'Brien, M. E. (2003). *Parish nursing: Healthcare ministry within the church*. Boston: Jones and Bartlett.

O'Brien, M. E. (1982). Religious faith and adjustment to long-term hemodialysis. *Journal of Religion and Health, 21*, 68–80.

Orem, D. E. (1995). *Nursing: Concepts of practice* (5th ed.). St. Louis: Mosby–Year Book.

Parse, R. R. (1998). *The human becoming school of thought: A perspective for nurses and other health care professionals*. Thousand Oaks, CA: Sage Publications.

Parsons, T. (1958). Definitions of health and illness in the light of American values and social structure. In E. G. Jaco (Ed.), *Patients, physicians, and illness*. New York: Free Press.

Peck, M. S. (1993). *Further along the road less traveled: The understanding journey toward spiritual growth*. New York: Simon & Schuster.

Pender, N. J., Murdaugh, C. L., & Parsons, M. A. (2002). *Health promotion in nursing practice* (4th ed.). Upper Saddle River, NJ: Prentice Hall.

Peterson, E. A. (1987). How to meet your clients' spiritual needs. *Journal of Psychosocial Nursing, 25*, 34–39.

Poling-Goldenne, M. (1998). You are generationally gifted. In R. S. Griener, D. Schmitz, & V. Zarth (Eds.), *Nurturing faith through the stages of life* (pp. 30, 31). Minneapolis: Augsburg Fortress.

Pruyser, P. (1976). *The minister as diagnostician*. Louisville, KY: Westminster John Knox Press.

Puchalski, C. & Romer, A. L. (2000). Taking a spiritual history allows clinicians to understand patients more fully. *Journal of Palliative Medicine, 3*(1), 129–137.

Reed, P. G. (1992). An emerging paradigm for the investigation of spirituality in nursing. *Research in Nursing and Health, 15*, 349–357.

Rethemeyers, A. & Wehling, B. A. (2004). How are we doing? Measuring the effectiveness of parish nursing. *Journal of Christian Nursing, 21*(2), 10–12.

Rogers, M. E. (1970). *An introduction to the theoretical basis of nursing*. Philadelphia: FA Davis.

Roy, C. & Andrews, H. A. (1999). *Roy adaptation model* (2nd ed.). Stamford, CT: Appleton & Lange.

Rupp, J. (Speaker). (1989). *Walking with those who hurt* (Cassette Recordings No. 0-87793-815-6). South Bend, IN: Ave Maria Press.

Savary, L. M. & Berne, P. H. (1988). *Kything: The art of spiritual presence*. New York: Paulist Press.

Sawatzky, R. & Pesut, B. (2005). Attributes of spiritual care in nursing practice. *Journal of Holistic Nursing, 23*(1), 19–33.

Saylor, C. (2004a). The circle of health: A health definition model. *Journal of Holistic Nursing, 22*(2), 98–115.

Saylor, F. (2004b). Health and spirituality fellowship named in Larson's honor. *Science & Theology News, 4*(9), 2.

Seeger, D. A. (2001). In C. Whitmire (Ed.), *Plain living: A Quaker path to simplicity* (p. 112). Notre Dame, IN: Sorin Books.

Shelly, J. A. & Miller, A. (1999). *Called to care: A Christian theology of nursing*. Downers Grove, IL: InterVarsity Press.

Smith, J. (1983). *The idea of health: Implications for the nursing profession*. New York: Teachers College Press.

Solari-Twadell, P. A. (1999). The emerging practice of parish nursing. In P. A. Solari-Twadell & M. A. McDermott (Eds.), *Parish nursing: Promoting whole person health within faith communities* (pp. 3–24). Thousand Oaks, CA: Sage Publications.

Stallwood, J. & Stoll, R. (1975). Spiritual dimensions of nursing practice. In I. L. Beland & J. Y. Passos (Eds.), *Clinical nursing: Pathophysiological and psychosocial approaches* (pp. 1086–1098). New York: Macmillan.

Starr, P. (1982). *The social transformation of American medicine*. New York: Basic Books Inc.

Stoll, R. I. (1989). The essence of spirituality. In V. B. Carson (Ed.), *Spiritual dimensions of nursing practice* (pp. 4–23). Philadelphia: WB Saunders.

Stoll, R. I. (1979). Guidelines for spiritual assessment. *American Journal of Nursing, 79*, 1574–1577.

Stuart, E., Deckro, J., & Mandle, C. (1989). Spirituality in health and healing: A clinical program. *Holistic Nursing Practice, 3*(3), 35–46.

Taylor, E. J. (2002). *Spiritual care: Nursing theory, research, and practice*. Upper Saddle River, NJ: Prentice Hall.

Tuck, I., Wallace, D., & Pullen, L. (2001). Spirituality and spiritual care provided by parish nurse. *Western Journal of Nursing Research, 23*(5), 441–453.

Vailot, M. C. (1970). The spiritual factors in nursing. *Journal of Practical Nursing, 20*, 30, 31.

Van Dover, L. J. & Bacon, J. M. (2001). Spiritual care in nursing practice: A close-up view. *Nursing Forum 36*(3), 18–30.

Ware, J. E., Kosinski, M., Gaandek, B., Aaronson, N. K., Apolone, G., Bech, P., et al. (1998). The factor structure of the SF-36 health survey in 10 countries: Results from the IQOLA project. International Quality of Life Assessment. *Journal of Clinical Epidemiology, 51*(11), 1159–1165.

Westberg, G. (1999). A personal historical perspective of whole person health and the congregation. In P. A. Solari-Twadell & M. A. McDermott (Eds.), *Parish nursing: Promoting whole person health within faith communities*. Thousand Oaks, CA: Sage Publications.

World Health Organization. (2004). WHO Constitution. [On-line.] Available: http://www.who.int./about/en.

Wylie, L. J. & Solari-Twadell, P. A. (1999). Health and the Congregation. In P. A. Solari-Twadell & M. A. McDermott (Eds.), *Parish nursing: Promoting whole person health within faith communities* (pp. 25–33). Thousand Oaks, CA: Sage Publications.

Additional Resources

Baldacchino, D. & Draper, P. (2001). Spiritual coping strategies: A review. *Journal of Advanced Nursing, 34,* 83.

Burkhardt, M. A. & Nagai-Jacobson, M. G. (2002). *Spirituality: Living our connectedness.* Albany, NY: Delmar.

Burkhart, L. & Solari-Twadell, P. A. (2001). Spirituality and religiousness: Differentiating the diagnoses through a review of the nursing literature. *Nursing Diagnosis, 12,* 45.

Carroll, B. (2001). A phenomenological exploration of the nature of spirituality and spiritual care. *Mortality, 6*(1), 81–98.

Carson, V. B. & Koenig, H. G. (2004). *Spiritual caregiving: Healthcare as a ministry.* Philadelphia: Templeton Foundation Press.

Cavendish, R., Konecny, L., Luise, B. K., & Lanza, M. (2004). Nurses enhance performance through prayer. *Holistic Nursing Practice, 18*(1), 26–31.

Chiu, L., Emblen, J. D., Van Hofwegen, L., Sawatzky, R., & Meyerhoo, H. (2004). An integrative review of the concept of spirituality in the health sciences. *Western Journal of Nursing Research, 26,* 405–428.

Dossey, L. (2001). *Healing beyond the body.* Boston: Shambhala.

Ebright, P. R. & Lyon, B. (2002). Understanding hope and factors that enhance hope in women with breast cancer. *Oncology Nursing Forum, 29*(3), 561–568.

Ellermann, C. R. & Reed, P. G. (2001). Self transcendence and depression in middle-aged adults. *Western Journal of Nursing Research, 23,* 698–713.

Ellis, M., Campbell, J., Detweiler-Breidenbach, A., & Hubbard, D. K. (2002). What do family physicians think about spirituality in clinical practice? *Journal of Family Practice, 51,* 249–254.

Emblen, J. & Pescut, B. (2001). Strengthening transcendent meaning: A model for the spiritual nursing care of patients experiencing suffering. *Journal of Holistic Nursing, 19,* 42–56.

Fitchett, G. (2000). *Assessing spiritual needs: A guidebook for caregivers.* Lima, OH: Academic Renewal Press.

Flannelly, L. T., Flannelly, K. J., & Weaver, A. J. (2002). Religious and spiritual variables in three major oncology nursing journals: 1990–1999. *Oncology Nursing Forum, 29,* 679–685.

Goldberg, B. (1998). Connection: An exploration of spirituality in nursing care. *Journal of Advanced Nursing, 27,* 836–842.

Hatch, R. L., Burg, M. A., Naberhause, D. S., & Hellmich, L. K. (1998). The spiritual involvement and beliefs scale: Development and testing of a new instrument. *Journal of Family Practice, 46,* 476–486.

Hawks, S., Hull, M., Thalman, R., & Ridhins, P. M. (1995). Review of spiritual health: Definition, role, & intervention strategies in health promotion. *American Journal of Health Promotion, 9*(5), 371–377.

Henery, N. (2003). Constructions of spirituality in contemporary nursing theory. *Journal of Advanced Nursing, 42,* 550–557.

Hermann, C. P. (2001). Spiritual needs of dying patients: A qualitative study. *Oncology Nursing Forum, 28,* 67–72.

Kendrick, K. D. & Robinson, S. (2000). Spirituality: Its relevance and purpose for clinical nursing in a new millennium. *Journal of Clinical Nursing, 9,* 701–705.

Kinney, A. Y., Emery, G., Dudley, W. N., & Croyle, R. T. (2002). Screening behaviors among African-American women at high risk for breast cancer. Do beliefs about God matter? *Oncology Nursing Forum, 29,* 835–843.

Kociszewski, C. (2003). A phenomenological pilot study of the nurses' experience providing spiritual care. *Journal of Holistic Nursing, 21*(2), 131–148.

Koenig, H. G. (2002). *Spirituality in patient care.* Radnor, PA: The Templeton Foundation Press.

Koenig, H. G., McCullough, M. E., & Larson, D. B. (2001). *The handbook of religion and health.* New York: Oxford University Press.

Larson, D. B., Sawyers, J. P., & McCullough, M. E. (1998). *Scientific research on spirituality and health: A report based on the scientific progress in spirituality conferences.* New York: John M. Templeton Foundation.

Lauver, D. (2000). Commonalities in women's spirituality and women's health. *Advances in Nursing Science, 22,* 76.

Lemone, P. (2001). Spiritual distress. In M. L. Maas, K. C. Buckwater, M. D. Hardy, T. Tripp-Reimer, M. G. Titler, & J. P. Specht (Eds.), *Nursing care of older adults: Diagnoses, outcomes and interventions* (Chapter 62). St. Louis: Mosby–Year Book.

Maddox, M. (2002). Spiritual assessment in primary care. *The Nurse Practitioner, 27*(2), 12, 14.

Malinski, V. M. (2002). Developing a nursing perspective on spirituality and healing. *Nursing Science Quarterly, 1*(5), 281–287.

Matthews, D. A. (1999). *The faith factor: Proof of the healing power of prayer.* New York: Penguin Books.

McKenzie, E. R., Rajagopal, D. E., Meilbolm, M., & Lavizzo-Mourey, R. (2000). Spiritual support and psychological well-being: Older adults' perceptions of religion and health connection. *Alternative Therapies in Health and Medicine, 6*(6), 37–45.

Meisenhelder, J. B. & Chandler, E. N. (2000). Prayer and health outcomes in church members. *Alternative Therapies in Health and Medicine, 6*(4), 56–60.

Meraviglia, M. C. (1999). Critical analysis of spirituality and its empirical indicators. Prayer and meaning in life. *Journal of Holistic Nursing, 47*(1), 18–33.

Morris, E. L. (2001). The relationship of spirituality to coronary artery disease. *Alternative Therapies, 7,* 96–98.

Narayanasamy, A. & Owens, J. (2001). A critical incident study of nurses' responses to the spiritual needs of their patients. *Journal of Advanced Nursing, 33*(4), 446–456.

O'Brien, M. E. (2001). *The nurse's calling: A Christian spirituality of caring for the sick.* Mahwah, NJ: Paulist Press.

O'Brien, M. E. (2004). *A nurse's handbook of spiritual care: Standing on holy ground.* Sudbury, MA: Jones and Bartlett.

O'Brien, M. E. (2003). *Prayer in nursing: The spirituality of compassionate caregiving.* Sudbury, MA: Jones and Bartlett.

O'Connor, C. I. (2001). Characteristics of spirituality, assessment, and prayer in holistic nursing. *Nursing Clinics of North America, 36,* 33–46.

Oldnall, A. (1996). A critical analysis of nursing: Meeting the spiritual needs of patients. *Journal of Advanced Nursing, 23,* 138–144.

O'Mathuna, D. P. (1999). Prayer research: What are we measuring? *Journal of Christian Nursing, 16*(3), 17–21.

Plante, T. C., Saucedo, B., & Rice, C. (2001). The association between strength of religious faith and coping with daily stress. *Pastoral Psychology, 49,* 291–300.

Sappington, J. Y. (2003). Nurturance: The spirit of holistic nursing. *Journal of Holistic Nursing, 21*(2), 8–19.

Sellers, S. C. & Haag, B. A. (1998). Spiritual nursing intervention. *Journal of Holistic Nursing, 16*(3), 338–354.

Sloan, R. P., Bagiella, E., VandeCreek, L., Hover, M., Casalone, C., Hirsh, T. J., Hasan, Y., Kreeger, R., & Poulos, P. (2000). Should physicians prescribe religious activities? *New England Journal of Medicine, 342,* 1913–1916.

Stoner, M. H. (1997). Measuring hope. In M. Frank-Stromborg & S. J. Olson (Eds.), *Instruments for clinical health-care research* (2nd ed., pp. 189–201). Sudbury, MA: Jones and Bartlett.

Stranahan, S. (2001). Spiritual perceptions, attitudes about spiritual care, and spiritual care practices among nurse practitioners. *Western Journal of Nursing Research, 23*(1), 90.

Tanyi, R. A. (2002). Towards a clarification of the meaning of spirituality. *Journal of Advanced Nursing, 39,* 500–509.

Taylor, E. J. (1997). The story behind the story: The use of story telling in spiritual caregiving. *Seminars in Oncology Nursing, 13*(4), 252.

Taylor, E. J., Highfield, M. F., & Amenta, M. O. (1999). Predictors of oncology and hospice nurses' spiritual care perspectives and practices. *Applied Nursing Research, 12*(1), 30–37.

Vandenbrink, R. A. (2001). Spiritual assessment: Comparing the tools. *Journal of Christian Nursing, 18*(3), 24–27.

Winslow, G. R. & Winslow, B. W. (2003). Examining the ethics of praying with patients. *Holistic Nursing Practice, 17*(4), 170–177.

Woodward, E. K. & Sowell, R. (2001). God in control: Women's perspectives on managing HIV infection. *Clinical Nursing Research, 10,* 233–250.

Wright, K. B. (1998). Clinical scholarship: Professional, ethical, and legal implications for spiritual care in nursing. *Image: The Journal of Nursing Scholarship, 30,* 81–83.

Wright, M. C. (2002). The essence of spiritual care: A phenomenological enquiry. *Palliative Medicine, 16*(2), 125–132.

→ Web Resources

http://www.aapc.org   American Association of Pastoral Counselors

http://www.ahna.org   American Holistic Nurses Association

http://www.Catholic.net   Catholic faith issues

http://www.catholic.org   Catholic Online

http://www.deaconess.org   Deaconess Foundation

http://www.geri.duke.edu   Duke University Center for the Study of Religion/Spirituality and Health

http://www.dcfl.org/eliz.htm   The Elizabeth Ministry

http://www.fetzer.org   Fetzer Institute (mind-body-spirit relationships)

http://www.gwish.org   George Washington Institute for Spirituality and Health

http://www.healthministriesassociation.org   Health Ministry Association

http://www.ihpnet.org   Interfaith Health Program—The Carter Center

http://www.icihs.org   International Center for the Integration of Health and Spirituality

http://www.mbmi   Mind Body Medical Institute

http://www.ivcf.org/ncf   Nurses Christian Fellowship

http://www.science-spirit.org   Science and Spirit magazine

http://www.spiritualityhealth.com   Spirituality and Health magazine

http://www.stephenminsirty.org   Stephen Ministries Foundation

http://www.templeton.org   John Templeton Foundation

http://www.vatican.va   Official Web site of the Vatican

II

Faith, Health, and the Community

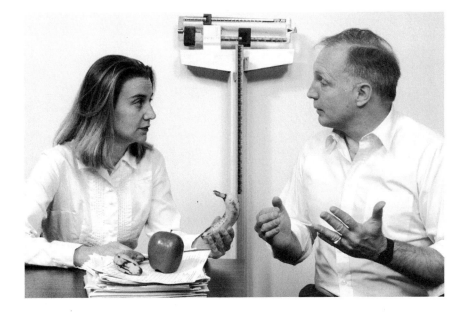

Working in a Faith Community

4

Faith community, or parish, nursing is a unique, evolving nursing specialty. Faith community nurses (FCNs) are licensed, registered professional nurses who serve as members of the staff within a faith community to promote health as wholeness of the faith community, its groups, families, and individual members, and the community it serves. It does this through the independent practice of nursing, as defined by the nurse practice act in the jurisdiction in which the nurse practices and the *Faith Community Nursing: Scope and Standards of Practice* (American Nurses Association and Health Ministries Association [ANA-HMA], 2005.) As an organized social structure, the faith community holds special challenges for the FCN. The faith community has a culture that needs to be learned and understood, if the FCN is to be successful. Equally essential is that FCNs are clear about the role they will play in the faith community and that they make this role clear and understood by all members. Faith communities are organized social systems (Richardson, 1996), and an FCN will want to know her or his place in that system.

Brudenell (2003) conducted a study to describe the development and effectiveness of parish nurse programs. A qualitative design, using the grounded theory method, was used to answer the following research questions:

- How do faith communities form parish nurse programs?
- What is the effect of parish nursing programs on health outcomes?

The subjects for this study were 13 nurses and 8 pastors, representing 13 congregations with parish nurse programs, 2 hospital chaplains, and 2 parish nurse coordinators ($n = 24$). Eight denominations were represented, and church membership ranged from 80 to 2,500 members and included rural, suburban, and urban areas. Findings of this study indicate that faith communities form parish nurse programs/health ministries in a developmental process. Strategies are used to move forward, dealing with transitions and limitations over time. The process involves knowing the congregation and the community. Brudenell (2003) describes four phases of the process:

1. A preliminary phase of finding out or thinking about parish nursing.
2. Knowing the faith community.
3. Being accepted as part of the congregation's ministry.
4. Becoming an ongoing ministry that distinguishes a congregation.

Beginning Steps

FCNs come to their positions in many ways. Some nurses are approached by their minister to look into the role for their faith community. Other nurses act as catalysts to start a program in their faith community, approaching their ministers with the idea and gathering information about similar programs throughout the area and, perhaps, in their own denomination. The growing number of parish nursing educational offerings of varying intensities allows nurses to learn about the role and to begin to think whether this is a potential role for them in their own faith community. Often, the nurse, as a member of the congregation, sees the problems that other members are facing and feels that with a little effort, much could be done for their community. Many nurses have been performing some functions of the parish nurse role as knowledgeable health care professionals. Other congregational members see the nurse as a trusted resource and a friendly face who helps to interpret the complex health care system. For many nurses, faith community nursing answers a calling to blend their spiritual lives with their professional lives in a way of service that they have not been able to do in previous health care settings. The FCN working in the faith community has the opportunity to work with and care for individuals and their family members on a longer, more intimate level than most nurses experience. The FCN understands health to be a dynamic process that embodies the spiritual, psychological, physical, and social dimensions of the person. The spiritual dimension is central to the FCN's practice (Solari-Twadell, 1999). "The relationship between the patient and the nurse is often closer when a nursing response includes spiritual interventions" (Schnorr, 1999, p. 51).

Patterson (2003) relates the concept of Christian diaconal ministry to faith community nursing. *Diakonia* is the Greek word for "service." Early in the development of the Christian church, service on behalf of the church to the community was recognized as ministry. Diaconal ministry is a fusion of care for the body and soul, done in the context of community and tied to the roots of worship. Theological frameworks support diaconal ministry following the example set by Christ, as an opportunity to serve as a witness for Christ, and that by serving those in need, provide service to Christ. Patterson states that, historically, diaconal ministries were faith-based responses to human needs at a time when governments had no organized response, and the Church could not respond through the work of the ordained pastoral clergy alone. FCNs of all faith traditions are following in sacred footsteps, doing holy work.

Brudenell (2003) describes the first phase of beginning a parish nurse program as the preliminary phase. In this phase—"thinking about parish nursing"—pastors and nurses recounted when they had first heard about a health and spirituality program. Several pastors heard about parish nursing programs at national conferences and were aware that their denominations had well-established health information and ministry programs. Three other pastors described experiences with parish nurses and recounted the resulting benefits to their congregations. Some pastors viewed health ministry as another way to connect congregational members with the health care system as well as the larger community. Having professionals available and willing was a deciding factor in developing a health ministry.

Chase-Ziolek (2003) raises the issue of rethinking our terms about health ministries. She states that the term *health ministry* serves as the umbrella term most commonly used to describe the church's role in health, with parish nursing as one aspect of health ministry. Other aspects might include lay health promoters, caring communities, and health ministry teams.

As the term *health ministry* joins two concepts—health and ministry—to form a new entity, while retaining aspects of each, the term has appeal to both health and ministry professionals. Chase-Ziolek believes that the time has come to talk about *ministries of health* rather than *health ministries.* She states that this language more clearly identifies the work as *ministry.* This language provides the perspective of how *ministries of health* fit into the culture and understanding of the congregation, rather than simply bringing health services to the church setting, and it ensures the future of the church's role in health and healing. Historically, the health care environment has been inconsistent about support for health ministries, and institutionally sponsored health ministry programs are continually vulnerable to budget cuts. However, when health promotion is understood as an essential ministry, the congregation will find a means to provide support for it.

Garity and Ryan (2002) believe that an advisory board can help nurses and congregations interested in starting or managing a parish nurse program to avoid five common pitfalls. The pitfalls were previously identified by Meyer (1996) and include: (a) no strategy, (b) poor planning, (c) weak organization, (d) ineffective leadership, and (e) lack of control. Garity and Ryan describe an advisory board of carefully recruited professionals with expertise in administration, nursing, education, social work, and theology. The purposes of the advisory board are to shape a philosophy for the program, to establish policy and program guidelines, and to provide mentoring to the parish nurse program coordinator. They report positive program outcomes using this approach.

Great diversity exists in the size, governance structures, and financial abilities of faith communities. A starting point for ministries of health in a faith community is the development of a health cabinet or health ministry team. Again, depending on the size and resources of the congregation, a health cabinet might be a small group of three or four health professionals or a larger interdisciplinary group with a focus on health. Having a committee of people establishing congregational health ministries endorses the concept as a congregational ministry as opposed to an individual's ministry. A health cabinet may be formed at the suggestion of the pastor, priest, rabbi, or imam; or congregational members may initiate the establishment of such a structure.

Once a health cabinet is in place, the members need to become informed about the possibilities for the ministry. This may involve Web-based research, visits to other congregations, and/or having speakers brought in. An abundance of current literature and research related to faith and health relationships is available, and materials about faith community nursing are readily available from the International Parish Nurse Resource Center (IPNRC). Health cabinet members will need to investigate the financial and logistic elements of starting a parish nursing program.

Several decisions need to be made at this stage of the process. Will the FCN serve as an internal resource, or would the health cabinet like to see the FCN doing community outreach work as well? Will the position be full-time or part-time, and will it be a paid position?

As discussed in Chapter 2, many opinions exist on whether or not the FCN can, will, or should be paid. Some parish nurse leaders, such as Rosemarie Matheus, have a bias for the paid model. She feels there is greater responsibility to maintain a documentation system and a set number of hours when the FCN is paid (Carson & Koenig, 2004). Patterson (2003) and Smith (2003) advocate for paid FCNs, although Patterson reports that over 65% of FCNs in the United States are doing health ministry on an unpaid basis. Briefly, the advantages of a paid position include:

- The recognition of the position as requiring professional education and credentials.
- Paid FCNs can be supervised as an employee and held to the standards of a position description and the *Faith Community Nursing: Scope and Standards of Practice* (ANA-HMA, 2005).
- Compensation provides an increased time commitment.
- A larger pool of potential job applicants.
- Increased program visibility.

Briefly, advantages and issues related to unpaid positions include:

- The unpaid FCN affirms the concept of a priesthood of all believers.
- Ease of program startup as fewer decisions about resources need to be made.
- Commitment of the individual to the program.
- Established presence in the congregation (although this can also be a disadvantage).
- Lower cost to the congregation.

Clear disadvantages of an unpaid model are the inability to supervise and evaluate a volunteer, decreased time given to the program, confidentiality issues, and whether or not the program can be sustained over time.

When a program proposal and budget has been developed, the cabinet will present the program proposal to the faith community leadership. The health cabinet must be prepared to conceptually connect the health ministry to the mission and theological position of the faith community. Depending on the structure, a congregation vote may be required to start the program.

Hiring a Faith Community Nurse

A first step in the hiring process of an FCN is the development of a position or job description. This important document outlines the functions and roles that the nurse will (and will not) play in the faith community. Congregations are not known for their clear descriptions of job responsibilities, but it is vitally important that the effort be taken at the beginning of a program. Solari-Twadell and McDermott (1999) feel that the following three questions need to be addressed in the job description:

1. What is the job?
2. To whom are you responsible?
3. Where do you fit in the overall ministry?

The following is an additional question that needs to be addressed in the process of developing the job description: Do the responsibilities outlined in the job description match the hours allotted to the program? Editing an existing description specific to the needs of the congregation is easier than creating a brand-new document. An example of a very thorough job description can be found in Box 4-1.

The IPNRC recommends that a parish nurse have a bachelor of science in nursing (BSN), with at least 5 years of clinical experience. Experience in medical surgical nursing and in community health nursing is desirable, as is theological and/or clinical pastoral education. A BSN is recommended because this preparation provides educational content and practice in community assessment and community health nursing experiences. Spiritual leadership experiences and the ability to function as part of a team are special job characteristics related to faith community nursing. Magilvy and Brown (1997) posit that parish nursing is an advanced practice role and that parish nurses should possess a master's degree because of the independent nature of the role. Needless to say, credentialing issues continue to plague the profession of nursing.

An understanding of both the Nurse Practice Act for one's state and the ANA-HMA *Faith Community Nursing: Scope and Standards of Practice* (2005) is needed so that the FCN is not practicing outside of the scope of his or her practice. Often these documents can aid the nurse to more clearly define his or her role. Members of the congregation may see the nurse role as the answer to many of the physical care problems facing them. Many members would love to have someone to give insulin, administer medications, and change wound dressings on a regular basis. However, these hands-on functions are not appropriate for the FCN. The role of the FCN as one that emphasizes the relationship between spiritual health and well-being requires congregational education. Many people still need to understand the benefit and science behind prevention and health.

The goal of faith community nursing activities is to enhance the holistic health and well-being of individuals and groups within the faith community. FCNs may assume one or more of the roles associated with the practice to achieve this (Berquist & King, 1994).

Once the decision is made to initiate a parish nurse program, the task of hiring the FCN must be addressed. Some programs linked with health care systems hire the nurse jointly,

BOX 4-1
Job Description for the Ministry of Faith Community Nursing Practice

This position is designed to provide whole person health promotion disease prevention services with an emphasis on spiritual care. The major accountabilities and job activities of the parish nurse role are integrator of faith and health, health educator, personal health counselor, referral agent, developer of support groups, trainer of volunteers, and health advocate.

I. Accountabilities

  A. Integrator of faith and health

    1. Assesses congregation's assets and needs incorporating an understanding of the relationship between faith and health.

    2. Participates as a staff member of the congregation, attending all meetings of the staff of the congregation.

    3. Identifies opportunities to enhance the understanding of the relationship of faith and health within the congregation.

    4. Fosters, promotes, and provides opportunities for spiritual care to be discussed and integrated into the parish nurse role documenting spiritual care of groups and individuals.

    5. Participates in the planning and providing of prayer and worship life of the congregation.

    6. Teaches and models the integration of faith and health into daily life.

  B. Personal Health Counselor

    1. Provides individual health counseling related to health maintenance, disease prevention, or illness patterns.

    2. Encourages the client through presence and spiritual support to express his or her faith beliefs and to use them regularly, especially in time of crisis and despair.

    3. Documents client assessment, nursing diagnosis, interventions, and outcomes while maintaining confidential client record in accordance with the policy on documentation.

    4. Makes visits to clients, as needed, providing health counseling, education, and spiritual presence/support.

    5. Promotes stewardship of the body, emphasizing self-care of the whole person.

    6. Collaborates with pastoral staff to plan for health education programming.

    7. Communicates with other health professionals, as needed, to meet the health needs of clients.

  C. Health Educator

    1. Uses information from asset and needs assessments of the congregation and surrounding community in planning for education programs.

    2. Prepares, develops, and/or coordinates educational programs based on identified needs for healthier lifestyles, early illness detection, and health resources.

    3. Maintains records of educational programs, including objectives, content, evaluation, attendance, and budget.

    4. Documents individual educational assessment diagnosis, interventions, and outcomes.

    5. Provides the pastor, health committee of the congregation, and other designated parties a summary evaluation of educational programs noting attendance and response of participants.

    6. Networks with appropriate resources in the community to secure educational program resources.

    7. Provides consultation and acts as a health resource to other staff of the congregation.

  D. Trainer of Volunteers

    1. Identifies and recruits professional and lay volunteers who can be available to respond to the health-related needs of members of the congregation.

(continued)

BOX 4-1
Job Description for the Ministry of Faith Community Nursing Practice *(continued)*

  2. Facilitates and, when appropriate, trains individuals to assume volunteer responsibilities to meet identified needs of the congregation.
  3. Works with staff, health committee, or others, focusing on the integration of health into the life of the congregation.
  E. Developer of Support Groups
  1. Develops and/or facilitates support groups based on identified needs and resources.
  2. Identifies available support groups in the community that could resource the congregation.
  3. Refers and documents client participation in designated support groups.
  F. Referral Agent
  1. Provides and documents referrals to health care services and resources within the congregation and external community.
  2. Collaborates with community leaders and agencies to facilitate effective working relationships while identifying new health resources.
  3. Develops community contacts to secure resources and services to meet the needs of members of the congregation.
  4. Networks with other FCNs and professionals.
  G. Health Advocate
  1. Encourages clients to avail themselves of services, which will enhance their overall well-being, assisting the clients in identifying values and choices, which encourage them to be more responsible for their health status.
  2. Assists client and client families in making decisions regarding their health, medical services, treatments, and care facilities as well as documenting assessments, diagnosis, interventions, and outcomes.
  3. Identifies, communicates, and works cooperatively with community leaders, elected officials, and agencies to meet health needs of members of the congregation and surrounding community.
II. Job Activities
  A. Management
  1. Prepares an operating budget for program development as needed.
  2. Develops reports regarding FCN activities as needed.
  3. Collaborates with others in developing and managing grant projects.
  4. Coordinates all faith community nursing programming in the congregation.
  B. Professional Development, Education, and Research
  1. Participates in continuing education programs to meet identified professional learning needs.
  2. Participates in regular personal spiritual formation.
  3. Acts as a preceptor to students from schools of nursing, seminaries, and other disciplines as requested.
  4. Develops and/or participates in research related to faith community nursing.
  5. Develops and submits articles for publication on experiences in faith community nursing.

with the congregation having the final vote. Some programs hire the nurse who was instrumental in initiating the program. The congregation can also hire the nurse who was asked to investigate establishing a parish nursing program. This brings the issue of hiring an FCN from within or someone new to the congregation.

BOX 4-1
Job Description for the Ministry of Faith Community Nursing
Practice *(continued)*

JOB REQUIREMENTS

COMPETENT LEVEL QUALIFICATIONS	MINIMUM LEVEL QUALIFICATIONS
Organizing skills	Excellent communication skills
Basic computer skills	Organizing skills
Excellent communication skills	
Ability to develop reports	
BSN required	BS preferred
5+ years experience in med-surg	5 years clinical nursing experience
Community health nursing experience desirable	Assessment skills
Ability to do community assessments	
Ability to do health counseling	
Current license as an RN in the state the congregation is located	Current license as an RN in the state the congregation is located
Completion of a basic preparation course in faith community nursing, based on the standard core curriculum endorsed through the International Parish Nurse Resource Center (IPNRC)	
Spiritual leadership as evidenced by experience in congregational ministries, lay leadership, theological education, and other related spiritual development	Works well independently and yet can function well as part of a team
Substantial weekend and evening work	Has a good understanding of spirituality and religiosity

Printed with permission of Deaconess Nurse Ministries, 1998–2002. St. Louis, MO.

Hiring the nurse from within the membership of the congregation brings someone who knows the faith community, knows the informal and formal leadership, committees, and history of the congregation. The challenge for the new FCN is that he or she must be comfortable taking on a new role in the congregation, and the members of the congregation must be comfortable in accepting that individual's new role.

Patterson (2003) recommends hiring a nurse from outside the congregation because a new nurse coming into the setting has no preconceived ideas about the church, no historical knowledge, and sees everything fresh. Some pastors prefer this, because they are bringing on a new program and a new face to run it. If the decision is made to hire from outside the congregation, the health cabinet will need to advertise for the position and review the résumés of the applicants. Only candidates with the required credentials should be considered. The top two or three candidates should be interviewed by a subcommittee of the health and faith community leader. All members of the subcommittee need to attend every interview and then make a recommendation as to which candidate should be offered the position.

Working with the Congregational Leader

Initiating a faith community nursing program into a congregation can be the biggest challenge that a new FCN faces, whether hired from within the congregation or from the community. An *essential* element to the success of a program is the support of the faith community leader. Also essential is for a potential FCN to possess a clear understanding of the church culture, both pastoral and theological, in which he or she will be serving. The pastoral leadership culture relates to the pastoral administrative style of the church in terms of power and decision-making (O'Brien, 2003). The relationship between a pastor and FCN is critical to the success of a program and must be built on trust, respect, and support. Trust between a pastor and an FCN is a key element in promoting a seamless initiation of the FCN program. For the program to flourish, an essential factor is that a pastor be kept informed and is supportive of all anticipated activities within his or her church (O'Brien). Without the support of the pastor or congregational leader, the FCN's work is much harder and may be destined to failure.

The relationship between the FCN and pastor is as professional colleagues. To work as colleagues, the FCN must understand the administrative structure of the congregation. The parish nurse must be aware of the formal and informal leaders of the faith community, as well as the pastor's passions and influences. The FCN and the congregational leadership must agree upon the goals of the program. Often the pastor asks the FCN to meet with the various committees of the congregation. This can be a perfect opportunity to introduce the concept of parish nursing and holistic health to active members of the congregation, as well as to begin to assess the needs of the faith community. If the pastor is supportive of the program, it can be anticipated that the committees will be supportive and will share the concept of the role of the FCN with others in the faith community. The FCN's understanding of the governance structure of the congregation is important. How decisions are made in the congregation is an important aspect of the culture of the congregation. Is the congregation formal, with committees with rigid rules and guidelines, or is it more informal, with general meetings open to the whole congregation? Is the ministry staff small or large? Is the ministry staff paid? Is the staff accessible? Where will the FCN fit in the organizational structure? Will she or he report directly to the leadership or to a health ministry committee? The answers to these questions allow the nurse to see where he or she will fit into the church's structure and culture.

The faith community is an organized social structure (Richardson, 1996), and the FCN needs to understand his or her place in that structure. As a resource in the community, the FCN needs to know the makeup of the membership, the distance that the members travel to the church, the congregation's associations with area agencies and area churches. This information is important as the FCN begins the journey of initiating a new program in the congregation.

Funding a Faith Community Nursing Program

Many creative plans are in existence to support the FCN in the faith community. One creative example is that the time the FCN volunteered was tithed to the church. Many nurses find it hard to put a dollar value on their work while working in the faith community. One nurse asked her congregation to pay her the same hourly rate that they pay the part-time police officer who directs traffic on Sunday! Most agree, whether paid or not, that a program should be explicit as to the number of hours that a nurse will work, and a plan to reevaluate the status in a specific time period should be developed. Some nurses will offer their services unpaid for a year, with an agreement with the church's leadership that after this time period, the topic of compensation will be addressed. Some congregations have plans by which the nurse is paid for a few hours and the hours paid gradually increase over time. A congregation can assess the hourly wage for the FCN by looking at the market rate of nurses in their community and comparing that to a rate that they may pay a temporary employee or an employee who works only a few hours a week, and who is not part of the church staff. Many churches have creative ways to compensate the parish nurse when the hourly rate is much smaller than the community standard. One church greatly reduced the tuition for a nurse's children to attend the church school. It seems understood that if a congregation does not give financially to a program, the contributions by the FCN will not be respected, even if the FCN role is fully integrated into the ministry of the congregation. Solari-Twadell and McDermott (1999) posit that it is more important how the chosen model is managed, integrated, rather than whether or not the nurse is paid.

In institutional models of faith community nursing practice, FCN coordinators may be paid to oversee volunteer FCNs, or FCNs may be paid by the institution to provide direct services to congregations. Schweitzer, Norberg, and Larson (2002) conducted a qualitative descriptive study to describe the role and functions of the parish nurse coordinator (PNC) charged with leadership of a group of parish nurses networked together as a parish nurse program. The IPNRC recommends that a PNC complete both the basic parish nurse preparation course and a second course focusing on parish nurse leadership development. Schweitzer et al. state that the PNC, in the leadership role, combines the skills of a professional nurse manager with a sense of spiritual direction to guide nurses in their practice within faith communities. In this leadership role, the PNC works with a group of parish nurses to plan and implement holistic health/wellness programs aimed at improving the health of communities of faith (2002).

This study identified the following parish nurse coordinator responsibilities:

- Evaluate parish nurses' performance.
- Establish informal agreement with the faith community.
- Establish a formal agreement with the faith community.
- Evaluate faith community participation.
- Teach parish nurses in partnership with college/university.
- Teach continuing education for parish nurse.
- Teach formal core curriculum for parish nurse education (Schweitzer et al., 2002).

In institutional models, the congregation is relieved of the "start-up" management of FCN programs and have the added benefits of the resources of the cooperating institution. However, the mission of the institution supersedes that of the congregation, because the nurses are employees of the institution. Incompatible missions will make this model unacceptable to some congregations.

Initiating a New Ministry

The biggest challenge facing an FCN is initiating a new program within a congregation (O'Brien, 2003). For many congregational members, this is a new and expanded role of the nurse. The first step of a new parish nurse program is to educate the congregation about parish nursing. This can be accomplished by clearly explaining the role and functions of the parish nurse, using the church bulletin, developing a brochure outlining services offered, or explaining from the pulpit. For many programs, an installation service is held to welcome the nurse into the ministry of the congregation. This service indicates the value placed on the role as well as the support of the leadership. Sometimes the FCN will speak from the pulpit on the role and function of the health ministry or parish nurse program during services. This example is a perfect opportunity to explain the goals and purpose of the program and reinforce the role of spirituality in one's wellness.

Often one aspect of the roles that an FCN can play is used as a foundation for the initial phase of the parish nurse program. When starting a new program it is best to start simply but thoroughly. This initial step is vitally important in a new program, so that the congregation does not expect things that the nurse cannot deliver. And early successes help to "sell" the new idea of having an FCN.

Pastor Granger Westberg (1987) feels that "every church with a parish nurse should have a health cabinet or committee that can become a true support for the nurse" (p. 26). Members of this committee should have an interest in advising and supporting a church's ministry (O'Brien, 2003). Health cabinet members should be representative members of the congregation and bring different perspectives to the ministry. The health cabinet members can act as ambassadors for the FCN, emphasizing the goals of the program and explaining the program to other members of the congregation, and educating the congregation about the importance of the FCN/health ministry activities (O'Brien).

Expectations of the Nurse, the Ministry Team, and the Congregation

Vital to the success of a new program is that the initial goals remain simple and clear. Clarity of the program, starting small, staying focused and within the scope and standards of the professional practice is critical. This approach allows the nurse to gain confidence, competence, and a strong foundation.

Brudenell (2003) describes the second phase of establishing a faith community nursing program as "knowing the faith community." Pastors and nurses must know their congregations and what they want and need for their health ministry. Strategies to increase knowledge of the health care needs of parishioners include health assessments. Using a community health nursing process to assess needs and to integrate knowledge about national public health standards and objectives will improve the efficacy of achieving congregational goals. Chapter 5 provides detailed information on conducting assessments and interest inventories.

After completing an assessment of the congregation and community, the nurse should ask the congregation to complete an interest survey. Based on the information gathered, the nurse can begin to plan the initial phase of the program. It should always be communicated to the congregation that programs are based on the interests they indicated and an assessment of their needs. One congregational nurse offered monthly health education programs for her congregation. The programs were based on the interest survey as well as her assessment of congregational needs. The programs were offered on the most popular night, but after a year of disappointing attendance, the programs were canceled. What was popular in this setting—and got a great deal of positive feedback—were the articles written in the church bulletin. The program change was communicated to the congregation, and the program took on a new focus during the second year. The FCN continued to write health articles for the church bulletin.

The research literature shows that different congregations place higher value on different parish nurse roles. Some faith communities prefer the FCN to focus on the more traditional nursing roles of health promoter, educator, and risk screener, whereas other congregations place higher value on the role of integrator of faith and health (Chase-Ziolek & Gruca, 2000; Mayhugh & Martens, 2001; Tuck, Wallace, & Pullen, 2001; Wallace, Tuck, Boland, & Witucki, 2002; Weis, Schank, Coenen, & Matheus, 2002). The amount of time, in hours per week, that the parish nurse is able to provide will also dictate which and how many role functions the nurse can realistically and successfully implement.

Brudenell (2003) identifies the third phase of establishing a parish nurse program as "being accepted as a faith community ministry." This occurs naturally over time as congregants learn about and accept the parish nursing program as an ongoing, caring activity. Another indicator of this phase is that the health ministry team functions well and becomes more independent from the pastor in making decisions and taking action. All pastors and nurses in this study described "being present" or visible—talking, praying, being involved in the community—as key to becoming accepted as a caring ministry. Mutual valuing—responding with reciprocal caring—was described as another dimension of accepting the parish nurse program.

A benefit of establishing a solid foundation for the program is that the nurse can enlist the aid of volunteers to the program. One parish nurse enlisted other health professionals in the congregation to write occasional health articles based on their areas of expertise. Using others in the faith community to grow the parish nurse program is a challenging but important aspect of the parish nurse role. It helps other members to see the value of the parish nurse program, and it shares their talents and gifts with other members. This creates a "win-win" situation, in which all participants "own the program" and everyone benefits from their participation.

Wuthnow (2004) reports that members of religious congregations are twice as likely to be involved in volunteer activities as nonmembers, and that people who attend religious services every week are about twice as likely to be involved as those who attend only a few times a year.

He states that doing volunteer work is reinforced by what he terms *spiritual practice*. Spiritual practice involves intentional activity concerned with strengthening one's relationship with God. Daily prayers, study of Scripture, meditation, and other efforts that nurture spiritual growth are common forms of spiritual practice. Research data suggest that these are people who are most likely to be involved in volunteering.

Volunteers are the backbone of the faith community. Enlisting the assistance of interested volunteers can help the parish nurse program grow as well as provide ambassadors to educate others about the benefits of the health ministry. Parker (2000) talks about a three-step process to motivate volunteers: inviting, igniting, and uniting—and feels that volunteers are uplifted on their own personal journey as a result of volunteering. Anyone who is interested in health ministry should have a place in the program.

Health professionals have an obvious role to play in a faith community nursing program, but others can all contribute their gifts to the program. For examples of volunteer job responsibilities see Box 4-2. Volunteer programs are as unique as the congregations they serve. Health care professionals can be called upon to share their expertise with other members.

Some older members might send caring cards to other members who are experiencing challenges in their life. Healing meals is a program one church organized for members who need short-term assistance with meals. Retired members are often drivers for others to medical appointments or errands.

By including volunteers in the FCN program, it is essential that each volunteer understand his or her role and job in the program. Some programs have developed simple job descriptions to clearly state expectations and avoid confusion. Volunteers can enhance a parish nursing program and expand the reach of the nurse. Essential is that the FCN recognize the work of the volunteers on a regular basis, and, if

---

BOX 4-2
Volunteer Possibilities

Health professionals
Blood pressure screeners
Facilitators of health education seminars
Disease specialists
Lawyers
    Living will/durable power-of-attorney
    Wills/estate planning
Educators
    Review health education articles/brochures
Lay members
    Shut-in reassurance
    Administrative assistance for programs
    Caring card program
    Healing meals

budgets allow, on a yearly basis either in the form of a lunch or recognition celebration. Simple things to acknowledge and appreciate the volunteers within a program reinforce everyone's input in positive ways. Early intervention when volunteer roles "take on a life of their own" can prevent future problems. Supervising volunteers can be a rewarding experience but also one that entails diplomacy and tact and sometimes conflict resolution skills. The case study illustrates the challenges of working with volunteers.

Challenges

From the perspective of the author, challenges in the FCN role are primarily time, energy, and vision. The vision and mission of the parish nurse program need to be periodically revisited and discussed within the strategic plan and vision for the congregation. Learning good time management skills is important to efficiently use the time allotted to the program.

Although the role of an FCN is rewarding and exciting, potential areas of concern to be aware of exist. Members of the faith community need to be reassured that their confidences are kept. A statement of confidentiality can be printed on the FCN brochure as well as posted on the church bulletin and in the nurse's office. Congregation members need to be assured that what they tell the FCN will not be shared with anyone, unless the individual gives the nurse permission to do so. This includes the pastor, priest, imam, or rabbi. The FCN and her immediate supervisor, either the pastor or a delegate, must understand the confidentiality aspect of this type of work. Essential is that the lines of communication remain open between the FCN and his or her supervisor. Regular times to discuss issues and working relationships prevent problems. Respecting each other as professionals, each with a valuable role in the faith community, benefits the entire congregation. Chapter 7 (Community Connections) addresses the collaborative nature of the ministry team.

Other challenges to FCNs are time management and prioritization of tasks. As previously stated, Patterson (2003) reports that 65% of FCNs work in a part-time capacity. She states that the optimal amount of time for an FCN to be employed by a congregation is at least 20 hours per week, with at least 2 Sundays per month in attendance at worship services. She cautions that churches having an FCN for fewer than 10 hours a week will probably provide few benefits to the congregation. Essential is that the nurse, in collaboration with the pastor or health ministry team, determine priorities and realistic expectations and outcomes for the program. These priorities and goals need to be communicated clearly to the congregation.

Program Management and Resources

At minimum, an FCN will need a desk, a telephone with an answering machine or voice mail, and a locking file for client records. Ideally, the parish nurse would have a separate office for privacy for consultation and counseling. A laptop computer with Internet access would be extremely helpful for both documentation and client-related research. Client-related files need to be kept in a locked cabinet in the nurse's office that only the nurse can access. Space for storing supplies and health education materials is also necessary. A dedicated space for the program indicates to the congregation the value that the leadership places on the role of the FCN and the importance of each member's health and well-being. Patterson (2003) suggests an operating budget, which excludes the previously mentioned items as $2,000 to $3,000 for the first year and $500 to $1,000 for subsequent years.

Working in an independent role, the FCN needs to establish record-keeping methods. Documentation of all activities is vital to help the nurse explain the range of activities to others in the congregation as well as to track the progress of clients. Documentation of an FCN's

BOX 4-3
Sample Budget, Volunteer Parish Nurse Program

EXPENSES	AMOUNT/ YEAR
Mileage reimbursement	$525
Based on the congregation's policy ($0.35 per mile/35 miles/week)	
Equipment	200
Stethoscope	
Blood pressure cuff	
Scale	
Office supplies	175
Postage, photocopying	
Office equipment	1,500
Locking file cabinet	
Computer	
Desk	
Health education literature	300
Pamphlets, videos, books	
Drug reference books	
Display rack	
Speaker fees	200
Professional fees	400
Association memberships	
Professional journals	
Health newsletters	
Professional education conference	
Miscellaneous expenses	500
Office space (heating, electricity, Internet)	
Secretarial support	
TOTAL	**$3,800**

BOX 4-4
Sample Budget, Paid Parish Nurse Program

EXPENSES	
Salary (# hours per week × hourly rate)	
Parish nurse	$26,000
Secretarial support	2,000
Benefits (12% of salary for insurance, retirement, taxes)	5,000
Office space	600
Office supplies	400
Mileage reimbursement ($0.34 × 30 miles/week)	510
TOTAL	**$34,510**

activities is important to protect the ministry as well as to provide "witness of the value and usefulness of the program and its impact on improving the quality of parishioners' lives" (O'Brien, 2003, p. 143). Documentation will be further addressed in Chapter 8.

Adequate fiscal resources are necessary to provide a successful faith community nursing program. Boxes 4-3 and 4-4 provide sample budgets for faith community nursing programs. Funding for faith community nursing programs and specific initiatives can be raised in various ways. Chapter 14 presents information related to the grant-writing process.

Professional Network

FCNs often work independently within a church structure where they may be the only health professional on staff. Add to this the independent nature of the role, and it becomes necessary for the FCN to find resources for problem solving, interpretation of the role, as well as continuing education. Often FCNs form their own local support networks; other times the support network is more structured, as when the nurses are organized through a health care system. Currently, an online Web site is available for parish nurses to share concerns, resources, and ideas. This support is vital for the independent nature of the parish nurse role. Chapter 7 presents content on collaborative relationships within the faith community and with the larger external community.

Personal/Professional Boundaries

The FCN may face many challenges in this new role. Examples of these challenges are the needs of the congregation members exceeding the boundaries and abilities of the FCN role and the needs of the congregation exceeding the time available.

The FCN must abide by the professional code of ethics and *Scope and Standards of Practice*. FCNs do not participate in dependent functions of nursing, such as invasive procedures. When the needs of the members of congregation require direct care, the parish nurse must use her or his assessment skills and refer the client to the appropriate community agency. He or she may teach family members or volunteers to deliver direct care and follow-up to ensure that the correct care is being carried out. In a qualitative study by Chase-Ziolek and Gruca (2000), patients seen in a congregation reported that the greatest impact came from the parish nurse serving as an advocate with the health community. Often the idea of a nurse not delivering hands-on care is initially difficult for congregational members to understand.

Congregations vary in their membership. In a congregation with older members where the medical needs may be complex, the needs of the members may exceed the time the nurse is available to the congregation. Having to set limits and boundaries can be very stressful. The nurse keeping to her time commitment is essential to prevent burnout. Often this struggle between the needs of the congregation and the time available may lead to seeking out volunteers to expand the program. The support of the pastor and leadership is essential in this example.

Parish nursing/faith community nursing was recently recognized as a subspecialty by the American Nurses Association (1998). Working in faith communities, the parish nurse has the potential to reach all ages and socioeconomic levels. Reaching individuals in a familiar and safe place, the parish nurse can assist individuals to understand the complex health care environment and assist them through complicated medical and social problems. "The roles of the parish nurse flow from the goal of enhancing quality of life for all community members" (Schank, Weis, & Matheus, 1996, p. 11).

Brudenell (2003) describes the final phase of establishing a parish nurse program as "parish nursing as an ongoing ministry." At this point, the faith community nursing program is recognized by the congregation as established and essential. Church members talk about being able to "count on the parish nurse" and "can't imagine managing without the parish nurse." Programs that have reached phase four are characterized by continuously reaching out to others both within and outside the congregation. Working relationships between the pastor, parish nurse, health ministry team, church staff, parishioners, and community agencies are evident and positive.

Most congregations should be able to establish a parish nursing program over a period of 18 to 24 months. The amount of parish nurse time allotted to the program and the needs of the congregation will dictate parish nurse role priorities and the extent of health programming. A formal evaluation process should be created, and parish nurse performance review should be conducted by the appropriate supervisor at least annually.

Summary

This chapter has provided beginning information about working in a faith community. The phases of forming a faith community nursing program were discussed in detail. Topical information was provided on the congregational leader and governance structures, initiating a new ministry, and the expectations of the parish nurse, the ministry team, and the congregation. Management of a faith community nursing program was discussed in relation to fiscal and human resources and the use of volunteers.

Reflect and Discuss

1. Identify challenges in initiating a new faith community nursing program.
2. Discuss ways a health cabinet can support a faith community nursing program.
3. Describe steps to forming a volunteer network for the faith community nursing program.
4. What are the advantages and disadvantages of a health care system-supported faith community nursing?
5. What strategies can be created to ensure documentation of activities of a faith community nursing?

Case Study

Mary is the FCN for a large congregation. This is her second year in the position; the first year she volunteered her time, but this year she is paid for 20 hours per week. She has five members of the congregation who are interested in volunteering in the health ministry. She is planning her first volunteer meeting. Mary's volunteers are two retired nurses, a stay-at-home mom, a teacher, and a widow whose husband recently died of cancer.

At the first meeting, Mary shares the goals for the program for the second year. She wants to expand the blood pressure screening to all services each week, as well as begin to offer health education programs for 10 months of the year. She wants to supplement the monthly bulletin with a health article.

The nurses of the group agree to participate in the Sunday blood pressure screenings and ask for further time to discuss the details of the program. They each bring years of valuable experience and are well respected in the congregation.

The stay-at-home mom is very interested in health care but postponed college to support her husband and raise her children. Her time is variable, but she is known in the congregation as a very reliable and organized woman. She is open to any job Mary has for her but is very interested in doing research for the bulletin articles.

The teacher is new to the congregation and is interested in the idea of holistic health. She is shy but also wants to contribute to the program. Mary doesn't yet have a specific job in mind for her.

The widow came to the volunteer meeting because she wants to start a bereavement group. She is not interested in any of the goals that Mary has for the year. Based on her recent loss she feels that she can run a group. She knows how people want to be treated and how to help them get what they want from health professionals. She is adamant that an ongoing bereavement group is what is needed in the church. Mary recognizes that the woman is still grieving her husband's death but knows that a bereavement group has not been identified as a need on the congregation's assessment. She wants to support the woman's interest but realizes that the woman is not qualified to handle a group. Mary asks if they can meet privately to discuss this large undertaking. Mary realizes that she needs to come up with a plan to support this woman and funnel her loss into constructive action. They agree to meet in a week's time.

Mary has the start of a volunteer program. She has volunteers who are interested and want to participate in the health ministry. She has also identified a new client who needs support and assistance.

References

American Nurses Association & Health Ministries Association. (2005). *Faith community nursing: Scope and standards of practice.* Silver Springs, MD: ANA.

Berquist, S., & King, J. (1994). Parish nursing. *Journal of Holistic Nursing, 6*(12), 155–171.

Brudenell, I. (2003). Parish nursing: Nurturing body, mind, spirit, and community. *Public Health Nursing, 20*(2), 85–94.

Carson, V. B., & Koenig, H. G. (2004). *Spiritual caregiving: Healthcare as minister.* Philadelphia: Templeton Foundation Press.

Chase-Ziolek. (2003). Rethinking our terms: Health ministry or ministry of health? *Journal of Christian Nursing, 20*(2), 21, 22.

Chase-Ziolek, M., & Gruca, J. (2000). Client's perceptions of distinctive aspects in nursing care received within a congregational setting. *Journal of Community Health Nursing, 17*(3), 171–183.

Garity, J., & Ryan, A. (2002). The impact of an advisory board on a parish nurse program. *Journal of Nursing Administration, 32*(12), 616–619.

Health Ministries Association, Inc, & American Nurses Association. (2005). *Faith community nursing: Scope and standards of practice* (2nd ed.). Washington, DC: American Nurses Publishing.

Magilvy, J. K., & Brown, N. J. (1997). Parish nursing: Advanced practice nursing model for healthier communities. *Advanced Practice Nursing Quarterly, 2,* 67–72.

Mayhugh, L. J., & Martens, K. H. (2001). What's a parish nurse to do? Congregational expectations. *Journal of Christian Nursing, 18*(3), 14–16.

McDermott, M. A., Solari-Twadell, P. A., & Matheus, R. (1999). Educational preparation. In P. A. Solari-Twadell & M. A. McDermott (Eds.), *Parish nursing: Promoting whole person health within faith communities* (pp. 269–275). Thousand Oaks, CA: Sage Publications.

Meyer, P. A. (1996). Management fundamentals for parish nurse programs. *Perspectives in Parish Nurse Practice, 1,* 3–6.

O'Brien, M. E. (2003). *Parish nursing healthcare ministry within the church.* Boston: Jones and Bartlett Publishers.

Parker, M. (2000, Summer). Mobilizing volunteers for service. *Healing Hearts and Hands, 4*(3), 1.

Patterson, D. L. (2003). *The essential parish nurse: ABCs for congregational health ministry.* Cleveland, OH: Pilgrim Press.

Richardson, R. (1996). *Creating a healthier church.* Minneapolis: Augsburg Fortress.

Schank, M. J., Weis, D., & Matheus, R. (1996). Parish nursing: Ministry of healing. *Geriatric Nurse, 17*(1), 11–13.

Schnorr, R. (1999). Parish nursing: Service and care within the faith community. Available online at: http://www.psna.org.

Schweitzer, R., Norberg, M., & Larson, L. (2002). The parish nurse coordinator: A bridge to spiritual health care leadership for the future. *Journal of Holistic Nursing, 20*(3), 212–231.

Smith, S. D. (2003). *Parish nursing: A handbook for the new millennium.* New York: The Haworth Press.

Solari-Twadell, P. A. (1999). The caring congregation: A healing place. *Journal of Christian Nursing, 14*(1), 4–9.

Solari-Twadell, P. A., & McDermott, M. A. (Eds.). (1999). *Parish nursing: Promoting whole person health within faith communities.* Thousand Oaks, CA: Sage Publications.

Tuck, I., Wallace, D., & Pullen, L. (2001). Spirituality and spiritual care provided by parish nurses. *Western Journal of Nursing Research, 23*(5), 441–453.

Wallace, D. C., Tuck, I., Boland, C. S., & Witucki, J. M. (2002). Client perceptions of parish nursing. *Public Health Nursing, 19*(2), 128–135.

Weis, D. M., Schank, M. J., Coenan, A., & Matheus, R. (2002). Parish nurse practice with client aggregates. *Journal of Community Health Nursing, 19*(2), 105–113.

Westberg, G. (1987). *The parish nurse: How to start a parish nurse program in your church* (2nd ed.). Park Ridge, IL: Parish Nurse Resource Center.

Wuthnow, R. (2004). *Saving America: Faith–based services and the future of civil society.* Princeton, NJ: Princeton University Press.

Additional Resources

Chase-Ziolek, M. (2000). Client's perception of distinctive aspects of nursing care received within a congregational setting. *Journal of Community Health Nursing, 17,* 171–183.

Chase-Ziolek, M. (1999). The meaning and experience of health ministry within the culture of a congregation. *Journal of Transcultural Nursing, 10*(1), 46–55.

Kociszewski, C. (2003). A phenomenological pilot study of nurses' experience providing spiritual care. *Journal of Holistic Nursing, 21*(2), 131–148.

Kuhn, J. (1997). A profile of parish nurses. *Journal of Christian Nursing, 14*(1), 26–28.

Rydholm, L. (1997). Patient-focused care in parish nursing. *Holistic Nursing Practice, 11*(3), 47–60.

Scott, L., & Sumner, J. (1993). How do parish nurses help people? A research perspective. *Journal of Christian Nursing, 10*(1), 16–19.

Tuck, L., Pullen, L., & Wallace, D. (2001). A comparative study of the spiritual perspectives and interventions of mental health and parish nurses. *Issues in Mental Health Nursing, 22*(6), 593–606.

Tuck, L., & Wallace, D. (2000). Exploring parish nursing from an ethnographic perspective. *Journal of Transcultural Nursing, 11*(4), 290–299.

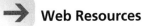 **Web Resources**

http://www.parishnurses.org   International Parish
   Nurse Resource Center
http://www.healthministriesassociation.org
   Grassroots organization supporting health ministry, an interfaith focus.

http://www.tdh.state.tx.us/library/nursing.htm
   Good bibliography of parish nursing resources
http://www.healthfinder.gov/library   Health
   Observances Calendar

5

Assessment of the Faith Community and Geopolitical Community

This chapter will present information on the assessment process. A community assessment is the process of examining a community's characteristics, assets and resources, liabilities, and needs, in collaboration with the community, to develop strategies that improve health and quality of life for the community (Carroll, 2004, p. 52). Content about assessing the faith community will be presented first, followed by assessment of the surrounding geopolitical community.

Standard I of the *Faith Community Nursing: Scope and Standards of Practice* (American Nurses Association-Health Ministries Association [ANA-HMA], 2005) document focuses on assessment. This standard states, "The faith community nurse (FCN) collects comprehensive data pertinent to the patient's wholistic health or the situaton" (p. 11). *Wholism* (or holism) is defined as the view that an integrated whole is a reality independent of and greater than the sum of its parts. Wholistic nursing supports the connectedness of mind, body and spirit (Dossey, Keegan, & Guzetta, 2005). Standard II states that, "The FCN analyzes the wholistic assessment data to determine the diagnoses or issues" (ANA-HMA, 2005, p. 12).

Because the focus of this chapter is on the assessment process, an appropriate place to begin the process is to identify *who* the client or patient is in the faith community setting. According to the glossary of the *Faith Community Nursing: Scope and Standards of Practice* (2005), "the faith community is an organization of groups, families and individuals who share common values, beliefs, and religious doctrine, and faith practices that influence their lives, such as a church, synagogue, or mosque, and that functions as a patient system, providing a setting for faith community nursing" (p. 36). From a systems perspective, the whole of the faith community is composed of the sum of the persons, environments, structures, values, and practices, and, as a whole, is more than and different from the sum of the parts. Because each part of the faith community system is interrelated, each part of the community affects and is affected by changes in every other part. Although communities of faith may have different names (church, temple, mosque, synagogue), each will demonstrate characteristics of faith, spirituality, theology, and religion that can be identified and assessed (Clark, 2000). Clark describes faith as "being in relationship with," spirituality as "an experience of being in relationship with," theology as "reflections on being in relationship with," and religion as "a community within which to share reflection and celebration around experiences of being in relationship with."

Definitions of community abound in the literature. Carroll (2004) states that the following three dimensions need to be included in any definition of community:

- *Status*—information about morbidity and mortality, life expectancy, crime rates, and education.
- *Structure*—the socioeconomic, age, gender, and ethnic distribution as well as resources available.
- *Process*—how the community operates; how it functions as a whole to solve problems. (p. 52)

Carroll (2004) also states that the process dimension includes the concept of *community competence*. She describes competence as the community's ability to effectively identify needs, to achieve working consensus on issues, to agree on ways to implement goals, and to work together to implement desired actions. She states that a community's *capacity* to get a particular issue resolved or to get a particular job done builds on the community's level of competence.

Blum (1974) describes several types of communities, including face-to-face, neighborhood, community of identifiable need, community of problem ecology, community of concern, community of political jurisdiction, community of special interest, and community of solution. Blum's types of communities infer both structural and functional aspects. A faith community may serve a neighborhood in an inner city, or it may serve persons who reside in several different towns. A faith community is always a community of special interests and may also often be a community of solution for its membership. The mission(s) of the faith community may steer the focus of assessment. For example, if there is a strong commitment to serve the youth of a community, it can steer the assessment process to focus on this age group.

Higgs and Gustafson (1985) describe the concept of "community as client" as a group or aggregate of people within a geopolitical boundary who comprise the unit of practice. This conceptualization of community arose from the early public health movement's aim to prevent communicable disease in a particular locale. "Faith community as client" refers to the concept of a faith community of people as the focus of nursing services.

Shuster and Goeppinger (2000) describe community as a "locality based entity, composed of systems of formal organizations reflecting societal institutions, informal groups and aggregates" (p. 307). They see the personal, geographic, and functional components of community as being interrelated. Although a faith community certainly contains formal and informal structures, whether or not it reflects societal institutions would depend on the faith tradition. Many faith traditions, by intent, have value systems that differ from societal institutions.

Anderson and McFarlane (2000) describe community as encompassing eight components: physical environment, education, safety and transportation, politics and government, health and social services, communication, economics, and recreation. These eight components conceptually surround the people of the community. This definition of community is more appropriate to geopolitical communities than to faith communities.

Ervin (2002) discusses the concept of "community as a relational experience" as a more complex idea than the previously presented conceptualizations of community. Here, community is defined as the everyday life experience of living and "being in" community. The experience of "being in" community is having a sense of connection, history, safe places to be, collective memories, hopes, and dreams. It is about the experience of having overlapping lives and interrelationships and the idea of shared emotional connections. The faith community is very much a relational community, although also a community with structure and function. Other examples of relational communities would include the extended family and religious communities (e.g., members of religious orders).

Anderson (1990) defines a faith community as an assembly of people (or congregation) whose beliefs about God combine with a common identity, shared history, regular worship, and common values to effect personal and social transformation. According to McKnight (1987), as a community association, a faith community identifies with the following characteristics:

- Communities are interdependent—to weaken one part of the community is to weaken all.
- The community environment is constructed around the recognition of fallibility rather than the ideal, thus there is room for many leaders.
- Such associations have the capacity to respond quickly because they do not have to move issues through an institutional, corporate structure before taking action.
- The development of community associations allows for the flowering of creative solutions.
- Community associations are usually small, face-to-face groups, so the relationship is very individualized, which results in "hand-tailored" responses.

- Communities can provide care that represents consent versus control.
- Community is a forum in which citizenship can be expressed. (p. 56)

The preceding discussions about the concept of community reinforce the idea that faith communities serve as places of holistic health promotion. Health ministry is a seamless garment, demonstrating that faith, health, and wholeness are one and cannot be separated. Health ministries are actualized by building caring communities that nurture each person in body, mind, and spirit; by promoting good stewardship of one's body; and by working for a just, equal, and effective system of health care (Health Ministries USA, 2004). Specifically, what persons make up the health ministry team, committee, or cabinet will be a function of the resources of the faith community. Larger faith communities tend to have more formal structures, whereas smaller faith communities with fewer resources tend to have more informal structures.

Assessment of the Faith Community

The purposes of assessing the faith community include: describing the attributes of the membership, learning its gifts and strengths, identifying its health and spiritual needs, identifying its health risk factors, and identifying its needs and interests in health-related services and programming. Inclusion of both quantitative and qualitative data will provide the most complete assessment. Data can be collected from the faith community membership in various ways. Trofino, Hughes, O'Brien, Mack, Marrinan, and Hay (2000) identify assessing congregational health needs as a critical component of establishing a faith community nursing partnership.

How the faith community defines its mission will influence what, how much, and when various health assessments are conducted. The size and structure of the faith community will determine who will conduct the assessment process. Larger faith communities with established health ministries or health ministry cabinets will have a structure in place for a committee to participate in the data collection and analysis aspects of the assessment process. Small faith communities operating with a worship leader and a part-time volunteer FCN may need to ask for volunteers to assist in the process, or they may choose to set up an ad hoc committee to assist with data collection and analysis. Ideally, the entire faith community will participate in the process. This creates a feeling of ownership and reinforces the faith community's role in the health promotion of its membership.

A good starting point in the faith community assessment is to do a "walk-about." A "walk-about" is a mini-assessment of a community carried out primarily by walking about and observing the faith community setting. It would be helpful to do the walk-about with the faith community leader and a member of the health ministry team. Each of these individuals will have information to add to the walk-about assessment. A "walk-about" is a smaller scale, walking version of the traditional community health nursing windshield assessment. Using this method, the FCN will collect data about the setting and structure of the congregational meeting place (church, temple, mosque), the services offered to the membership, the size and nature of both the clerical and lay staff, and ways that the membership participates in the faith community worship services and other congregational activities. See Box 5-1, How to Conduct a Walk-about Assessment.

Once the FCN and health ministry cabinet have observed the faith community, a review of the available data about the congregation is the next logical step of the assessment process. Many congregations keep a computerized database of the demographic properties of the membership. Such a database usually includes names, addresses, telephone numbers, e-mail addresses, and birth dates of the members, and may also contain an inventory of the members' talents and gifts and areas where they are willing to serve as volunteers. Some congregational databases provide information about membership participation in the worship activities. If this information is readily available to the FCN, it will provide a wonderful starting point for the assessment of the faith community. Inviting a member of the health ministry team to

BOX 5-1
How to Conduct a Walk-about Assessment

As the faith community nurse makes observations of the faith community, the following areas and related questions should be considered:

SETTING

What is this place called?

What is the structure of the place of worship? Is it free standing or within another structure?

Approximately how many persons could occupy the worship area?

Is it structure accessible to people with disabilities?

Are there spaces in the building for religious education? Child care areas? Offices for staff? Are the spaces of adequate size and number?

What messages are communicated through bulletin boards, banners, signs, and/or posted announcements?

Is there a library? Are there telephones and/or computers available?

Are there kitchen facilities?

Are there any apparent safety hazards?

Is there parking available, and is it adequate to meet membership needs?

Is the place of worship accessible by public transportation?

What is the neighborhood surrounding the place of worship like?

Are the properties well maintained?

Are people out and about? Ages?

Are the streets clean and free of trash and debris?

Do you feel safe walking in this neighborhood in both the day and the evening? Why or why not?

Are there any unusual odors evident?

MEMBER SERVICES

How many worship services are held per week?

Is religious education available? For which age groups?

Is child care available during worship services?

What ministries exist in the faith community? Music? Youth? Outreach?

What services exist for homebound members?

MEMBER PARTICIPATION

Are worship services attended by the majority of the membership?

Are certain age-groups overrepresented or underrepresented?

Is the physical setting adequate for the number of participants?

Do members volunteer to provide direct services such as child care and/or serve on faith community committees?

Do you feel welcome in this place?

assist in reviewing these data adds perspective to the process. Looking at the sensitive elements of these data—for example, the ages and family composition of the membership—will help the FCN plan and prioritize programs and services. For example, if the mean age of the membership is over 55 years, planning and programming for seniors would be a likely priority. Other important descriptive information would include cultural diversity, use of languages other than the dominant tongue, and literacy level. If this information is not available to the FCN, collecting it would become part of the first step of the data collection process.

The next area of assessment to consider is the administrative structure of the faith community. Questions to ask and answer in this area include the following:

- Who are considered to be the faith community leaders?
- Who comprises the ministry staff, and what is the hierarchy?
- What areas of responsibility does each staff member have?
- What is the mission(s) of the faith community?
- What is the governing body of the faith community? Is it elected or appointed by the clergy?
- How are decisions made in the faith community? Who must be consulted to approve plans and programs?
- Do both men and women serve in all roles, or are roles gender-based?
- Is there an existing committee structure? Does it include a health ministry? What services does it currently provide?
- Who develops and manages the faith community budget?
- Are the human and financial resources adequate to meet community needs?

If the congregation has an existing committee structure, these committees can be used as *focus groups* for data collection. *Focus groups* are small groups of people brought together to solicit their opinions about a specific idea or issue. A focus group approach to data collection puts the FCN in face-to-face contact with key decision-making persons in the faith community. In providing these individuals with information and an opportunity to shape the evolving FCN program, the nurse optimally gains advocates for the program as well as information. Clark, Cary, Diemert, Ceballos, Sifuentes, Atteberry, Vue, and Trieu (2003) state that focus groups provide an effective means of incorporating the perspectives of "hidden" populations in a community.

The FCN would need to request a portion of each committee's agenda to present the faith community nursing concept and to gather assessment data. When beginning a faith community nursing program, many members of the congregation may be unaware of the potential programs and services that a health ministry can provide to them. Congregation members won't know—what they don't know, about faith community nursing. If the church is large with an extensive committee structure, the FCN (with guidance from the health ministry team) may choose to meet with only some of the committees.

The focus group setting is an important and opportune venue to promote awareness of the faith community as a place to access health promotion services and to provide health education programming. Prefacing the data collection part of the focus group meeting with a brief presentation of the "possibles" of the faith community nursing program is important. The range of what these "possibles" might be will have been (and should be) discussed at the health ministry team level prior to discussion with congregation members.

Data about specific kinds of programming and services that the congregation wants and is willing to participate in are the required key data elements. Swinney, Anson-Wonkka, Maki, and Corneau (2001) suggest the following questions to guide focus group discussions:

1. What are some of the things about your health or your family's health that concern you at this time?
2. When you are not feeling well, with whom do you usually speak?
3. Do you believe the church has a role in helping to meet the health needs of church members? In your opinion, how important is this?
4. What type of services would you like to see the church and FCN work to establish to help you to better meet your health needs?

5. Do you know someone in the church community who may be having trouble obtaining health care when needed?

6. The church wants to do its part in helping promote and maintain the health of people in its faith community. Are there health problems in our community of which you are aware? (p. 42)

Although focus groups can provide the FCN with valuable data, they are time-consuming to conduct, and they provide contact with relatively small numbers of people. Focus groups may be tape-recorded (with the permission of the participants) to review the discussion for patterns of content.

Another method of data collection is one-on-one interviews with opinion leaders in the congregation. The FCN may know who these individuals are from history with the congregation, or the nurse may need to be referred to opinion leaders identified by other members of the pastoral staff or health ministry team. Individual interviews are time-consuming; however, they do help the FCN to form relationships with key informants in the faith community. Once again, this approach may create both an advocate and an ally for the FCN, as well as provide insider information.

Survey data may also be helpful to the FCN. Paper and pencil questionnaires have time-saving advantages and can provide a large quantity of data. Another advantage to this data collection method is that the respondent can choose to be anonymous—an individual can provide information without disclosing one's identity. A disadvantage of this method is that the responses are limited to what data people are willing to share—if they are willing to participate at all. The biggest drawback to using questionnaires is that many people do not complete and return them. A response rate of over 60% is usually considered to be acceptable for survey research purposes (Polit & Beck, 2004), but this percentage clearly leaves a significant data gap about a faith community. The response rate for a survey will be higher, if the survey form is distributed during a worship service (and collected at the end of the service), than if the forms were mailed to homes (Thomas & King, 2000). Unless supplemented with a mailed survey, this approach will limit participation to those members who attend worship services.

Many congregational questionnaire forms are available in the literature. Later in this chapter Boxes 5-2 and 5-3 provide samples that can be modified to meet faith community needs. Customizing a questionnaire for a specific faith community is advisable and will increase the response rate. When designing a questionnaire, be sure to carefully consider the content of the survey items. Ask *only* for information that will be used and that has direct relevance to the FCN's role(s) in the faith community. In the introductory paragraph of the questionnaire, tell the respondents how the information that they provide will be used. Also consider the level of intrusiveness of the questions. Individuals will choose, not disclose, what they consider to be private information and may resent being questioned about private or sensitive topics. Also, do consider both the ethical and legal aspects of health information and personal privacy.

The tone of the questionnaire should be positive in nature. Give the respondents opportunities to identify their positive health behaviors as well as solicit their areas of health information interest. Asking people to consider learning more about a topic is much more self-affirming than asking people to identify their weaknesses so that they can be "fixed" or "corrected." Providing checklists of potential topics for programs is helpful so that respondents can indicate their areas of interest. Also helpful is to ask respondents to indicate the day and times they would prefer that programming occur.

Data collected from all assessment sources should be recorded in an organized and retrievable manner. The most efficient way to do this is by entering the data into either a spreadsheet or database computer program; however, a three-ring notebook will suffice if a computer is not available to the nurse. Depending on the type of data collected, varying levels of security will be required to maintain respondent confidentiality. See Chapter 8 for a discussion of legal issues in record keeping.

Mayhugh and Martens (2001) describe the results of a congregational survey to determine faith community nursing outcomes. They report that the services most preferred (80%) were educational, with content about staying well and health screening. Over half of the respondents wanted FCNs to visit members who were terminally ill, post-hospitalization, or in a nursing home. Chi square analysis determined that respondents younger than age 60 preferred that the FCN visit after births and during and after hospitalization, significantly more than persons greater than age 60 ($p = <0.05$).

Research conducted by Gottlieb and Allen (1997) identifies eight categories of health-related issues about which people seek nursing expertise. These categories provide the FCN with themes about which people seek nursing advice and expertise. These researchers found that people consult nurses when their family experiences changes in family size, composition, roles, and relationships. Second, families seek out nurses when learning to function in the social system—for example, when people need help negotiating the health care system or planning for a role change. The third category of family situations involved interaction between environmental conditions and development of health promotive behaviors, such as weight loss or beginning an exercise program. Fourth, they found that nurses help persons experiencing biophysiologic changes related to growth and development. Fifth, families consult nurses to learn how to cope with chronic illnesses in a healthful way. Sixth, nurses are consulted when families encounter episodes of acute illness or injury. Seventh, nurses are sought out by families adapting to economic changes. And, finally, nurses are consulted when families are trying to maintain interpersonal relations or to resolve conflict. These themes can be used to structure a congregational assessment survey.

Analysis of the Faith Community Data

Once the FCN has collected data from the faith community, the data are then analyzed for descriptive elements about the congregation, for common threads in programming and service requests, as well as for gaps or areas of missing data. For example, if congregational committees consisting of mostly retired persons are surveyed, yet the membership data base identifies a large number of young families, the committee members are not representative of the young families. This would represent a data gap. Gaps in the data direct the parish nurse to collect additional data.

As the FCN analyzes data about the faith community, assets and areas of health risk for the community will emerge. Assets can be written in the form of a list and usually do not need any type of prioritizing. Areas of risk or need are written in the form of a nursing diagnosis and should be prioritized. As the taxonomies for nursing diagnosis are written for the individual patients rather than aggregates, Shuster and Goeppinger (2000) suggest using a version of a three-part nursing diagnosis format proposed by Muecke (1984). The diagnostic statement is written as, "Risk of _____ among _____ related to _____." "Risk of" identifies a problem or health risk faced by the community. "Among" specifies with whom the nurse will be working in relation to the problem or risk, and "related to" describes possible causative factors or characteristics of the community identified in the assessment. For example, a diagnostic statement in this format would read "Risk of hypertension among African American men related to high sodium diets."

An important aspect of data analysis is priority setting. High priority items are those program or service requests identified by the largest number of respondents. High priority items are also those to which the FCN and health ministry can most readily and appropriately respond. Planning for *early* (even if small) successes is important when introducing new programs. Early successful programs provide positive credibility and publicity to the faith community nursing program. The interpretation of data will reveal a significant congregational need that is out of the scope of nursing, such as a need for more parking, or a need for taxi services for elders. When these needs are identified, the FCN should refer them to the appropriate person or committee. The case study presents a community assessment and analysis of data.

Assessment of the Geopolitical Community

Assessment of the larger geopolitical community will provide a context for understanding the faith community's relationships to it. This level of assessment will provide a wide angle or big-picture view of what structures exist in the community and how they function with each other—or not. In planning, it is very important for the FCN to learn whether the faith community is representative of the larger community and/or how it differs from the larger community. Olson (2000) states that to become knowledgeable in the function of referral agent and liaison with congregational and community resources, the FCN should undertake a comprehensive community assessment. This involves assessing the resources and needs within the congregation, as well as those that exist in the larger community. Olson cautions that although the assessment process is ongoing, once it has begun, the FCN is in position to fulfill the role of referral agent and liaison with the congregation and the community. She points out that a continuous assessment process provides the FCN with an awareness of new resources in the community, and through the exchange of information, the health ministries of the faith community become known to outside agencies. This two-way communication process fosters positive partnerships between the faith community and the larger community (2000).

The health ministry cabinet may elect to personally conduct a community assessment of the geopolitical community in which the faith community resides or may look to other sources for this information. Many communities conduct periodic community assessments for various reasons. Regions that are served by health departments will have a good source of health-related biostatistical data about the community. Health department assessments may cover many aspects of the community or may be limited to specific health information. Local development councils or chambers of commerce conduct community assessments that focus on the business and economic resources of communities. The U.S. Census is a national assessment carried out by the federal government every 10 years. Federal census data available on the Web (www.census.gov) document demographic and economic data at the community, state, and national levels. Regional and local universities are also good resources for locating recently completed community assessment projects. A telephone call to a university's department of nursing or public health may provide the FCN with a direct source of a current community assessment. Locating such a document will be a time-saver for the FCN.

A comprehensive community assessment may take several months to a year to complete. The scope of the community assessment is determined by the purpose of the assessment and by the complexity of the community. The FCN is interested in attaining an overall flavor and context of the community, where the faith community resides, to understand the resources and concern in the greater community. Therefore, the assessment should focus on data that are highly sensitive—data that carry significant meaning in achieving the purpose of gaining community context. Important to note early in the process is that *data standing alone have little or no value* and merely describe what exists. Data should be *compared* to regional and state means or to other standards to have actual relevance and meaning for the community being studied. They also need to be interpreted in terms of the mission of the faith community and its health ministry goals.

Community assessment data can be collected by seven different methods: informant interviews, observation, secondary analysis of existing data, constructed surveys, focus groups, community forums, and windshield surveys (Allender & Spradley, 2005; Lundy & Barton, 2001; Porche, 2004). Levy, Anderson, Issel, Willis, Dancy, and Jacobson (2004) report that multiple sources of data yield useful information for program planning and a better understanding of cultural differences and similarities. If a health ministry team structure is in place, members of the team can assist the FCN in data collection. For the purpose of gaining community context, and in the interest of expediency, a windshield survey, observation, secondary data analysis, and informant interviews are recommended to the FCN as usually preferred data collection methods.

Data Collection

The community assessment process can be done in an in-depth format or as a community overview. The depth of assessment information the FCN will need is dependent on the nurse's familiarity with the community in question. Obviously, a lifelong resident or a nurse with community health nursing experience in the community of interest will have a different frame of reference than a newcomer. For either individual, a good place to start the data collection process is with a windshield survey.

Windshield Survey

A windshield survey is a directed observation of a community through the windshield of one's automobile. Helpful (but not necessary) is to have someone drive the FCN around the community, so that the FCN can focus on observing and recording, rather than on driving. An FCN who is new to the community might invite a member of the health ministry team or a congregant to accompany her or him (or drive her or him) on the windshield survey. This person can highlight historical elements and recent changes and plans of the community. This experience helps both the nurse and health ministry member understand the community in refreshed ways. As you pass through the streets and neighborhoods of the community, think about your five senses.

First, think about what you see. Where are people congregating? What are the racial/ethnic characteristics of the people that you see? Are they young or elderly? Do the ages of the people vary with the neighborhoods? What does the housing look like? Are the majority of the homes single-family or multi-family dwellings? Are the homes in good repair? Are there yards or green spaces near the homes? Do you see senior citizen housing or retirement communities? Do you see playgrounds, theaters, libraries, pools, tennis courts, and other recreational areas? Are there retail shopping and health care facilities available in the community? Are these services accessible? Do you see churches and other places of worship? Do they represent diverse faith traditions? Do you see any evidence of public transportation and police and fire services? Are the community's streets free of trash? Are animals on the loose? Are there industries in the community? Are they located near residential areas? Do you see schools, preschools, and senior centers? Are there any overt signs of pollution or other environmental hazards?

Next, use your other senses. Do you notice any types of odors as you drive around the community? What is the noise level? What is there to taste in this community? Is there a variety of restaurants? How does this community feel to you? Would you be comfortable walking alone in all of the neighborhoods of this community? Do they feel friendly to you?

Data collected in the windshield survey give the FCN a starting point in gaining an overall picture of the community. Usually, a windshield survey raises several questions about the community that will require further data collection. The data collected from the windshield survey should be documented and can be stored in the first section of a large three-ring binder, accordion file, or in a computer file. Using a three-ring binder or an accordion file is also helpful for the storage of brochures and flyers related to the various areas of assessment.

In a formal community assessment, data are collected about the various aspects or subsystems of the larger community. In the *analysis* of these data, conclusions are drawn about the competence of the community by identifying community assets, strengths, or resources, as well as community deficits and areas of need or concern. Community competence has been described by many authors (Cottrell, 1976; Minkler & Wellerstein, 1997; Wallerstein, 1992). A competent community is described as one where members participate collaboratively to identify community problems and needs and work together to set goals, prioritize, and implement solutions. Newspaper articles and minutes of community meetings are examples of sources that would document community competence (or lack of it).

Kretzmann and McKnight (1993) introduced the idea of a community assets assessment (instead of an assessment of needs or deficits). This approach focuses on identifying and addressing the strengths and capacities that can serve as a foundation for community intervention. These authors believe that the key to community regeneration is to identify all available assets and to begin connecting them to one another to multiply power and effectiveness. They point out that the most accessible community assets are those located at, and controlled by, local residents (1997). These assets include both individual and organizational assets and capacities. The next most accessible assets are those located locally but controlled by an outside authority. The least accessible assets or resources are those both located and controlled outside the community. Identifying faith community assets provides the FCN and health ministry cabinet with both starting points for building on community strengths and resources. For example, if you discover that you have a large number of health care professionals in the membership, it will extend the potential abilities of a health ministry.

Ammerman and Parks (1998) describe the assets assessment approach as empowering for both the nurse and the community. The assets assessment process identifies what individuals and organizations can contribute to the community, rather than focus on what is lacking. It does require more time and interaction with the community than the more traditional community deficits approach.

If a formal community assessment is not available to the FCN from another source, the FCN may elect to conduct one. Data will be collected about each of the following community subsystems: population demographics, economics, education, health and social services, transportation, communication, politics and government, physical environment, safety and protective services, spiritual resources, and recreation. Extensive amounts of secondary data about each of these subsystems are available to the FCN on the Internet. Novices at the community assessment process often believe that the more data one can collect, the better or more complete the community assessment. However, not all data are created equally—some data provide highly sensitive and significant information about a community and some tell very little. In the discussion of data collection for each of the subsystems, the more sensitive data areas will be highlighted for the reader. When data are contradictory or conflicting, it is helpful to clarify or validate secondary data with community representatives.

Each of the following subsystems should have a separate section in a large three-ring binder or a separate computer file. Each section will contain the data collected and end with an analysis of the data for that subsystem. Having more than one person review the data and participate in each analysis is important. If time and resources allow, health cabinet meeting time can be allotted for discussion and analysis of each major section of the assessment.

Population Demographics and Vital Statistics

Population demographics describe the characteristics of the population of the target community. A wealth of information is available about population demographics on the federal census Web site (www.census.gov). Sensitive data for this subsystem include: total population, age distribution in years, marital status, racial/ethnic composition, number of households (by size), literacy level, homeless rate, and educational achievement levels. These data will tell you who your community members are in terms of these categories. You then need to *compare* your community's data with the county and state figures to determine what the numbers actually mean.

For example, if you find that your community has a Latino population that is 25% of the total population, this percentage would be considered very high in southern Vermont but not unusual in southern Texas. Identification of diverse cultures within a faith community would also guide event planning and provision of materials in the appropriate languages.

Vital statistics about the population of the community are available on the Web sites of the state and local health departments as well as the vital statistics system of the National Center for Health Statistics (NCHS). Morbidity and mortality data are usually provided at the county level and are often compared to the *Healthy People 2010* objectives (USDHHS, 2000). Sensitive data include: birth and death rates, maternal and infant death rates, incidence of low birth weight (LBW), number of births to adolescents, percentage of mothers receiving prenatal care, causes of death, Behavioral Risk Factor Surveillance System (BRFSS) data, and communicable disease incidence.

Economics

Economic data will give you a picture of the economic success (or lack of success) of the community. These data are available on the U.S. Census Web site and in publications and Web sites of the local chamber of commerce and/or development council. Key or sensitive data include: employment/unemployment rates, annual household income (mean and median), number of families below the poverty level, number of individuals/families on public assistance, food stamps, Medicaid and WIC, percentages of white collar, blue collar, and agricultural workers, and major employers. Once again, discussion of the economic assets or areas of concern needs to be related to how the community compares to the region and to the state.

Education

A good source of information about this subsystem will be the public school district's Web site. Sensitive data for this subsystem include: high school graduation rate, dropout rate, mean SAT scores, percentage of graduates going to college, per-pupil spending in dollars, and the percentages of the school-age population attending public and private schools. These data should be compared with regional and state data to provide an understanding of their meaning.

Health and Social Services

This subsystem addresses the health and social service resources available in the community. Key data pieces for health services include: acute care hospitals (number of beds per population), mental health services, long-term and rehabilitative services, number of physicians, dentists and registered nurses, health department services, home health services, and complementary and alternative health providers. Key data pieces for social service agencies include: accessibility of welfare, Social Security and Medicare offices, the presence/absence of child protective services, homeless shelter, domestic violence services, meals-on-wheels programs, adult day care, and substance abuse programs. Adequacy of the services and manpower are analyzed based on population size, age, and health care needs.

From data collected in this subsystem, the FCN should develop a resource file. It can be computer-based or a card file that lists the agency name, type of services provided, eligibility criteria, address, telephone, fax, and Web site information, fees, insurances honored, a contact person, and whether or not a physician's referral is required.

Transportation

Adequate transportation is vital to the growth and health of communities. The U.S. Census provides information about how people get to work and how long they travel to their place of employment. Accessibility to public transportation (road, rail, and air), number of households without automobiles, taxi services, and transportation services for the elderly are key data to collect for this subsystem. Analysis of transportation data should address the adequacy (or inadequacy) of transportation.

Availability and accessibility of transportation modes provide the FCN with information about how easily members of the faith community can get to worship services and to health care services.

Communication

Data on a community's communication systems provide information about how the community is linked to the rest of the world. Key data for this subsystem include: local radio and television stations, local newspapers/publications, percentage of housing units with telephones, Internet availability to homeowners, and availability of public-use computers. Data analysis should include the strengths and weaknesses of the communication subsystem.

How people receive information has implications as to how the health ministry will provide information to faith community members and how services can be publicized.

Politics and Government

The politics and government of a community are important because they provide the formal structures that affect health and social welfare. Key data for this subsystem include: structure of the local government, level of voter registration and participation, identification of the decision-making process. A review of the community's annual report and reading the local newspaper will provide information about issues considered important to the community. Attending and participating in community meetings over time will help the FCN and health ministry team members identify local opinion leaders and key political decision makers.

Physical Environment

The physical environment subsystem encompasses location and boundaries of the community, topography, climate, housing, sanitation, air and water quality, sewage, solid waste, and vector control. Key data regarding topography and climate include: risk for flooding and earthquake and the need for shelter services. Key data related to housing include: average value of real estate, percentage of vacant homes, percentage of homes with lead-based paint, numbers of single- and multi-dwelling homes, the number of owners and renters, and the population density. Analysis of these data should include the strengths and weaknesses of the topography, climate-related risks, and adequacy of housing.

Data and quality standards related to air and water quality and hazardous waste monitoring can be retrieved from the U.S. Environmental Protection Agency (EPA). Data related to wastewater and solid waste disposal are available from the U.S. Census and from local health departments. Key elements in this area would be that the community has met or surpassed acceptable quality standards.

Safety and Protective Services

The safety subsystem includes fire and police protection, and emergency and disaster services. The key element in this subsystem is that the community services are adequate to meet the community safety needs. Other sensitive data for this subsystem are the overall crime rate in the community (in large communities, a breakdown of neighborhood crime activity) and whether or not the protective services provide any community education programming.

Spiritual Resources

The spiritual subsystem describes the resources for spiritual and religious worship and activities in the community. Key elements in assessing this subsystem include the number and diversity of places of worship and spiritual activity, existence of other health ministries, and whether any types of religious coalitions or collaborations exist in the community.

Recreation

This subsystem addresses the recreational resources in the community for individuals across the life span. It includes park and playgrounds, theaters, athletics facilities, swimming pools and lakes, galleries, libraries, restaurants, and museums. Local universities may also provide the community with recreational and cultural events.

Key elements in this subsystem include whether or not recreational opportunities exist in the community, whether activities are public or private, and whether they are free of charge or at a cost to the participant.

Data Analysis

Although community data collection is always an ongoing process, the data need to be analyzed to have meaning and context for the target community. As the data are reviewed for each subsystem, the health ministry team will identify strengths or assets as well as areas of weakness or concern and list them in writing at the end of the section. Then consider the community as a whole in terms of its assets and areas of need or concern. Assets should be listed and areas of concern should be expressed in a community diagnosis statement. For the purposes of community planning and/or grant writing, the next step in the process of community assessment is priority setting. An important consideration is that priorities be *community* priorities. Community priorities may not necessarily be the same as those of the FCN or the clergy.

For the FCN and the health ministry team, the purpose of the assessment is to gain a broad understanding of the community from a "bottom-up" perspective. One outcome of this process that the FCN will learn is whether the faith community is representative of the larger community and/or how it differs from the larger community. However, the most important outcome is that the assessment provides the base of information upon which a health ministry program can be developed.

Summary

This chapter has provided the FCN with methods to assess both the faith community and the geopolitical community in which the faith community resides. Where resources permit, including the health ministry committee/cabinet or an ad hoc task force in the process of data collection and analysis is positive. It helps a larger constituency of the membership own the assessment process and understand how the base from a health ministry program will be shaped.

Collection and analysis of data from multiple sources provide the FCN and the health ministry team with an understanding of the structure and functions of both the faith and the geopolitical communities. The prioritization of faith community diagnoses is potentially a political process. Considering the priorities that emerge from the community data and putting aside personal opinions of what one thinks should be priorities is very important. Health team ministry and congregational participation in the assessment process reinforce the faith community as a "health place." It also reinforces importance of the ministry of health and serves a platform for program planning and implementation.

Reflect and Discuss

1. Discuss how the FCN gains entry to a faith community and fosters a community-as-partner climate?
2. What advantages or disadvantages involve faith community members in the assessment process?
3. What commonalities do faith communities and geopolitical communities have?
4. Identify the community commonalities that would be considered assets.
5. How might knowledge of community assets support health in the wider community?

Case Study

Marcy Scott is a new faith community nurse at Trinity Church, a 500-member suburban Christian church. Marcy was particularly interested in determining what this community does to maintain its health and what areas of interest the congregation has for health programming. To gather data about these two areas, she used questions 5 and 6 of the Congregational Assessment—Long Form (Box 5-2) to gather data from the faith community. She distributed and collected the questionnaires at two worship services. This method yielded 198 completed questionnaires.

Data Analysis
The responses to question 5 were varied, but themes did emerge from the data. Respondents indicated that they maintain their health by:
- Seeing their physician (89)
- Eating well (64)
- Following a prescribed medication regime (59)
- Taking vitamins (53)
- Praying (36)

Many other respondents wrote down what they believed they should be doing to maintain their health—but were not doing. These responses included:
- I don't exercise enough. (90)
- I should lose weight. (78)
- I should eat better. (71)
- I should quit smoking. (32)

Marcy reviews this data and draws the following conclusions:

1. The majority of the respondents indicate that they seek medical care and follow their prescribed treatment regimes.
2. A third of the respondents correlate their spiritual life with health maintenance.
3. The respondents have preconceived ideas about what they should be doing in terms of exercise, weight control, and smoking cessation, but have indicated that they have motivational issues about following through on these activities.
4. There is conflict between "eating well" and "should eat better" because some respondents made both statements.

As Marcy analyzes the data from question 6, she notes high degrees of interest in health promotion topics about exercise (134), parenting (65), weight control (126), stress reduction (99), conflict resolution (78), and adolescent health issues (58). Marcy also notes that weight control and exercise are areas that appear in the responses to both questions. This information could be used as the starting point for her program planning, or she can attempt to collect additional data. Because the rate of return for her survey is below 60% of the congregation, the data may not be as representative of the whole congregation as one would like. She may choose to supplement this survey with a mailed survey.

BOX 5-2
Congregational Assessment—Long Form

KEY TERMS

Health—physical, emotional, spiritual, and relational well-being of a person or institution.
Health Care—all of the ways we promote and develop good health.
Medical Care—ways we treat illness.
Using this broader view of health, please answer the following questions. Signing your name is optional, but *please return the completed survey to the Health Ministry mailbox.*

1. What health and medical problems do you have, or do you know of in your family, congregation, and community? Check all that apply.

Individual/Family

___Can't afford medical care	___Problems in relationships with others
___Problems with stress	___Barriers to raising healthy children
___Persons ill at home	___Need for spiritual renewal and focus
___Substance abuse problems	___Chronic illness or disability
___Problems with sexuality	___Primary caregiver for another person
___Under/uninsured persons	___Need for personal counseling
___Poor health habits	___Need for personal counseling
___Loneliness, isolation	___Financial, legal, housing, job problems
___Grief and/or loss	___End-of-life issues
___Physical/emotional abuse or neglect	___Other_____

Congregation

___Need to be more inclusive	___Leadership/decision-making circle small
___Problems in resolving conflicts	___Humor/laughter occurs infrequently
___Lack of vision or purpose	___Resistance to exploring possible change
___Need for support groups	___Intolerance of spiritual questioning
___Clergy and staff overworked	___No regular process for evaluation of staff
___Need for confession and healing	___Lack of outreach ministries
___Other_____	

Community

___Poverty	___Lack of medical services
___Inadequate sanitation	___High infant mortality rate
___Too few doctors/hospitals	___Substandard housing/homelessness
___Hard to get to medical services	___Environmental health risks
___Inadequate health education	___Racism, sexism, ageism
___Inadequate social services	___Other_____

(continued)

BOX 5-2
Congregational Assessment—Long Form *(continued)*

2. In your congregation's meetings, classes, worship, and sermons—about how often do you hear or talk about each of the following from a faith perspective? Please rate as (1) Almost never, (2) Seldom, (3) Often, or (4) Very often.

___Physical health   ___Social/relational health
___Medical care issues   ___Emotional health issues
___Spiritual health

3. How much interest do you and your congregation have in learning more and taking some active steps to improve health at each of these levels? Please rate (1) Little interest, (2) Some interest, or (3) High interest.

	Myself	Congregation
Individual health issues	___	___
Family health issues	___	___
Congregational health	___	___
Health in our community	___	___
Health in our state	___	___

4. How much interest is there in learning more about and taking active steps to improve medical care at the same levels? Please rate each as (1) Little interest, (2) Some interest, or (3) High interest.

	Myself	Congregation
Individual health issues	___	___
Family health issues	___	___
Congregational health	___	___
Health in our community	___	___
Health in our state	___	___

5. What do you do to keep yourself as healthy as possible?

_____

_____

_____

6. Specific health-related activities in which you have a high interest/low interest:

	HIGH INTEREST	LOW INTEREST
Observe Health Awareness Week	___	___
Observe an annual Health Care Sabbath	___	___
Health fair	___	___
Exercise program	___	___
Weight control program	___	___
Smoking cessation program	___	___
Illness/disability support groups	___	___
Alcohol substance abuse support groups	___	___
Optional healthy snacks at meetings	___	___
Congregational care teams	___	___
Faith Community Nurse Program	___	___
Health Ministry	___	___

BOX 5-2
Congregational Assessment—Long Form *(continued)*

	HIGH INTEREST	LOW INTEREST
Study groups on health issues	—	—
Services of prayer and healing	—	—
Parenting skills classes	—	—
Health issues for children	—	—
Health issues of adolescents	—	—
Visit people who are ill at home	—	—
Medical or dental clinic	—	—
Spiritual renewal programs	—	—
Support for persons with mental illness	—	—
Advocacy for better local medical services	—	—
Transportation help to medical services	—	—
Stress management classes	—	—
Conflict management skills classes	—	—
Illness screening: blood pressure/diabetes	—	—
Education for youth about HIV/AIDS	—	—
Adult/child day care	—	—
Ministry to persons affected by HIV/AIDS	—	—
Food pantry	—	—
Library of books/videos on health issues	—	—
Hospice services	—	—
Advance directives/ Living wills	—	—
Advocacy for state health issues	—	—
Annual clergy/staff evaluation	—	—

7. List any resources you know of in your congregation or community that might help develop and carry out any of the above activities.

_____

_____

_____

8. Do you need additional information concerning specific health/medical topics or issues? Please list below. If you would like special assistance for yourself, a family member, or your congregation, please specify.

_____

_____

_____

9. Please indicate your preferred day and time for health programming:
   ____After worship services   ____Evenings   ____Day of the week

_____

Print your name on the above line (optional)

_____

Adapted from Health Ministries USA. (2004). *Beginning and implementing parish nursing and health ministry.* Available online at: http://www.pcusa.org/health/usa.

BOX 5-3
Congregational Health Survey—Short Form

DEAR (CONGREGANT, PARISHIONER, SISTERS AND BROTHERS)

Please assist us in planning for health screenings and health promotion programs for our faith community by answering the following questions. There is no need to sign your name—and all information provided is confidential.

Please put an *X* by your answer.

I would have an interest in attending the following types of health screening programs:

____Blood pressure (Hypertension screening)   ____Stroke prevention screening

____Blood sugar (Diabetic screening)   ____Other_____

I would be interested in learning more about:

____Adolescent health issues   ____Exercise and health

____Addictions   ____Grief and loss

____Advance directives/Living wills   ____Heart disease

____Alternative/complementary therapies   ____Hypertension

____Alzheimer's disease   ____Medication management

____Anxiety disorders   ____Menopause

____Arthritis   ____Men's health issues

____Cancer   ____Pain management

____CPR   ____Respiratory diseases

____Caring for aging parents   ____Sleep disorders

____Depression   ____Smoking cessation

____Diabetes   ____Weight control

____Eating disorders   ____Women's health issues

Which day of the week and time would you be interested in attending a program?

____Monday   ____Tuesday   ____Wednesday   ____Thursday   ____Friday

____Saturday   ____Sunday

____Morning   ____Afternoon   ____Evening

Thank You!

References

Allender, J., & Spradley, B. (2005). The community as client: Community assessment and diagnosis. In *Community health nursing: Promoting and protecting the public's health* (6th ed.). Philadelphia: Lippincott Williams & Wilkins.

American Nurses Association and Health Ministries Association. (2005). *Faith community nursing: Scope and Standards of Practice.* Silver Springs, MD: ANA.

Ammerman, A., & Parks, C. (1998). Preparing students for more effective community interventions: Assets assessment. *Family & Community Health, 21*(1), 32–45.

Anderson, E., & McFarlane, J. (2000). *Community as Partner: Theory and Practice in Nursing* (3rd ed.). Philadelphia: Lippincott Williams & Wilkins.

Anderson, H. (1990). The congregation as a healing resource. In D. S. Browning, T. Job, & I. S. Evinson (Eds.), *Religious and ethical factors in psychiatric practice* (pp. 264–287). Chicago: Nelson-Hall in association with the Park Ridge Center for the Study of Health, Faith and Ethics.

Blum, H. L. (1974). *Planning for health.* New York: Human Services Press.

Carroll, P. L. (2004). *Community health nursing: A practical guide.* Clifton Park, NY: Delmar.

Clark, M. B. (2000). Characteristics of faith communities. In M. B. Clark. & J. K. Olson (Eds.), *Nursing within a faith community: Promoting health in times of transition* (pp.17–29). Thousand Oaks, CA: Sage Publications.

Clark, M. J., Cary, S., Diemert, G., Ceballos, R., Sifuentes, M., Atteberry, I., et al. (2003). Involving communities in community assessment. *Public Health Nursing, 29*(6), 456–463.

Cottrell, L. S. (1976). The competent community. In B. Kaplan, R. Wilson, & A. Leighton (Eds.), *Further explorations in social psychiatry*. New York: Basic Books.

Dossey, B. M., Keegan, L., & Guzetta, C. E. (2005). *Holistic nursing: A handbook for practice* (4th ed.). Sudbury, MA: Jones and Bartlett.

Ervin, N. E. (2002). *Advanced community health nursing practice: Population-focused care*. Upper Saddle River, NJ: Prentice Hall.

Gottlieb, L., & Allen, M. (1997). Developing a classification system to examine a model of nursing in primary care settings. In L. Gottlieb & H. Ezer (Eds.), *A perspective on health, family, learning and collaborative nursing: A collection of writing on the McGill model of nursing* (pp. 18–31). Montreal, Quebec: McGill University School of Nursing.

Health Ministries USA. (2004). *A congregational guide to beginning and implementing parish nursing health ministry*. Available online at: http://www.pcusa.org/health/usa.

Higgs, Z. R., & Gustafson, D. D. (1985). *Community as client: Assessment and diagnosis*. Philadelphia: FA Davis.

Kretzmann, J., & McKnight, J. (1993). *Building communities from the inside out: A path toward finding and mobilizing a community's assets*. Chicago: Center for Urban Affairs and Policy Research, Northwestern University.

Levy, S. R., Anderson E. E., Issel L. M., Willis M. A., Dancy B. L., & Jacobson K. M., et al. (2004). Using multilevel, multisource needs assessment data for planning community interventions. *Health Promotion Practice, 5*(1), 59–68.

Lundy, K. S., & Barton, J. A. (2001). Community and population health: Assessment and intervention. In K. S. Lundy & S. Janes (Eds.), *Community health nursing: Caring for the public's health*. Boston: Jones and Bartlett.

Mayhugh, L. J., & Martens, K. (2001). What's a parish nurse to do? Congregational expectations. *Journal of Christian Nursing, 18*(3), 14–16.

McKnight, J. L. (1987). Regenerating community. *Social Policy, Winter*, 54–58.

McKnight, J. L., & Kretzmann, J. P. (1997). Mapping community capacity. In M. Minkler (Ed.), *Community organizing and community building for health* (pp. 157–172). New Brunswick, NJ: Rutgers University Press.

Minkler, M., & Wallerstein, N. (1997). Improving health through community organization and community building. In K. Glanz, F. Marcus Lewis, & B. K. Rimer (Eds.), *Health behavior and health education: Theory, research, and practice* (2nd ed.). San Francisco: Jossey-Bass.

Muecke, M. A. (1984). Community health diagnosis in nursing. *Public Health Nursing, 1*(1), 23.

Olson, J. K. (2000). Functions of the nurse as health promoter in a faith community. In M. B. Clark & J. K. Olson (Eds.), *Nursing within a faith community:*

Promoting health in times of transition (pp. 141–155). Thousand Oaks, CA: Sage Publications.

Polit, D. F., & Beck, C. T. (2004). *Nursing research: Principles and methods* (7th ed.). Philadelphia: Lippincott Williams & Wilkins.

Porche, D. J. (2004). *Public and community health nursing practice: A population-based approach*. Thousand Oaks, CA: Sage Publications.

Shuster, G. F., & Goeppinger, J. (2000). Community as client: Using the nursing process to promote health. In M. Stanhope & J. Lancaster (Eds.), *Community & public health nursing* (5th ed.). St Louis, MO: Mosby.

Swinney, J., Anson-Wonkka, C., Maki, E., & Corneau, J. (2001). Community assessment: A church community and the parish nurse. *Public Health Nursing, 18*(1), 40–44.

Thomas, D. J., & King, M. A. (2000). Parish nursing assessment: What should you know? *Home Healthcare Nurse Manager, 4*(5), 11–13.

Trofino, J., Hughes, C. B., O'Brien, B. L., Mack, J., Marrinan, & Hay, K. M. (2000). Primary care parish nursing: Academic, service, and parish partnership. *Nursing Administration Quarterly, 25*(1), 59–74.

U.S. Department of Health and Human Services (USDHHS). (2000). *Healthy people 2010*. Washington, DC: Author.

Wallerstein, N. (1992). Powerlessness, empowerment, and health: Implications for health promotion programs. *American Journal of Health Promotion, 6*(3), 197–205.

World Health Organization. (1978). *Primary health care: Report of the international conference on primary health care, Alma Alta, USSR, 6–12 September 1978*. Geneva, Switzerland: Author.

Additional Resources

Asbury, J. (1995). Overview of focus group research. *Qualitative Health Research, 5*(4), 414–420.

Hildebrandt, E. (1999). Focus groups and vulnerable populations: Insight into client strengths and needs. *Nursing and Health Care Perspectives, 20*(6), 256–259.

Matteson, M., Reilly, M., & Moseley, M. (2000). Needs assessment of homebound elders in a parish church: Implications for parish nursing. *Geriatric Nursing, 21*(3), 144–147.

Miskelly, S. (1995). A parish nursing model: Applying the community health nursing process in a church community. *Journal of Community Health Nursing, 12*(1), 1–14.

Nardi, D. A., & Petr, J. M. (Eds.). (2003). *Community health and wellness needs assessment: A step-by-step guide*. Clifton Park, NY: Delmar Learning.

Scott, L., & Sumner, J. (1993). How do parish nurses help people? A research perspective. *Journal of Christian Nursing, 10*(1), 16–19.

Thomas, D., & King, M. (2000). Parish nursing assessment—What should you know? *Home Healthcare Nurse Manager, 4*(5), 11–13.

→ Web Resources

http://www.apha.org   American Public Health Association

http://www.bahm.org   Bay Area Health Ministries

http://www.cdc.gov   Centers for Disease Control

http://www.hcwp.org/resourcescommhrealth/index.asp   Community Health Assessment: Tools of the Trade (State of Pennsylvania)

http://www.search-institute.org   Developmental Assets of Children

http://www.hc-sc.gc.ca/english/index.html   Health Online Canada

http://www.chp-pcs.gc.ca.CHP   Health Canada Portal

http://www.hc-sc.gc.ca/english/lifestyles/index/html   Healthy Living

http://www.healthypeople.gov   Healthy People 2010

http://www.cddc.gov/mmwr   Morbidity & Mortality Weekly

http://www.nachc.com   National Association of Community Health Centers

http://www.info@naccho.org   National Association of County & City Health Officials

http://www.statcan.gc.ca   Statistics Canada

http://www.census.gov   U.S. Census

http://www.epibiostat.ucsf.edu   WWW Virtual Library on Epidemiology

6

Diverse Faith Traditions

This chapter presents an overview, doctrines, and health-related customs of the major faith traditions present today in American culture. The reader should be aware that diversity exists *within* faith traditions, and that not all members of a given faith tradition practice their faith in the same way. Careful and sensitive assessment is necessary to understand the personal meaning(s) one has about one's faith. Congregational nurses in all settings should allow the clients the opportunity to share their beliefs, traditions, and customs rather than make assumptions. Only then can culturally competent and congruent care take place.

Ebersole (2000) reports that the roots of faith community nursing are as old as ancient civilizations. From the beginning of human records, the cleanliness of the body, the interpretation of natural phenomena, birth, death, cure, and healing have been considered to be aspects of the spiritual leader's role. In the development of scientific thought, the division between church and state, nature and nurture, body and soul, and medicine and health occurred. Ebersole says we have now come full circle as churches and temples are recognizing and reclaiming their role in integrating holy and holistic health.

According to Miskelly (1995), the faith community nurse (FCN) role is supported by religious leaders of various denominations because it integrates their vision of the religious institution as a historical facilitator of healing and health with modern-day health promotion goals. Weis, Matheus, and Schank (1997) state that the doctrines of the major world religions contain a clear relationship between their God and their physical, mental, and spiritual state. Writing in *Health and Medicine in the Jewish Tradition,* the Jewish code authored by Maimonides, the rabbi physician of the 12th century states, "One should aim to maintain physical health and vigor in order that his soul may be upright, in order to know God" (Feldman, 1986, p. 15). The Muslims view people *holistically*—as spiritual, psychological, and physical beings. The Qur'an (26:30) states, "And I sicken, Allah heals me" (Ali, Hussain, & Sakr, 1985, p. 7). In Christian Scripture, Luke states, "And he called the twelve together and gave them power and authority over all demons and to cure diseases, and he sent them out to preach the kingdom of God and to heal (9:1–2).

Complementing the religious goals for wellness and healthful living are governmental goals. In contemporary America, *Healthy People 2010* (USDHHS, 2000) is the framework that guides federal health initiatives. *Healthy People 2010* is an agenda for action for the first decade of the 21st century. The purpose of *Healthy People 2010* is described as promoting health and preventing illness, disability, and premature death. The two overarching goals of *Healthy People 2010* are to increase quality and years of healthy life and to eliminate health disparities. The goals are supported by 467 measurable objectives in 28 focus areas. The Healthy People initiatives represent a paradigm shift from an illness-driven to wellness-driven society. Americans are focusing on improving, protecting, and enhancing their health through lifestyle modification, and they are recognizing that health promotion and disease prevention will save valuable resources (Trofino, Hughes, O'Brien, Mack, Marrinan, & Hay, 2000).

Diversity and Culture

Chase-Ziolek and Holst (1999) state that although parish nursing began in mainline Protestant and Roman Catholic churches, it has grown to include increasingly diverse denominations and ethnic groups. For faith community nurses this means an increased exposure to people of different cultures and faith traditions.

Heritage consistency is a concept that was developed by Estes and Zitzow (1980) to describe the extent to which one's lifestyle reflects his or her respective tribal culture. The theory has been expanded to study the degree to which a person's lifestyle reflects his or her traditional culture. The values indicating heritage consistency exist on a continuum, and a person can possess value characteristics of both a consistent heritage (traditional) and an inconsistent heritage (acculturated). The concept of a cultural continuum allows for individual differences within cultures and negates the idea of cultural stereotypes. Heritage consistency includes a determination of one's cultural, ethnic, and religious background.

The following definitions were developed by the Office of Minority Health (2001):

- *Culture*—thoughts, communications, actions, customs, beliefs, values, and institutions of racial, ethnic, religious, or social groups. (p. 131)
- *Ethnicity*—a group of people who share a common and distinctive racial, national, religious, linguistic, or cultural heritage. (p. 131)
- *Religion*—a set of beliefs, values, and practices based on the teachings of a spiritual leader. (p. 132)

Spector (2004) reminds us that religious teachings in relation to health help present a meaningful philosophy and set of practices within a system of social controls having specific values, norms, and ethics. These are related to health in that adherence to a religious code is conducive to health and spiritual harmony (p. 12). Different cultural backgrounds create different attitudes and reactions to illness and affect how people express themselves both orally and nonverbally. Culture also guides the way an ill person is defined and treated. Illness may be viewed as a punishment for the violation of a religious code or for sinful behavior. Religion also determines the role that faith plays in the person's response to treatments and to the recovery process.

Faith communities can be culturally homogeneous or culturally diverse. An FCN in a culturally diverse faith community will need to understand the cultures of the congregation and make cultural assessments prior to providing health education (see Chapter 5 for assessment tools). An advantage of a faith community setting is the common bond of a shared belief system; however, culturally congruent communication will be essential to health education.

Leininger is a nurse theorist who focuses on transcultural nursing care. She defines *culturally competent* and *congruent care,* as "the use of culturally based care knowledge that is used in assistive, facilitative, sensitive, creative, safe and meaningful ways to individuals and groups for beneficial and satisfying health and well-being or to face death, disabilities, or difficult human life conditions" (2002, p. 128). Her definition is holistic and focuses on the complex interrelationships of lifeways, religion, kinship, politics, law, education, technology, language, environmental context, and worldview.

All of these variables need to be considered in providing culturally competent nursing care.

Judaism

Farlee (1999) states that *Judaism* is a term that includes many facets, all of which overlap. A full description of contemporary Jews must take into account the following:

- A monotheistic religious identity that draws its roots in sacred Scripture.
- A "rabbinic" tradition of ongoing interpretation.

- Adverse history of experiences of living among other, dominant cultures.
- A complex literature of lore, law, and ritual practice; a modern national identity linked to Israel and its culture.
- A diverse sense of ethnicity that allows for "secular" Jews.

Although Judaism's date of origin is not certain, significant early events include the call of Abraham (who can be credited with founding Christianity and Islam, as well as Judaism), God giving Jews the Ten Commandments and the Torah at Mt. Sinai, and covenanting them as his chosen people. The Torah refers explicitly to the five books of Moses, called the Pentateuch. In a broader sense, the written Torah refers to the Old Testament as well as to authoritative rabbinic teachings over centuries, which have been codified in the Talmud and other codes of Jewish law. Scripture provides 613 Mitzvoth, or commandments, that are continually interpreted by rabbinic authority in every age. Although Scripture provides the original commandment, rabbinic interpretation defines specific behaviors.

Judaism has various cultural and ethnic differences. *Ashkenazic* Jews come from Central and Eastern Europe and constitute the majority, whereas *Sephardic* Jews are Western Europeans, Spanish, North African, and native-born Israelis. Each of these groups has many separate and specific dialects, rituals, and liturgical identities.

Doctrines of Judaism

The way of the covenant became known as *Torah*, which may be translated as Law, Path, Way, and Revelation. Torah is law in the sense of basic principle, the basic order of reality. God made a covenant with the children of Abraham because he sought to bring people back to the basic order of things. The Torah became those principles by means of which the covenant between God and humanity is restored and maintained. The Hebrew religious way is a rich tradition of ethical and ritual principles that are necessary to the way of the covenant. The Jewish way is a continuing tradition, with rabbinic commentary and interpretation of the Torah in relation to the changing times (Wentz, 2003).

Common to all observant Jews is the high reverence for the Torah, the celebration of the major religious festivals, and the importance of, and respect for the weekly *Shabbat* (Sabbath)—from sundown on Friday to sundown on Saturday. Dietary laws, strict adherence to rabbinic tradition and law are binding to certain branches of Judaism. The fall cycle of holy days begins with *Rosh Hashanah* (New Year), continues with the Ten Days of Repentance, and ends with *Yom Kippur* (Day of Atonement). These are called the High Holy Days. *Hanukkah,* the Feast of Lights, commemorates an ancient military victory. It occurs in December. *Pesach,* or Passover, is observed with a Seder meal and retelling of the story of Exodus. During the 8-day festival, Jews do not eat any leavened products and consume specially blessed Passover foods. Two observances that link Jews to their modern history are *Yom Hashaoh*—the Holocaust Memorial Day, and *Yom Haatzmaut*—Israeli Independence Day. Both emphasize the importance of the ethnic link that most Jews have with these events.

Branches of Judaism

ORTHODOX JUDAISM

To be orthodox about anything is to be concerned for the most complete manifestation of it. Orthodox is assumed to be *right* (ortho) *thinking* (doxos). However, the "thinking" is an orthodoxy of a mind that seeks to show something for what it truly is, to "give glory." The "rightness" of the thinking has to do with its fullness, not its narrowness (Wentz, 2003). Orthodox Judaism is distinguished by a literal belief in the Torah as the ultimate word of God and in the Talmud.

CONSERVATIVE JUDAISM

Conservative Judaism is a scholarly movement that retains the use of the Hebrew language in both worship and life. Conservative Jews are bound by the laws of the Torah and Talmud, but they interpret the laws in the context of current times. Conservative Judaism has been ordaining female rabbis since 1986 (Grundmann & Truemper, 2004c).

RECONSTRUCTIONIST JUDAISM

Reconstructionist Judaism is the movement developed in reaction to the earlier conservative movement. To the Reconstructionists, the Torah and the Talmud are important but not just as religious documents. They are important as sources for determining Jewish culture and tradition.

   This branch of Judaism believes that Jews should reconstruct their lives in a new cultural covenant on the foundation of their existence as a historical people, for which the existence of the state of Israel is of vital importance. Reconstructionist Jews nurture a sense of belonging to an old and well-established cultural body of global dimensions, while practicing a fairly liberal religious attitude toward modern changes (Grundmann & Truemper, 2004c).

REFORM JUDAISM

The largest, one branch of Judaism is Reform Judaism. It began in the early 19th century. The binding force of Jewish ritual law was declared void, and the use of the Hebrew language was restricted to certain liturgical prayers. The reform movement declared that Jews should not expect to return to Palestine, and the liturgy was changed accordingly. The Torah and Talmud are sources to be consulted, but they are not understood as the final and authoritative word of God. Jews of the Reform movement are the most liberal and modern (Grundmann & Truemper, 2004c).

Health and Judaism

The Jewish belief that the body is created by God and given on loan for lifetime stewardship provides a strong base for health promotion and disease activities in the synagogue. Cleanliness and purity are valued for hygienic reasons and as a religious duty to honor God's creation (Grundmann & Truemper, 2004c).

   Congregational nurses need to be familiar with Jewish dietary laws. Orthodox and Conservative Jews will keep a kosher home, meaning that all food served will be prepared according to the Jewish religious code. Meat and dairy products are prepared and served separately, using designated cooking vessels and serving dishes. Shellfish and all pork products are banned.

   Although all branches of Judaism revere the Sabbath, Orthodox and Conservative Jews will be more restrictive of activities during the Sabbath. Businesses will be closed on Saturdays, and automobiles and use of telephones may be avoided.

   Orthodox and Conservative Jews name their sons on the eighth day after delivery, when the ritual circumcision is performed by a *mohel* (a person qualified to circumcise). A female receives her name on either the eighth day of life or on the next Sabbath following her birth, during a reading of the Torah. Until the naming ceremonies occur, the baby is referred to as a son or a daughter.

   Visiting the sick is regarded as an important religious duty and as a factor contributing to healing and comfort. Large congregations often have Visiting Societies who organize visits to congregants. The congregational nurse will work closely with the Visiting Society and will refer congregants to them as needed.

Jews believe that dying persons should be surrounded by their people, and a dead body is never left alone. The bodies of deceased Orthodox Jews are washed and prepared by members of the congregation's Burial Society, and burial is immediate. When a death occurs on the Sabbath, these activities will be postponed until the following day.

The Shleimut Institute is a fairly new, national initiative dedicated to training and supporting community-based care teams who work to promote health in the Jewish community. Shleimut provides continuing education programs to health and social service professionals, rabbis, and lay people through affiliates around the nation. Shleimut is funded by a network of Jewish academic and social services institutions. *Shleimut* is a Hebrew word meaning wholeness and completeness. The goal of the Institute is to create a health care model that incorporates Jewish traditions of health, healing, and community. "Shleimut professionals provide holistic, accessible, practical responses that weave together the awesome, everyday powers of community, prayer, service, study, caring, relationship and presence" (Shleimut Institute, 2004). The Institute provides courses and workshops in health and healing in the Jewish tradition that incorporate practical skills in health ministry and program development. Schweitzer (2004) reports that the International Parish Nurse Resource Center (IP-NRC) lent support to Shleimut's development by sharing their parish nurse curriculum. Shleimut now offers its own course in congregational nursing. The Shleimut Institute Web site (www.shleimut.org) provides a resource center with links to related sites. This institute will be a valuable resource for Jewish nurses working with their congregations.

Another resource for the Jewish congregational nurse is the Reform Jewish Nurses Network. This organization was created under the auspices of the Union of American Hebrew Congregations (UAHC), Department of Family Concerns. It publishes a quarterly newsletter and maintains a Web site (www.uahc.org/jfc/rjnn.shtml). This organization meets biennially in cooperation with the Biennial UAHC meetings.

Christianity

Christianity dates its origin to the life and ministry of Jesus of Nazareth, who after his resurrection, was acknowledged as the Christ (John 1:41). Christ's resurrection from the dead is interpreted as the promise of eternal life for all who believe (John 11:25; Romans 6–9). By the time the Bible was finalized in the 4th century, Christianity had become the official religion of the Roman Empire. From this time forward the church was regarded as "catholic" (universal) (Grundmann & Truemper, 2004a).

The Roman Catholic Church and the Eastern Orthodox Church

In 1054 C.E. the Latin church and the Eastern church broke apart by formally and mutually excommunicating each other. Following this break, the churches developed independently. The Roman Catholic Church became the dominant church of the West, whereas Orthodoxy became the dominant church of the East. The Roman Catholic Church developed the papacy as its central leadership. Orthodox churches affiliated with the national leadership, which brought about the Russian, Greek, Serbian, and Ethiopian Orthodox Churches, respectively.

The Lutheran Church

In 1517, Martin Luther, an Augustinian monk, hung his *95 Theses* on indulgences on the door of the Castle Church in Wittenberg, Germany, beginning the Reformation. Luther's Augsburg Confession of 1530 provided a clear account of the differences in core matters of faith, doctrine, and practice between the beliefs of Roman Catholics and Lutherans. One of Luther's key doctrinal issues was justification by faith, that salvation is based on one's faith in God not on one's good works. This Confession, along with the subsequent religious and political conflicts that followed, set the stage for emergence of the Lutheran Church and other Protestant denominations in other countries in Western Europe.

Other Protestant Traditions

The reformed tradition emerged in Switzerland in 1536 and was led by John Calvin and Hulreich Zwingli. They expressed their views in the *Confessio Helvetica* (Swiss Confession). The Calvinists, as those of the Reformed tradition were called, evolved into Congregationalists and Presbyterians in England, Ireland, and Scotland.

In 1563, King Henry VIII of England replaced the Pope as the head of the Church of England or Anglican Church (Episcopal Church in America). In the 17th century, the Puritans challenged the Church of England, and many immigrated to America for religious freedom.

In the Netherlands, Mennonites, descendants of Anabaptists, were followers of a Dutch priest named Menno Simons. He opposed any authority in the church other than God. The Hutterian Brethren and the Amish church were founded later, but they belong to this faith tradition as well.

UNITARIAN UNIVERSALISTS

The Unitarian denomination originated in Europe in the 16th century. This group believes that there is not a biblical basis for the doctrine of the Trinity. Persecution followed the Unitarians, and in some areas of Europe this group was suppressed. In America, Unitarians evolved from the Calvinist churches of New England, and the Unitarian Society was established in Boston in 1825. At the same time, in three different geographical areas, Universalism emerged based on the doctrine of God's loving redemption of all. Universalism was more evangelical than Unitarianism, and this faith tradition spread across North America and Canada. Both groups became active participants in social justice movements in the 19th and 20th centuries. Dorothea Dix and Clara Barton are representative of these groups. To have a stronger liberal religious voice, these two groups merged in 1961 to form the Unitarian Universalist Association (Harris, 2004).

QUAKERS

The Society of Friends, or Quakers, began as an offshoot of the Puritans, and they did away with all church governing structures, liturgy, and ministers to provide for the working of the Holy Spirit in their members. Quakers gather to worship in meeting houses, where they sit in silence until the Holy Spirit moves a member to speak. Quakers are known for their social and pacifist concerns.

THE METHODIST TRADITION

In 18th-century England, John Wesley and his brother Charles adopted a new method of ministry in which they went out to people where they lived and worked, preaching the Gospel to them in the open air. Although first conceived as an arm of the Church of England, Methodism formally broke away in 1795. Active missionary work brought Methodism to America in the late 18th century, and by the middle of the 19th century Methodism was the nation's largest denomination. By the end of the 19th century, the Holiness Movement separated from the Methodists, and parts of this movement, together with some independent Pentecostal congregations, formed the Church of the Nazarene (Grundmann & Truemper, 2004a).

Church of Latter-day Saints

The origin of the Church of Latter-day Saints dates to 1830, the year Joseph Smith published *The Book of Mormon* in upstate New York. In this book, Smith relates the history of the people of God to the people of America, both indigenous and colonist. The book is based on information Smith received on gold plates that an angel directed him to find. This religious group moved westward to find a place of undisturbed living, with the largest group settling in Utah in 1847, under the leadership of Brigham Young. Mormons today belong to one of five different denominations, the largest of which is the Church of Latter-day Saints, with a membership of 4.5 million. They regard *The Book of Mormon* as a sequel to the Bible and the authority of church leadership as divinely inspired. Mormons practice celestial marriages—marriages sealed for eternity—and baptism of the dead; and all males are expected to do missionary work. Mormons focus on healthy lifestyles and avoid alcohol, tobacco, and stimulants (Grundmann & Truemper, 2004a).

Jehovah's Witnesses

After the Civil War, Charles Taze Russell, a former Presbyterian haberdasher of Pittsburgh, became convinced that the Bible reveals God's plan for the end of the world.

"Pastor Russell" predicted the end of the world to occur in 1914, after which Christ would rule God's kingdom on Earth. Preaching of Christ's millennial reign became Russell's vocation, as it is for all of the more than 6 million Jehovah's Witnesses today. Every Witness does fieldwork by personally telling others about God's kingdom as perceived by the church's teaching and by distributing its official magazines, *Watchtower* and *Awake!* Witnesses do not form churches or build churches but Kingdom Halls. No ordained ministry or hierarchy exists in this denomination. Elders and servants lead the teaching of the congregations without pay. Witnesses renounce the Trinity but do practice baptism by immersion. Witnesses refuse to salute the flag, vote, or join the military. They refuse blood transfusions and do not donate blood (Grundmann & Truemper, 2004a).

Christian Scientists

Christian Scientists are members of the Church of Christ Scientist, which was founded in Boston in 1879 by Mary Baker Eddy. Her book, *Science and Health with a Key to the Scriptures,* is revered as the authoritative interpretation of the Bible and is considered Holy Scripture by Christian Scientists. Christian Science "practitioners" are members who engage in mental healing and are used by members who are ill. Christian Scientists avoid alcohol, tobacco, drugs of all forms, and they refuse immunizations (Grundmann & Truemper, 2004a).

Other Traditions

Pentecostalism, a revivalist relative of the Holiness Movement, emerged early in the 20th century. Its name refers to the first Pentecost where the church was given the gifts of the Holy Spirit. According to Pentecostals, all Christians should seek the gifts of the Holy Spirit, which manifest as speaking in tongues, healing, and prophesying.

Another branch of Christianity that has gained much influence and prominence are the *evangelicals* or *fundamentalists*. These groups believe in the infallibility of the Bible. They accept neither biblical interpretations nor biblical critique.

Adventists represent a cluster of several groups, among which the Seventh-day Adventists and the Worldwide Church of God are prominent today. Like Jews, they observe a Saturday (seventh day) Sabbath and day of worship, regarded as speeding the "advent" or second coming of Christ. Adventists believe that the faithful should be prepared for final judgment in body, mind, and spirit. They advocate a healthy lifestyle, avoid alcohol, tobacco, coffee, and tea. They encourage exercise. Some are strict vegetarians, whereas others restrict only pork. Adventists generally comply with medical treatment and do not approve of faith healing (Grundmann & Truemper, 2004b). Box 6-1 details membership information about the Christian denominations in America.

Although Christianity is the largest religion in the world, with more than 2 billion adherents (Barrett & Johnson, 2002), Grundmann and Truemper (2004) comment that Christianity consists of highly diverse groups of denominations suffering from extreme individualism. Yet despite this individualism, which can also be considered divisiveness, the Ecumenical Movement of the 20th century represents a conscious effort toward unity. The establishment of the World Council of Churches in 1948 in the Netherlands represents an organized ecumenical effort.

Doctrines of Christianity

Most Christians believe in three dimensions of God, or a Trinity known traditionally as the Father, Son (Jesus), and Holy Spirit. Jesus is considered to have been simultaneously divine and human in nature during his life on Earth. Christians believe in the virgin birth of Jesus and that those who have faith in Jesus, his death and resurrection, will be saved and reconciled with God, the Father, in heaven.

Christians regard the Bible, both the Old and New Testaments as sacred, inspired Scripture. In its Protestant branches, Christianity shows a higher concern for scriptural in-

---

BOX 6-1
Christian Denominations in the United States

RELIGION	MEMBERSHIP
African Methodist Episcopal	4,581,000
Baptist (All branches)	28,241,000
Churches of Christ (including Disciples of Christ and United Church of Christ)	10,269,000
Eastern Orthodox (All)	3,297,000
Episcopal	2,311,000
Jehovah's Witnesses	998,000
Latter-day Saints (All)	5,209,000
Lutheran (All)	8,452,000
Mennonite, Church of the Brethren, and Amish	419,000
Methodist	8,464,000
Pentecostals and Holiness (including Assemblies of God, Free Methodist, Church of the Nazarene, Salvation Army)	
Presbyterian and Reformed	5,488,000
Roman Catholic	63,683,000
Seventh-day Adventist	881,000
Unitarian Universalist	220,000

U. S. Census Bureau. (2002). *Statistical abstract of the United States 2002* (p. 55).

terpretation and theological debate than do other religions. The community of believers—the church and communal worship—are important elements of Christianity.

Although the Roman Catholic Church recognizes more than two sacraments, most Protestant churches recognize the sacraments of baptism and Holy Communion. Depending upon the denomination, infants or adults are baptized by applying blessed water to the head or by immersion in water. Holy Communion is offered at every Roman Catholic Mass and at certain Protestant worship services. In Protestant churches, Holy Communion, or the Eucharist, is the ingestion of bread and wine as symbols of the body and blood of Christ. In Roman Catholic churches, Holy Communion is believed to be the body and blood of Christ. Box 6-2 provides denominational traditions.

Health in the Christian Church

Jesus of Nazareth was renowned for his miraculous healing and charged his disciples to care for the sick unconditionally. The parables of the Good Samaritan (Luke 10:25–36) illustrate this charge. According to Christians, caring for the sick is a divine calling that glorifies God. This calling is a hallmark of Christianity and has been the doctrinal basis for religious denominations to establish hospitals.

Christians, like Jews, believe that they are beings created by God and therefore accountable to God for the stewardship of their bodies. This belief provides a strong base upon which to build health promotion and disease prevention efforts in faith communities.

Because Christian denominations are so diverse, parish nurses need to be very familiar with the traditions, rituals, symbols, ceremonies, and practices of the faith community or communities served. Box 6-2 provides information about the traditions of selected denominations.

African American Christians

Historical Perspective

Understanding the importance of Christianity and the faith community for African Americans is best related historically. "African American religion developed within the larger context of American capitalism. It emerged initially under slavery and mercantile capitalism during the antebellum period" (Baer & Singer, 2002, p. ix). Within slave communities spanning the South, men and women covertly met for prayer and worship. Gathering together for religious services served as an excellent vehicle for communication. It did not matter whether the services were *white approved* or secretive. They served the same purposes. They allowed slaves an opportunity to socialize, encouraged fellowship, provided support for each other during such difficult times, and built a strong sense of community. As time passed, African Americans developed a distinctive "form of Christianity that stressed a belief in spiritual equality as well as freedom and happiness in the hereafter . . . and discarded those parts of Anglo Christianity that portrayed them as inferior" (http://www.bchm.org/wrr/recon/p17.html). Following the Civil War, 1861 to 1865, African American religions started to take shape, "in the form of a wide array of independent-organized sects and denominations" (Baer & Singer, 2002, p. ix). These faith communities offered purpose and strength to the African American community and were "second only to the family in building a solid foundation from which they fought for political, economic and social justice" (http://www.bchm.org/wrr/recon/p17.html). Important to note is that "The content, structure, and variability of black religion derive primarily from three sources: (1) African cultures; (2) religious patterns in Euro-American culture; and (3) religious responses on the part of Blacks to their minority status in American society" (Baer & Singer, 1981, p. 7).

BOX 6-2
Christian Denominational Traditions

DENOMINATION	TRADITION
Baptist	Believers baptism by immersion Holy Communion No alcohol or tobacco Strict church discipline and lifestyle regimen
Christian Science	No blood products are used Oppose abortion Abstain from caffeine, alcohol, and tobacco Use healing ministers
Church of Latter-day Saints	Oppose birth control and abortion Abstain from alcohol, caffeine, and tobacco Anointing of the sick, healing, praying Baptize older children by immersion
Episcopal	Infant baptism Holy Communion Ministrations and prayers for the sick
Jehovah's Witnesses	Baptism in lakes and streams Abortion and artificial insemination forbidden Blood products forbidden Abstain from alcohol, moderate use of alcohol Faith healing and organ donation forbidden Missionary zeal Refuse to vote, serve in the military, salute the flag Do not celebrate Christmas or Easter Meet in "Kingdom Halls," not churches
Lutheran	Infant baptism Holy Communion Anointing of the sick Ask regarding organ donation
Mennonites	Folk medicine called powwowing Anointing the sick Dedicate infants—baptize young adults Wear a traditional head covering Oppose abortion
Methodists	Infant baptism Holy Communion Receptive to organ donation Anointing the sick
Nazarene	Alcohol/tobacco forbidden May baptize infants if ill Believers baptism
Orthodox	Infant baptism by 40th day of life by immersion Holy Communion Anointing the sick and Last Rites May refuse autopsy, organ donation, abortion, and cremation

BOX 6-2
Christian Denominational Traditions *(continued)*

DENOMINATION	TRADITION
Pentecostal	Faith healing Prayer and anointing Prohibit alcohol and tobacco Believers baptism
Presbyterian/Reformed	Open to medical advancements Prayer and laying on of hands Infant baptism
Quaker	No sacraments/no clergy
Roman Catholic	Early infant baptism Anointing of the sick Holy Communion Meatless Fridays during Lent Use of religious artifacts, such as crosses and rosary beads Birth control, abortion, artificial insemination unacceptable
Seventh-day Adventist	Saturday Sabbath Dietary restrictions—some are vegetarian, all avoid pork, caffeine, alcohol, and tobacco Do not approve of faith healing Oppose hypnotism
Unitarian Universalist	Infant baptism Oppose faith healing

AFRICAN AMERICAN CHURCHES

Most African American Christians are affiliated with the Baptist and Methodist denominations. Reflecting their history, African American Baptist and Methodist churches maintain doctrines similar to other Baptist and Methodist bodies. They are Trinitarian, looking to God as the creator, Jesus Christ as the son of God and redeemer of humanity, and the Holy Spirit as the sanctifier. They teach the sinfulness of humans and their need for repentance as well as God's grace for salvation (Farlee, 1999). However, many other denominations are represented in the African American community. These include African Methodist Episcopal, Jehovah's Witnesses, Church of God in Christ, Seventh-Day Adventists, Pentecostal, Apostolic, Presbyterian, Lutheran, and Roman Catholic (Glanville, 2003). The church is an important social structure in the African American community, and prayer is the means to communicate with God in all situations.

African American churches have a tradition of providing nursing services (including spiritual care) to members during worship services. Nurses, dressed in their white uniforms, would provide services as needed, often in a health room.

African American faith communities today continue to play an important role both culturally and socially; but introducing new ministries, such as parish nurse programs, need extensive planning to be successful. The pros far outweigh the cons, however, and it is no wonder then that African American faith communities are a natural site for parish nurse programs. Although African American churches represent an array of different denominations, they share tradition and cultural roots that offer a wonderful base for a parish nurse program to be built upon.

HEALTH ISSUES IN AFRICAN AMERICAN CHURCHES

African American churches are no different from other faith communities in determining a fit for parish nursing. Unique to the situation is the impact that race and ethnicity have on health. One only needs to look to the *National Center for Health Statistics* in Box 6-3 to identify the top 10 leading causes of death for African Americans in the United States. This information is a starting point for planning parish nurse ministry programming. Additional indicators include, but are not limited to, the six priority areas identified by the Racial and

---

BOX 6-3
Leading Causes of Death For African Americans 2001

ALL CAUSES	**287,709**
Diseases of the heart	77,674
Malignant neoplasms	62,170
Cerebrovascular diseases	19,002
Unintended injuries	12,462
Diabetes mellitus	12,305
Homicide	8,226
Human immunodeficiency virus (HIV)	7,844
Chronic lower respiratory disease	7,589
Nephritis, nephritic syndrome, and nephrosis	7,274
Septicemia	5,880
MEN	
All causes	145,908
Diseases of the heart	37,016
Malignant neoplasms	32,679
Unintentional injuries	8,537
Cerebrovascular diseases	7,907
Homicide	6,780
HIV	5,328
Diabetes mellitus	5,049
Chronic lower respiratory diseases	4,187
Nephritis, nephritic syndrome, and nephrosis	3,186
Influenza and pneumonia	2,813
WOMEN	
All causes	141,801
Diseases of the heart	40,658
Cerebrovascular diseases	11,095
Diabetes mellitus	7,256
Nephritis, nephrotic syndrome, and nephrosis	4,088
Unintentional injuries	3,925
Chronic lower respiratory disease	3,402
Septicemia	3,245
Influenza and pneumonia	2,958
HIV	2,516

Adapted from Anderson, R. N., & Smith, B. I. (2003). Deaths: Leading causes for 2001. *National Vital Statistics Reports, 52*(9).

Ethnic Approaches to Community Health (REACH) 2010, which is an initiative of the National Center for Chronic Disease Prevention and Health Promotion. REACH 2010 is a *cornerstone* of the CDC's efforts to eliminate ethnic and racial disparities in health. These six areas include: infant mortality, deficits in breast and cervical cancer screening and management, cardiovascular disease, diabetes mellitus, AIDS/HIV, and child and adult immunizations (http://www.cdc.gov/nccdphp/aag/pdf/aag_reach2004.pdf).

Islam

The Islamic faith is the second largest religion in the world, with approximately 1.2 billion followers, and it is the fastest growing religion (Ohm, 2003). Although Islam originated in Arabia, it moved out of the Arabian peninsula in all directions to embrace many cultural groups. Although 28% of Muslims reside in the Middle East, other areas have large Muslim populations: sub-Saharan Africa (20%), Southeast Asia (17%), and the Indian subcontinent (25%) (Rassool, 2000). Indonesia has the largest concentration, followed by Pakistan, India, and Bangladesh. More than 1 billion Muslims live in the world, and approximately 8 million Muslims are in the United States, with at least 3 to 4 million being African Americans (Ohm, 2003; Sahkoor-Abdullah, 2002).

Islam means *peace and submission to the will of Allah.* Muslims believe in one God (Allah) and the last messenger, Muhammad. They also believe in all of the other prophets from Adam to Jesus, all of the books revealed to Muhammad, the angels, and the "last day" (Athar, 2004). Islamic teachings incorporate much of the teachings of Judaism and Christianity, with a few fundamental differences. Although all three religions believe in one divine omnipotent deity, the Islamic faith does not endorse the Trinity (Admed, 1999). Although the virgin birth of Jesus is acknowledged as a miracle, Jesus is considered to be a prophet not the Son of God; the Qur'an states, "It is not befitting to (the majesty of) God that he should beget a son" (19:35). Islam does not support the concept of original sin, and Muslims do not consider themselves to be a "chosen people." The Prophet Muhammad was explicit about the equality of all mankind (Ohm, 2003).

Wentz (2003) states that the heart of Islam is the Qur'an, a sacred text revealed to a man known as Muhammad early in the 7th century. The Qur'an was delivered to him one night by a voice from heaven as he meditated in a cave. The angel Gabriel directed Muhammad that he must "recite" and he must "cry" the power of God. "La Illa'ha Illa'lah"—*There is no god but the God (Allah)*—is the first word. The second is "Muhammadar rasulu'llah!—*Muhammad is the messenger of Allah!* Together these two elements make up what is known as the *shahada,* the first of the five pillars of Islam. The *shahada* means "witness," and the faithful Muslim will witness regularly to the truths. Five times a day, Muslims answer the call to prayer, which is heard from the minarets of mosques. The ritual prayer is said after having cleansed oneself by washing feet, hands, and face.

The elements of the practical expression of religion that hold up the Islam world are the five pillars. *Shahada,* or witness, is the first pillar. The second is *Salat,* the performance of the five daily prayers, done while facing in the direction of Mecca. At midday on Fridays, the people assemble at the mosque for these prayers and a sermon. Islam has no priesthood; Islamic scholars assume the role of *Imam,* or leader, of the prayer. The third pillar is *Zakat,* the giving of alms for those who are less fortunate. The fourth is *Siyam,* or fasting. Although fasting may be performed at any time, it is required during the ninth month of Ramadan. One fasts each day, refraining from food, drink, and sexual relations from just before sunrise to just after sunset. During this time, Muslims eat no meat of land animals and eat only an evening meal. Small children, pregnant women, and those who are ill are exempt from this practice (Spector, 2004). The fifth pillar is the *Hajj,* or pilgrimage, to Mecca that should be made by Muslims at least once in their lifetime. This pilgrimage is made from the beginning of the 10th month until the middle of the 12th month. Upon reaching Mecca, all pilgrims wear white seamless garments. All traces of rank, wealth, and other social distinctions are removed. A person who maintains the five pillars of Islam is a Muslim, knows *Allahu akbar,* that "God is the greatest," and surrenders to God. In this submission, the Muslim finds peace (Wentz, 2003).

Elements of Faith

In addition to the five pillars of faith, five elements of faith exist upon which the faith is founded. They are faith in God, in the reality of angels, in God's messengers (Adam, Abraham, Moses, and Jesus), holy books (the Qur'an and hadith, the sayings and behaviors of the Prophet), and faith in the day of resurrection and judgment, which addresses the afterlife (Smith, 1999, p. 6).

BRANCHES OF ISLAM

The verbal and practical expressions of Islam include extra-Qur'anic tradition (*hadith*) that is attributed to the Prophet Muhammad. The hadith consists of authoritative books about the sayings and actions of the Prophet Muhammad and is used for decision making and as a reference. This tradition is the *Sunna,* and the main body of Islamic following (90%) is known as *Sunni.* A minority (10%) of Muslims are known as *Shiites,* who are supporters of the spiritual leadership of the descendants of Ali, cousin and son-in-law of Muhammad. Shiites are found in Iran, Iraq, and parts of other Islamic countries as well as the United States. Shiite leadership tends to combine their teaching authority with strong political and social authority, because the will of God should be evident in all human affairs (Wentz, 2003).

Although these groups adhere to different interpretations of the Qur'an, the mystics, or *Sufis,* have added the dimension of personal piety and affectionate love for God and the prophet to Muslim life. Emerging in the late 8th century, Sufism flourished in the Middle Ages, at the end of which various orders and brotherhoods had formed that are still in existence today. The Sufis continue to have enormous influence on larger populations through their spiritual instruction, and they are responsible for large-scale missionary activities worldwide (Grundmann & Truemper, 2004b).

CENTRAL CONCEPTS OF ISLAM

The concept of *jihad*, or struggle, is an expectation of one's realization of the Islamic Path or *Shariah.* Sometimes the concept of jihad is interpreted to mean external struggles on behalf of Islam to defend it from its enemies. Another important concept of Islam is *umma,* the concept of community, the center of which is Allah. Umma is the social expression of Islam, and the individual derives his or her identity and meaning as a part of the umma. Wentz states that it is this insight that helps non-Muslims to understand why Muslims engage in external jihad to maintain and preserve the umma, which is the foundation of meaningful existence (2003).

ISLAM AND AFRICAN AMERICANS

Islam arrived in North America in the 1700s with North African slaves. It was not generally visible until the media brought Islam notoriety through coverage of the Moorish Science Temple, led by Noble Drew Ali. This was the first organized movement to introduce the Islamic faith to Black Americans. Established in 1913, the Moorish Science Temple established a connection between African Americans and their Moroccan ancestors. Loosely based on the Islamic faith, love, truth, peace, freedom, and justice were emphasized. The movement was considered to be a nationalistic response to the racism (Ohm, 2003).

The Black Muslim movement was formally organized by Elijah Muhammad, the self-proclaimed Prophet of Islam for Black Americans. He shared the news of W. D. Fard, the founder of the Nation of Islam, who was considered an incarnation of Allah. The movement gained considerable momentum after World War II, spurred by the rise of black consciousness and the emergence of Malcolm X as its most articulate representative (Grundmann & Truemper, 2004b). It was a product of Black experience in America, and it combined ideas of Black separatism and Black supremacy with certain Islamic teachings. It was a militant movement, providing a sense of worth for many Black persons, and it helped them to assume responsibility for their economic and social well-being. After his pilgrimage to Mecca in 1964, Malcolm X acknowledged the superiority of Orthodox Islam and organized the rival Muslim Mosque, Inc., which he led until his assassination in 1965. This conformity to Orthodox Islam continued when Elijah Muhammad died in 1975. His son Wallace D. Muhammad assumed leadership of the nation of Islam. W. D. Muhammad renounced the "God in Person" status of W. D. Fard and the position of Elijah Muhammad as the Prophet of God (Ohm, 2003). The Black Islam movement is now known as the World Community of Islam (Wentz, 2003) or the Muslim American Society (Sahkoor-Abdullah, 2002). Louis Farrakhan adopted the name "Nation of Islam" for a smaller group of African Americans continuing the original teachings of Elijah Muhammad, but it is Orthodox Islam that predominates in the African American community with 3 to 4 million members (Ohm, 2003).

Health and Islam

Yousif (2002) reports that contemporary Muslim approaches to medicine range from a total reliance on folk/spiritual medicine to a total reliance on modern medicine. He states, however, that the majority of Muslims fall somewhere between these two extremes, believing in prayer, supplications, and Qur'anic recitation, as well as recognizing the benefits of modern medicine. Islamic medicine has always been holistic, with attention to the spirit and the mind as well as the body. Medical personnel are expected to assist their patients to the best of their abilities and to leave the rest to Allah. The crescent is the symbol of medical and nursing care in Islamic societies (Rassool, 2000).

Diet

Cleanliness is considered "half of the faith." The Qur'an prohibits eating pork or pork products, meat of improperly slain animals, blood, and all intoxicants—all of which are considered to be unclean. Animals are slaughtered in an Islamic manner, which renders the meat to be "halal." Muslim law teaches that certain foods affect the way a person thinks and behaves, so one's diet should consist of foods that have a clean, positive effect. Beans are avoided because they are difficult to digest and considered to be animal fodder. Alcohol is avoided because it dulls the senses and causes illness (Spector, 2004).

In Muslim homes lunch is the main meal of the day. Food is eaten with the right hand because it is regarded as clean. Although traditional dishes differ from country to country, general characteristics are shared. Familiar spices and herbs, such as cinnamon, allspice, cloves, ginger, cumin, mint, parsley, bay leaves, garlic, and onions, are frequently used. Skewered cooking and slow simmering are typical modes of food preparation. All countries have rice and wheat dishes, stuffed vegetables, nut-filled pastries, and fritters soaked in syrup. Dishes are garnished with raisins and nuts. Favorite fruits and vegetables include dates, figs, apricots, mango, melon, papaya, bananas, citrus, guava, carrots, spinach, tomatoes, cucumbers, and grape leaves. Lamb and chicken are the most popular meats, and they are cooked to well-done temperatures. Bread is served at every meal, and olive oil is widely used. Foods are prepared "from scratch," so consumption of additives and preservatives is limited (Kulwicki, 2003, p. 97).

Muslims fast during the month of Ramadan. The belief is that it brings rest to the body, which has medical value.

HEALTH PRACTICES

Meditation and prayer bring psychological tranquility. Muslims accept illness and death with patience and prayers. They consider illness as atonement for their sins and death as the journey to meet Allah. Muslims are strongly encouraged to seek care for illness (Athar, 2004). Illness is considered a time of exception to the normally strict religious regulations (such as fasting), more so for women than for men. Women enjoy more lenience because of their menses, which is regarded as a time of ritual uncleanness that makes women unfit for religious observances. The lessening of religious duties means that woman do not have to comply with the usual practices of daily ritual prayer and fasting and diet (with the exception of consumption of pork). Nurses should be alert to clients who choose to omit oral medications during Ramadan.

Congregational nurses may encounter Muslim clients who believe that only God can cure them and may refuse medical treatment or be noncompliant with recommended medical treatment. This attitude is based on the verse in the Qur'an that states: "And when I am ill, it is He who cures me" (26:80). Nurses should be mindful that the Qur'an is touched only with clean hands.

Community and Customs

Farlee (1999) points out that Muslims do not consider Islam to be a religion in the sense of something separate from the rest of life, rather Islam is for them a complete system of life, encompassing all of existence. This includes the physical, mental, social, spiritual, and academic aspects. He cautions that it is important not to be confused with cultural traditions and values, because Islam is found in many cultures. To associate a cultural tradition with Islam is incorrect, but it is easy to do.

FAMILY

Islam recognizes that the foundation of society is the family. Marriage, which is ordained by Allah, dignifies society and preserves proper human relations. The Muslim family is both an extended family and a patriarchal one. When any important health issues occur within the family, the male head of the household is the final authority and is always consulted in a formal manner. Behind the scenes, however, the wife has tremendous influence regarding the home and children.

When entering a Muslim home, the absence of artwork on the eastern walls (the direction of Mecca) is noted. However, verses from the Qur'an may be displayed on this wall. Cleanliness is highly apparent; people remove shoes when entering a home, and house pets are rare (Ohm, 2003).

Muslim women are directed by the Qur'an to be modest and not to attract attention to themselves. Their dress ranges from the most conservative to modest clothing and a head covering (*hijab*). Although they prefer female health care providers, decisions cannot be made without consulting the husband, father, or brother as appropriate. Arab American women, in particular, have low rates for breast cancer screening, which may be related to modesty (Kulwicki, 2003).

American Muslim women assume professional pursuits (Ohm, 2003). Prophet Muhammad's first wife, Khadja, is held as an example for Muslim women. She was a successful businesswoman, politician, and spiritual authority (Smith, 1999).

WOMEN'S HEALTH

The various branches of Islam have different ideas about birth control and abortion. In general, high fertility rates are favored and large families are prized. A fetus having matured beyond 30 days postconception is considered to be a human being. Irreversible forms of birth control, such as tubal ligation and vasectomy, are not permitted. Abortion is usually not permitted except to save a mother's life.

Muslim births are attended by a traditional birth attendant, and the father is not usually present for the delivery. After delivery, a newborn child is bathed immediately and silently and then handed to the parents who will whisper the call to prayer to the infant, the first words the infant will hear. Muslim infants are almost universally breast-fed for a 2-year period, and amulets may be placed on the baby or in the room. Some Muslims observe a postpartum confinement period of up to 40 days. Islam prescribes male circumcision for purpose of cleanliness. The procedure is done without ceremony at a time of convenience (Kulwicki, 2003).

DEATH AND DYING

When death is imminent, the extended family and the imam (prayer leader of the mosque) are in attendance. The bed is moved so that the Muslim client is facing in the direction of Mecca, and prayers are said by all present. After a death occurs, the body is washed three times by Muslims of the same sex, preferably family members who wear gloves so as not to impart impurity on the "property of Allah." Because Muslims believe that the body belongs to God, organ donation and autopsy are unacceptable. What belongs to God should be returned to God and as soon as possible. For this reason, burial (never cremation) in a grave facing Mecca takes place within 24 hours after a death (Grundmann & Truemper, 2004b).

Resources

The Muslim American Society Health Alliance (MASHA) is a group of health practitioners committed to addressing health needs and concerns. Its members develop and coordinate programs that emphasize prevention, holistic health, and health awareness. MASHA believes that it is their divinely given responsibility to improve public health and create an environment conducive to wellness. It works cooperatively with others who are similarly committed. MASHA believes that good health is Allah's desire for mankind (Sahkoor-Abdullah, 2002). MASHA is a resource to nurses serving Muslim faith communities.

Hinduism

The religion known as Hinduism encompasses many different spiritual practices, unified by their reliance on ancient texts called the *Vedas*. The Vedas are considered to be timeless truths revealed to anonymous sages at least 4,000 years ago. The word *Veda* means "knowledge" in Sanskrit. Four Vedas exist, each with four parts, the last and most philosophical of each is the *Upanishads*.

The three main schools of Hindu philosophy are categorized according to whether God (Brahman) and humanity are understood as separate (dualism); humanity is the parts, God is the whole (qualified nondualism); or God and humanity are united (nondualism). Each school attempts to address the relationship between God and humanity (Farlee, 1999).

Use of the term *Brahman* is analogous to the Christian concept of God. According to Hindu philosophy, the goal of life is to establish a pure and eternal relationship with this ultimate reality.

The two basic ideas underlying the Vedas are Satya (truth) and Rta (eternal order). The Vedas explain the two great objects of the human life: duty, and liberation. The relationship between religion and social structure is complex. Religion provides the legitimacy and ideology for social and economic practices, whereas social structures produce particular religious beliefs, hence Hinduism is both a religion and a social system (Jambunathan, 2003).

Hindus believe in the authority of the Vedas and other sacred writings of the ancient sages, the immortality of the soul and a future life, the existence of a Supreme God, the theory of karma and rebirth, ancestor worship, the caste system, the theory of the four stages of life, and the theory of four *purusarthas,* or ends of human existence.

Caste System

The orthodox Hindu position is that society has been divinely ordained on the basis of the four castes or social categories. *Brahmanas* (priests and scholars), *Kshtriyas* (warriors), *Vaisyas,* (merchants), and *Sudras* (menials). The essential principles of the caste system are unchangeable inequality based on birth, the gradation of professions and their inequality, and restrictions on marriage outside one's own group. (Jambunathan, 2003, p. 95).

The *purusartha,* the four ends of man, underlie Hindu daily conduct. The first of these is *dharma,* which is characterized by righteousness, duty, and virtue. This virtue is considered the basis for social and moral order because it is a comprehensive doctrine of an individual's rights and responsibilities in an ideal world. *Artha,* or material gain, relates to activities a person does to gain something for himself or herself or to pursue pleasures. *Kama* is love or pleasure. *Moksa,* the fourth end, involves the renunciation of the other ends to devote oneself to religious or spiritual activities for liberation from a worldly life (Jambunathan, 2003, p. 96).

Spirituality and Worship

De (1996) describes four "kinetic ideas," which he says make up the core of Hindu spirituality: karma, maya, nirvana, and yoga. These ideas appear in the Upanishads. *Karma* is the law of universal causality, which connects man with the cosmos and condemns him to the cycle of birth-death-rebirth indefinitely, ascending or descending on the ladder of a given hierarchy, depending on the nature of one's life deeds. *Maya* refers to cosmic illusion—the mysterious process that gives rise to phenomena and maintains the cosmos. According to this idea, the world is not simply what it seems to the human senses—a view with which 20th-century scientists agree. Absolute reality is situated somewhere beyond the cosmic illusion, woven by maya and beyond human experience as conditioned by karma. *Nirvana* is the state of absolute blessedness, characterized by a release from the cycle of reincarnation; freedom from the pain and care of the world; bliss; and union with God or Atman. *Yoga* implies integration, the bringing of all faculties of the psyche under the control of the self. The word *yoga* is loosely applied to any program or technique that leads toward union with God or Atman. The five principal kinds of yoga include: Hatha (physical), Jnana (the way or path of knowledge), Bhakti (the way or path of love and devotion), karma (the way or path of action and work), and raja (mystical experience).

Hinduism recognizes that different people have different spiritual capacities because of their place in the rebirth cycle as this affects their mind/body. The *Bhagavad-Gita* (14:5–18) teaches that three universal *gunas,* or qualities, pervade all creation: *sattva* (light, spirit, clarity), *rajas* (movement, passion), and *tamas* (inertia, dullness, darkness). Because of past karma, each person is born with a specific configuration of the gunas and, therefore, with different spiritual capabilities. Varied spiritual paths are available to meet the needs of everyone. The more spiritually advanced follow the jnana yoga, with disciplines of study, meditation, and withdrawal from society. The majority of Hindus follow the karma yoga, which provides them with a means of spiritual advancement while they fulfill their roles in family and society. Performing one's actions out of duty, according to one's dharma, builds up good karma and leads to happiness in life and higher rebirth in the next life. Hindus believe that fulfilling one's proper role in life, as determined by caste and gender, is a spiritual path that brings blessings and wholeness for both the individual and the community (Ludwig, 2004b).

The third path, bhakti-yoga, the path of devotion to one's God, presents the highest path, and one open to all castes and both genders. This path permits devotion to many gods and has colorful rituals, festivals, music, and dance as a part of the tradition (Ludwig, 2004).

Approximately 1.3 million Hindus reside in North America, where worship may take different forms within the Hindu religious tradition (Andrews & Hanson, 2003). Hindus may privately carry out their worship in their homes. A household shrine containing representations of one or more deities is an aid rather than a requirement for worship. A traditional form of worship is *puja,* worship of a deity after calling for its presence and offering services or gifts. The two great gods for most Hindus are *Vishnu* and *Shiva.* Vishnu is the creator and preserver of the world. Hindus also worship Vishnu through his consort, Lakshmi, and through *Rama* and *Krishna*, Vishnu's incarnated forms or *avatara.* The other great god is Shiva, whose cosmic dance continually creates and destroys the world and who embodies male and female generative powers. Shiva is the supreme yogin who keeps the world operating through the power of his meditation. Shiva's female form (Shakti) is often worshiped as his wife. Hinduism allows for many gods—over 330 million of them, because the divine source can be seen in all living things. Most Hindus follow their family traditions and devote themselves to one of the several great gods/goddesses, together with their associated gods (Ludwig, 2004b).

Hindu temples serve as important institutions for the practice of the Hindu religion. The Hindu temple, and the invocation of God into its center, makes God present in that place, and land becomes holy. Worship may include praying, singing, hymns, reciting scripture, and repeating the names of gods. For some Hindus, worship is the merging of the inner self with the ultimate reality or *Brahman.* When Hindu people live far away from the temple, they can request blessings and make offerings by mail (Jambunathan, 2003).

Hindu Traditions

FAMILY

The most important structure for Hindus is the family. The Hindu family is a patriarchal structure, with the oldest man having the greatest authority. Men are considered to be superior over women. In India, family property is owned jointly by the men and is inheritable only to male heirs (although it is to be shared equally among male and female offspring). A submissive and acquiescent role is expected of women in the first years of married life, with little participation in decision making. Although Westernization has changed much about the status and roles of Hindu women, most remain subservient to their closest male relatives. Direct eye contact with elders and authority figures (including health care providers) is considered a sign of disrespect for women (Jambunathan, 2003).

In America, Hindu parents want their children to be successful and strongly encourage and emphasize scholastic achievement. Status indicators, such as education, income, and occupational leadership, replace ascribed social status. However, conflicts between the values of the West and those of the East continue for these families, which is especially true in regard to marriage. Although first-generation Hindus are familiar with arranged marriages, Hindus raised in the West may be unwilling to agree to this. Marriage is an important Hindu sacrament and is considered indissoluble.

Dietary Practices

Dietary practices differ according to country of origin; however, most Hindus do not eat meat because doing so involves harming a living creature. Hindus believe that foods have either hot or cold properties and therefore should only be eaten during certain seasons and not in combination. Because of the dramatic climate differences in India, many foods considered hot in the north are not considered so in the south. The hot/cold properties of foods are based on how they are thought to affect body functions. Failure to observe dietary rules will result in illness. Women generally cook and serve food but may eat separately from the men. Women are not permitted to prepare food during their menstrual periods (Jambunathan, 2003).

In a study of the dietary habits of 73 Asian Indians in relation to their length of residence in the United States, Raj, Ganganna, and Bowering (1999) found that in contrast to recent immigrants (less than 10 years), longtime immigrants reported eating mostly Indian foods for dinner and weekend meals. The authors also found that consumption of white bread, roots, tubers, vegetable oils, legumes, and tea changed little in the longtime resident group. The authors concluded that despite the small sample size, Asian Indians living in America do eat American foods, and they also continue to eat many traditional Indian foods.

Rituals

The Hindu life cycle is defined by special ritual times called *samskaras,* sacraments of passage. Birth rituals include a naming rite that occurs 10 days after birth and the first haircut at about 3 years. An important step for boys of the three upper classes is initiation into the student stage of life. The boy's head is shaved and a sacred cord is placed over the left shoulder, and he is taught the words of the Vedas. Marriage is a key family event and is celebrated over several days. The last samskara, the death ritual, involves cremation of the body while a prayer is said. The bones are gathered and placed in a river, and the final ritual of offering water and rice cakes is made (Ludwig, 2004b).

Health and Health Care Practices

Hindus in America use Western medicine or Ayurvedic medicine, or both. *Ayurveda* means "knowledge of life," and its roots are in the Vedas; it is based on the idea that everything in the world operates through the interaction of the three gunas or qualities: *Sattva* is white and bright, bringing clarity of perceptions; *rajas* is red, causing passion, emotion, sensation, and movement; and *tams* is dark, causing heaviness, inertia, and confusion. Human temperaments are classified according to the dominant guna (Ludwig, 2004b).

No restrictions are practiced for the use of medications and blood products for Hindus. All forms of birth control are acceptable, and no policy exists regarding abortion. Organ transplantation is permissible (Andrews & Hanson, 2003). Jambunathan (2003) reports that self-medication is a potential problem among Hindus. Many medications that require a prescription in the United States are sold over-the-counter in India.

The Ayurvedic System

The Ayurvedic system is based on the Tridosha theory, which states that the functioning of the body is governed by three doshas or biologic energy forces: *vata* (from space and air), *pitta* (from fire and water), and *kapha* (from earth). These three energy forces are present in every cell and differ in their combinations in each person. The Ayurvedic concept of health is a balanced state between the three doshas, seven tissues, and waste products; as well as mental temperament and functioning of the five elements in the process of nourishment. A balance between three elements or humors—phlegm or mucus, bile, and wind correspond to three different types of food required by the body: heat-producing, cold-producing, and gas-producing. The five elements include: space, air, fire, water, earth. Space, synaptic and cellular, permits the flow of information between cells. Air is *prana,* the vital life force related to all sensory stimuli and motor responses. Synaptic and cellular space in the body permits the flow of information between cells. Fire *(agni)* regulates body temperature and is responsible for digestion, absorption, and assimilation of food, and is active in each organ and each cell. Water exists in all body fluids and carries energy between cells. Earth *(kapha)* is present in all solid structures and cells. Any imbalance between these elements causes illness (Ludwig, 2004b).

Although the body is made up of five elements, the functioning of the body is governed by the three *doshas.* The doshas or biological energy forces are *vata* (from space and air), *pitta* (from fire and water), and *kapha* (from earth). Vata is the energy of movement, pitta is the energy of digestion or metabolism, and kapha is the energy that forms the body's structure. The three energy forms are present in every cell and structure of the body and differ in their combinations in each person. Ayurveda distinguishes seven basic body types: monotypes, with three qualities dominant; dual types, with two qualities combined; or equal, with the three doshas in equal proportions (Ludwig, 2004b).

Vata qualities are dry, light, cold, mobile, active, astringent, and dispersing. All of these qualities are found in persons in whom vata is dominant. People with unbalanced vata are susceptible to diseases involving air, such as emphysema, pneumonia, and arthritis, or nervous system disorders and mental confusion. Pitta qualities are hot, sharp, light, liquid, sour, oily, spreading, and having a strong smell and bitter taste. People with unbalanced pitta tend to have diseases involving the fire element, such as fevers, inflammatory diseases, jaundice, skin rashes, ulcers, colitis, and sore throats. Kapha qualities are heavy, slow, cool, oily, liquid, dense, thick, static, cloudy, sweet, and salty. People with unbalanced kapha tend to have diseases connected with water element, such as influenza, sinus congestion, diabetes, excess weight, and headaches (Ludwig, 2004b).

The Ayurvedic concept of health is the balance of the body matrix, a holistic conceptualization of health, including physical, mental, social, emotional, and spiritual well-being. Internal or external disturbances that lead to imbalances can cause toxins to build up and, if not corrected, will lead to disease. Internal and external disturbances may include lack of exercise, improper diet, use of tobacco, or emotional upset. Maintaining a healthy balance is the basis for any health promotion activities the congregational nurse might undertake.

WOMEN'S HEALTH

Elderly women, especially grandmothers, mothers, and mothers-in-law, are considered to have expert knowledge about pregnancy and childbirth. Pregnancy rituals to protect the pregnant mother and the unborn child from evil spirits are performed during specific months of pregnancy. Pregnancy rites called *Valakappu, Puchtutal,* or *Saddha,* according to the region of India, are performed in the woman's home during the fifth month of pregnancy. The husband performs another ritual called *Simantam,* during the eighth month (Duvvurry, 1991). Pregnant women wear a bangle bracelet, call *valai or valayal* (meaning to surround), to create a barrier that will prevent evil spirits from approaching (Duvvurry). Hindu women are modest and are used to female care providers. Female relatives traditionally attend the mother during labor and childbirth (Jambunathan, 2003).

Pregnancy is considered to be a hot condition, therefore hot foods, such as animal products, eggs, fruit, chilies, spices and ginger and gas-producing foods, are avoided. Hot foods are believed to cause overexcitement, inflammatory reactions, sweating, and fatigue. Hindu women believe that if hot foods are eaten early in pregnancy, fetal anomalies or a miscarriage will result. Conversely, cold foods, such as milk products and butter, are believed to strengthen and calm the pregnant woman (Lauderdale, 2003). Anemia may be a concern because of the practice of reducing the intake of green leafy vegetables to avoid producing a dark-skinned baby (Jambunathan, 2003).

The birth of a son is considered a blessing because a son carries the family name and will care for his parents in their old age. Birth of a daughter may be a concern because of the traditions and expense associated with a dowry (Jambunathan, 2003).

Following a birth, both mother and baby undergo purification rites on the 11th day postpartum. During the postpartum period, the mother is considered impure and is confined to her room. After the 10th day, a ritual bath is taken and a religious ceremony is performed by a priest, ending the period of confinement. The baby is officially named on the 11th day during the "cradle ceremony," and rituals are performed to prevent evil spirits from harming the infant. During the postpartum period, hot foods are considered to be good for lactation, whereas cold foods are thought to produce diarrhea and indigestion in the baby. Breast-feeding is the norm and may be supplemented with cow's milk and diluted with sugar water (Jambunathan, 2003).

ILLNESS BEHAVIORS

Hindus have a fatalistic attitude toward health and illness causation because of their religious belief in karma. The belief that illness is God's will or a punishment from God may be a barrier for the Hindu client to access care or to follow a therapeutic regimen. Individuals are first cared for by the family and seek professional help only when family and traditional healing has not provided symptom relief. A prevailing belief is that time will heal, and this belief may deter Hindus from seeking early medical assistance.

Because Hindus believe that death is a step toward the next life, they prefer to die in full possession of their mental faculties. For this reason, they may refuse pain medication or nourishment when they believe that death is near. Cremation is the most common form of body disposal. Ashes are collected and disposed of in holy rivers (Andrews & Hanson, 2003).

Buddhism

Buddhism arose in northeast India in the 6th century. It broke with Hindu social structure, by accepting men and women equally and by abolishing the traditional distinctions between classes and castes (Ludwig, 2004a). Farlee (1999) says that trying to describe Buddhism is like trying to describe a snowflake. The fact that there are so many forms of Buddhism led to a tendency to absorb local cultures and religious forms as it spread outward from India to Southeast Asia, China, Korea, Japan, and Tibet. Its adaptability has made Buddhism very successful. More than half of the world's population live in areas where Buddhism has been dominant at some time.

Buddhism came to America with the Chinese immigrants who worked on the railroads and in the gold mines of the West in the mid-19th century. The first Buddhist temple in the United States was opened in San Francisco in 1853. It was further strengthened with Japanese immigration to Hawaii and the West Coast at the turn of the 20th century. The Japanese community started the Buddhist Mission of North America in 1899, which later became the Buddhist Churches of America. In the 1950s and 1960s Japanese teachers brought Zen Buddhism, a sect of the Mahayana branch to America, where it was embraced by counterculture writers.

All forms of Buddhism have a basis in the Buddhist path that was taught by Siddhartha Gautama, the Buddha (the enlightened one), as the solution to the suffering of life (dukkha).

The Buddha spent his life teaching the *dharma* (truth). The concept of suffering was related to psychological/mental symptoms, such as anxiety, anguish, and unhappiness. The Buddha described himself as a physician, one who diagnoses people's sufferings and prescribes a solution for wholeness of life. The Buddha taught the interdependence of mind, body, and spirit, which affects wellness. The path to nirvana involves health and wholeness for the complete person.

All forms of Buddhism accept the Four Noble Truths and the Eightfold Path. The first sermon that the Buddha preached presented the *Four Noble Truths*. The *First Noble Truth* is of suffering; all of life is permeated with *dukkha,* suffering, or sorrow, recognition that anxiety and discontent underlie all aspects of life. Change, loss, illness, and dying are all experienced as suffering. The *Second Noble Truth* reveals the cause of suffering: clinging or attachment. The *Third Noble Truth* concerns the cessation of suffering. By eliminating clinging, suffering is eliminated, and perfect health or nirvana results. The *Fourth Noble Truth* is the Noble Eightfold Path, the way of life that will bring cessation of clinging and thus cessation of suffering. It consists of the right understanding, right intention, right speech, right action, right livelihood, right effort, right mindfulness, and right concentration (Ludwig, 2004a).

Underlying the Four Noble Truths is the vision of reality expressed in the teaching of the Three Marks of Existence: suffering, impermanence, and no-self. Suffering as a mark of existence is expressed in the First Noble Truth. Impermanence is also a mark of existence because nothing is permanent. The truth of *pratitya samutpada* is the fundamental truth about reality, dependent co-arising. This means that all occurrences are related, arising from something prior in an interrelated process. Every condition contributes to the next and is itself affected by other conditions. From this central truth arises the third mark of existence—that all aspects of reality have no atman, no self-standing and permanently existing self or soul. (Ludwig, 2004a).

The Buddha taught that a person is made up of five aggregates: bodily matter, sensations, perceptions, mental formations, and bits of consciousness. These aggregates are constantly changing, brought together in a lifetime by karma from previous lifetimes, dissipating again when death occurs. The karmic formations built in that lifetime cause another birth and another lifetime, and the cycle continues. Because everything is impermanent, nothing is there to cling to; when this is realized, suffering is eliminated and nirvana results. Achieving nirvana is the spiritual goal of the Buddhist path, but it may be many lifetimes away. The Buddhist path has practices appropriate for people at every stage along the way, which bring spiritual benefits and enhancement to life (Ludwig, 2004a).

The Eightfold Path can be arranged under three subheadings: wisdom, morality, and concentration.

Wisdom

- *Right views*—understanding the Buddha's teachings and truth/reality.
- *Right aspirations*—high and noble aims.

Morality

- *Right speech*—speaking kind words and truth; not lying, gossiping, or being verbally abusive.
- *Right conduct*—good, moral, compassionate behavior.
- *Right livelihood*—having an honest living that does not cause suffering to others.

Concentration

- *Right effort*—perseverance in goodness and clearing the mind.
- *Right mindfulness*—attentiveness to reality and present moment.

- *Right meditation*—concentration on Buddha and the *Dharma* (Buddha's teachings and the basic truth of things); using meditation as an instrument to attain enlightenment (Farlee, 1999).

The elements of The Eightfold Path need to be practiced simultaneously; no progression occurs, but each practice clearly reinforces and deepens the others.

The Buddha's teachings represent the Dharma, the truth, which is to be accepted and lived. Buddha's disciples collected his teachings in the *Tripitaka* (Three Baskets), a scriptural source. Those who devote their lives to following and living out the Dharma make up the *sangha,* the community of monks and nuns together with the lay people. A common formula that Buddhists use in prayer is the Three Refuge formula: "I take refuge in the Buddha, I take refuge in the Dharma, I take refuge in the Sangha" (Ludwig, 2004a).

Branches of Buddhism

Buddhism's three main divisions all originated and were developed in India: *Theravada, Mahayana,* and *Vajrayana.* Theravada Buddhists (way of the elders) consider themselves to be closest to the original teachings of Buddha. The Mahayana (greater vehicle) followers adopted some newer, broader teachings and practices. The Vajrayana (thunderbolt vehicle) adherents incorporate esoteric, Tantric practices into the basic Mahayana belief system. Theravada is the dominant branch in South Asia and Southeast Asia; Mahayana predominates in East Asia; and Vajrayana exists in Tibet and Japan (Ludwig, 2004a).

THERAVADA BUDDHISM

According to Theravada teaching, the Buddha is not to be worshiped as a god or savior. Rather, the life of the Buddha serves as an important model for Buddhists, who follow his path of detachment and meditation to reach nirvana.

For monks and nuns, who have reached higher levels of spiritual perfection, the practices are more intense and are designed to eliminate all attachments. The Buddha set up monastic orders for men and women guided by his Ten Precepts (Box 6-4) and more than 200 rules for the religious life. The rules are rigorous and include total celibacy, meditation, having no possessions, depending on others for support (begging), and the practice of loving kindness. The ultimate goal is to completely attain the state of nirvana, called *arhant.* When an arhant's life ends, there is no rebirth, only the permanent state of nirvana (Ludwig, 2004a).

Lay followers of Buddhism are encouraged to follow basic ethical principles and engage in devotion and meditation. Lay persons follow the Five Precepts: refraining from taking life,

---

BOX 6-4

The Ten Precepts

1. Refrain from taking life
2. Refrain from taking what is not given
3. Refrain from sexual activity
4. Refrain from lying
5. Refrain from using drugs and liquor
6. Refrain from eating after noon
7. Refrain from watching shows, singing, or dancing
8. Refrain from the use of perfumes, adornments, or ointments
9. Refrain from sleeping in a broad, high bed
10. Refrain from handling gold or silver

From Ludwig, T. M. (2004). Buddhist traditions. In K. L. Mauk & N. K. Schmidt (Eds.), *Spiritual care in nursing practice* (pp. 151–163). Philadelphia: Lippincott Williams & Wilkins.

taking what is not given, wrong sexual relations, lying, and drugs and alcohol. These precepts provide direction for living an ethical life and lead away from self-centered acts to acts of compassion and kindness. Lay people renew their commitment to the Buddhist path through daily rituals and devotions or by going to the temple on the fortnightly holy day and by participating in festivals. They build up merit by supporting monastic communities. Through such activities, lay people hope to achieve a peaceful and whole life and a future lifetime at a higher level of existence. Six realms of rebirth exist; in the hells, as animals, as wandering ghosts, as humans, as demigods, or as gods. The quality of karma acquired in the current lifetime determines the realm of rebirth.

Mahayana Buddhism

The term *Mahayana* means "larger vehicle," and this tradition of Buddhism developed broader, expanded teachings and practices. This branch believes that the Theravadins overstress the monastic class as being spiritually elite. Mahayanas believe that lay people can achieve nirvana. They accept a larger number of sutras or scriptures than only those contained in the Tripitaka and ascribe all as the "Word of Buddha."

For Theravadins, the Buddha is Siddhartha Gautama, the human being who reached enlightenment and became the teacher of Dharma. Although images of Buddha are venerated, the Buddha is not worshiped or prayed to. Mahayana Buddhists, however, take an expanded view of Buddha and describe three dimensions of the Buddha: the universal Buddha nature, the human forms of Buddha, and the heavenly Buddha. The fundamental dimension is universal Buddha nature, the eternal inner essence of all reality. It can be experienced at the human level and at the heavenly level. Siddhartha Gautama was a human form of Buddha to guide humans to enlightenment. The *Lotus Sutra* posits that there have been countless other Buddhas, in all worlds and in all ages that have taught humans about enlightenment. Heavenly Buddhas are widely worshiped in the Mahayana Buddhist world, almost as saviors. These cosmic Buddhas are believed to grant physical well-being as well as spiritual help.

Another Mahayana emphasis is on the *bodhisattva* (one who is becoming a Buddha) as the ideal goal of the Buddhist path. A bodhisattva is one who reaches nirvana but out of great compassion chooses to stay in the samsara cycles of death and rebirth, to help others spiritually and physically. The bodhisattvas are available to help all who call on them in times of distress. One such bodhisattva worshiped all over the Mahayana world is Avalokiteshvara, who is praised in the Lotus Sutra as an omnipresent savior deity. In East Asian Buddhism, this deity is often represented in the feminine form as a goddess of compassion. She has a special following among women, who desire her help during pregnancy, and among the elderly, who pray for a peaceful old age free from senility (Ludwig, 2004a).

This branch of Buddhism has developed special schools that put emphasis on one of the central themes of Mahayana. Thus, in understanding Mahayana Buddhism, it is important to know to which school or sect a worshiper belongs. Some of the divisions include: Tiantai (Japanese Tendai), Huayan (Japanese Kegon), Pure Land, Chan (Zen), and Nichiren Buddhism. Some sects focus on a savior deity, whereas others focus on a self-power approach through meditation (Ludwig, 2004a).

Vajrayana Buddhism

Vajrayana Buddhism, the thunderbolt vehicle, is prevalent in Tibet. It draws on the idea of the universal Buddha nature and the identification of samsara and nirvana. Vajrayana developed elaborate rituals and practices of meditation that lead to the experience of being a

Buddha in one's own body. The Dalai Lama, believed to be the reincarnation of the previous Dalai Lama, is one of the best known Vajrayana Buddhists in the world.

Buddhism in America

Approximately 780,000 Buddhists are in North America (Andrews & Hanson, 2003). White American Buddhists tend to follow one of three Buddhist traditions—Zen, Tibetan, or Vipassana Buddhism. All of these sects emphasize meditation as the path to enlightenment. Farlee (1999) says that the emphasis that these sects place on self reliance, meditation, and enlightenment as a goal, all appeal to competitive and individualistic Americans.

Another prevalent form of Buddhism in America is Shin Buddhism. This form emphasizes that the key to nirvana is faith rather than any rigorous ritual or strict aesthetic practice. This form is Japanese and is practiced by the Buddhist Churches of America, a nationwide organization of temples.

Health and Buddhist Congregations

Ludwig (2004a) reports that the diversity and multiethnic nature of Buddhism prevented a single medical tradition from developing. In India, Buddhists contributed to the development of *Ayurvedic* medicine, so traditional medicine is influenced by Ayurveda in Tibet, Sri Lanka, and parts of Southeast Asia. In East Asia, Buddhists have lived with and helped to shape traditional Chinese medicine. In all Buddhist lands, the ethnic folk practices are combined with the medical tradition.

Buddhism does not restrict dietary practices, so diet will reflect the culture of the Buddhist person. Because Buddhists believe that illness and suffering are a part of life and have spiritual benefits, they may not see illness as something that has to be or should be prevented or cured once it exists. Different sects and cultures will assign their own meanings to illness and its treatment. No religious restrictions are practiced on the use of blood and blood products, healing practices, or the use of medication. Artificial insemination and birth control are acceptable practices.

Western medical practices of concern to Buddhists include such issues as abortion, euthanasia, organ transplantation, and definitions of brain death. Harming or taking a life is contrary to the first precept, so Buddhists would not permit abortion (unless the life of the mother was threatened) or euthanasia. Organ donation would be considered an act of mercy, if there is no hope for recovery.

Buddhists consider a calm, peaceful mind to be important at one's death because it minimizes the karma that propels the rebirth cycle onward. Thus, Buddhist meditation and other religious rituals are considered important to help one face dying with calmness and detachment. Buddhists will avoid analgesics and sedatives as they approach death, so that their mind can be filled with wholesome thoughts. Cremation is preferred over burial.

Summary

This chapter examines the major faith traditions that exist in America today. An overview of religious doctrines, health traditions, and practices has been described for each. Key to the use of this information is the concept of cultural competence, assessing, and understanding what are important religious traditions to individuals and their families. Individualized assessment is critical because people within the major faith traditions are diverse and may not hold "textbook" belief or practice all of the rites, rituals, and traditions of their religion.

Reflect and Discuss

1. Is your faith congregation ethnically diverse? What accommodations are made to meet the needs of ethnically diverse persons?
2. What are the important rituals associated with your faith tradition?
3. How is illness viewed in your faith tradition.
4. In what ways does your faith tradition support healthful living?
5. How can the FCN provide culturally competent nursing care?

References

African American Christianity. Available online at: http://www.bchm.org/wrr/recon/p17.html.

Ahmed, A. S. (1999). *Islam today: A short introduction to the Muslim world.* London: IB Tauris Publishers.

Ali, Z., Hussain, S., & Sakr, A. (1985). *Natural therapeutics of medicine in Islam.* Chicago: Kazi Publications.

Andrews, M. M., & Hanson, P. A. (2003). Religion, culture, and nursing. In M. M. Andrews & J. S. Boyle (Eds.), *Transcultural concepts in nursing care* (pp. 432–502). Philadelphia: Lippincott Williams & Wilkins.

Athar, S. (2004). Information for health care providers when dealing with a Muslim patient. Available online at: http://www.islam-usa.com/e40.html.

Baer, H. A., & Singer, M. (2002). *African American religion: Varieties of protest and accommodation* (2nd ed.). Knoxville, TN: The University of Tennessee Press.

Baer, H. A., & Singer, M. (1981). Toward a typology of black sectarianism as a response to racial stratification. *Anthropological Quarterly, 54,* 1–14.

Barrett, D. B., & Johnson, T. M. (2002). Worldwide adherents of all religions by six continental areas, mid-2001. In 2002 *Britannica book of the year* (pp. 302, 303). Chicago: Encyclopedia Britannica, Inc.

Chase-Ziolek, M., & Holst, L. E. (1999). Parish nursing in diverse traditions. In P. A. Solari-Twadell & M. A. McDermott (Eds.), *Parish nursing: Promoting whole person health with faith communities* (pp. 195–204). Thousand Oaks, CA: Sage Publications.

De, S. (1996). The historical context of the Bhagavad-Gita and its relation to Indian religious doctrines. Available online at: http://www.eawc.evansville.edu/essays/de.htm.

Duvvurry, V. K. (1991). *Play, symbolism, and ritual.* New York: Peter Lang.

Ebersole, P. (2000). Parish nurse leaders. *Geriatric Nursing, 21*(3), 148, 149.

Estes, G. & Zitzow, D. (1980, November). Heritage consistency as a consideration in counseling Native Americans. Paper read at the National Indian Education Association Convention, Dallas, TX.

Farlee, R. B. (1999). *Honoring our neighbor's faith.* Minneapolis: Augsburg Fortress.

Feldman, D. (1986). *Health and medicine in the Jewish tradition.* New York: Crossroad Publishing Co.

Glanville, C. L. (2003). People of African American heritage. In L. Purnell & B. Paulanka, *Transcultural health care* (2nd ed.). Philadelphia: FA Davis.

Grundmann, C. H., & Truemper, D. G. (2004a). Christianity and its branches. In K. L. Mauk & N. K. Schmidt (Eds.), *Spiritual care in nursing practice* (pp. 75–82). Philadelphia: Lippincott Williams & Wilkins.

Grundmann, C. H., & Truemper, D. G. (2004b). Islam and its branches. In K. L. Mauk & N. K. Schmidt (Eds.), *Spiritual care in nursing practice* (pp. 75–82). Philadelphia: Lippincott Williams & Wilkins.

Grundmann, C. H., & Truemper, D. G. (2004c). Judaism and its branches. In K. L. Mauk & N. K. Schmidt (Eds.), *Spiritual care in nursing practice* (pp. 75–82). Philadelphia: Lippincott Williams & Wilkins.

Harris, M. W. (2004). Unitarian Universalist origins—our historic faith. Available online at: http://www.uua.org/info/origins.html.

Jambunathan, J. (2003). People of Hindu heritage. In L. D. Purnell & B. J. Paulanka (Eds.), *Transcultural health care: A culturally competent approach* (2nd ed.; CD-ROM, pp. 85–100). Philadelphia: FA Davis.

Kulwicki, A. D. (2003). People of Arab heritage. In L. D. Purnell & B. J. Paulanka (Eds.), *Transcultural health care: A culturally competent approach* (2nd ed., pp. 90–105). Philadelphia: FA Davis.

Lauderdale, J. (2003). Transcultural perspectives in childbearing. In M. M. Andrews & J. S. Boyle (Eds.), *Transcultural concepts in nursing care* (pp. 95–132). Philadelphia: Lippincott Williams & Wilkins.

Leininger, M. (2002). Culture care assessments for congruent competency practices. In M. Leininger & M. R. McFarland (Eds.), *Transcultural nursing: Concepts, theories, research, and practices* (pp. 117–143). New York: McGraw-Hill.

Ludwig, T. M. (2004a). Buddhist traditions. In K. L. Mauk & N. K. Schmidt (Eds.), *Spiritual care in nursing practice* (pp. 151–163). Philadelphia: Lippincott Williams & Wilkins.

Ludwig, T. M. (2004b). South Asian traditions. In K. L. Mauk & N. K. Schmidt (Eds.), *Spiritual care in nursing practice* (pp. 131–150). Philadelphia: Lippincott Williams & Wilkins.

Miskelly, S. (1995). A parish nursing model: Applying the community health nursing process in a church community. *Journal of Community Health Nursing, 12*(11), 1–14.

Ohm, R. (2003). The African American experience in the Islamic faith. *Public Health Nursing, 20*(6), 478–486.

Raj, S., Ganganna, P., & Bowering, J. (1999). Dietary habits of Asian Indians in relation to length of residence in the United States. *Journal of the American Dietetic Association, 99*(9), 1106–1108.

Rassool, G. H. (2000). The crescent and Islam: Healing, nursing and the spiritual dimension. Some considerations towards an understanding of the Islamic perspectives on caring. *Journal of Advanced Nursing, 32*(6), 1476–1485.

Sahkoor-Abdullah, B. (2002). Muslim American Society. *The Park Ridge Center Bulletin, 25.* Available online at: http://www.parkridgecenter.org/Page1949.html.

Schleimut Institute. (2004). About us—Our vision. Available online at: http://www.shleimut.org/AboutUs_Vision.htm.

Schweitzer, R. (2004). Schleimut: A multidisciplinary approach to Jewish health, healing, and wholeness. *Parish Nurse Perspectives, 3*(1), 7–8.

Smith, J. (1999). *Islam in America.* New York: Columbia University Press.

Spector, R. E. (2004). *Cultural diversity in health and illness* (6th ed.). Upper Saddle River, NJ: Prentice Hall.

Trofino, J., Hughes, C. B., O'Brien, B. L., Mack, J., Marrinan, M. A., & Hay, K. M. (2000). Primary care parish nursing: Academic, service, and parish partnership. *Nursing Administration Quarterly, 25*(1), 59–74.

U. S. Census. (2002). *Statistical abstract of the United States 2002.* Washington, DC: Author.

U. S. Department of Health & Human Services. (2000). *Healthy People 2010: Understanding and improving health* (2nd ed.). Washington, DC: U. S. Government Printing Office.

Weis, D., Matheus, R., & Schank, M. J. (1997). Health care delivery in faith communities: The parish nurse model. *Public Health Nursing, 14*(6), 368–372.

Wentz, R. E. (2003). *American religious traditions: The shaping of religion in the United States.* Minneapolis, MN: Fortress Press.

Yousif, A. F. (2002). Islamic medicine and health care. *The Park Ridge Center Bulletin, 25.* Available online at: http://www.parkridgecenter.org?Page1946.html.

Additional Resources

Baldwin, K., Humbles, P., Armmer, F., & Cramer, M. (2001). Perceived health needs of urban African-American church congregants. *Public Health Nursing, 18*(5), 295–303.

Bhaskarananda, S. (1994). *The essentials of Hinduism.* Seattle: Viveka Press.

Bukhari, A. H. (2004). *Muslim's place in the American public square: Hopes, fears, and aspirations.* Lanham, MD: Alta Mira Press.

Chaves, M. (2004). *Congregations in America.* Cambridge, MA: Harvard University Press.

Chen, Y. C. (2000). Chinese values, health, and nursing. *Journal of Advanced Nursing, 36*(2), 270–273.

da Costa Nunez, R. (2004). *A shelter is not a home or is it?* New York: White Tiger Press.

DiCaroli, R. (2004). *Haunting the Buddha: Indian popular religion and the formation of Buddhism.* New York: Oxford University Press.

Dosick, W. (1995). *Living Judaism.* San Francisco: Harper.

Gillum, R. F., Mussolino, M. E., Madans, J. H. (1998). Coronary heart disease risk factors and attributable risks in African-American women and men: NHANES I epidemiologic follow-up study. *American Journal of Public Health, 88*(6), 918–923.

Haight, W. (1998). "Gathering the spirit" at First Baptist Church: Spirituality as a protective factor in the lives of African American children. *Social Work, 43*(3), 213–222.

Hedayat, K. M. (2001). Issues in Islamic biomedical ethics: A primer for the pediatrician. *Pediatrics, 108*(4), 965–971.

Jacobson, S. F., Booton-Hiser, D., Moore, J. H., Edwards, K. A., Pryor, S., & Campbell, J. M. (1998). Diabetes research in an American Indian community. *Image, 30*(2), 161–166.

Jeung, R. (2005). *Faithful generations: Race and new Asian American churches.* New Brunswick, NJ: Rutgers University Press.

Kirdli, S. A. (2002). Health beliefs and practices among Arab women. *American Journal of Maternal Child Nursing, 27*(3), 178–182.

Lowe, J. (2002). Cherokee self-reliance. *Journal of Transcultural Nursing, 13,* 287–295.

Mendelson, C. (2002). Health perceptions of Mexican American women. *Journal of Transcultural Nursing, 13,* 210–217.

Musgrave, C. F., Allen, C. E., & Allen, G. (2002). Spirituality and health for people of color. *American Journal of Public Health, 92*(4), 557–560.

Nelson, T. J. (2004). *Every time I feel the spirit: Religious experience and ritual in an African American church.* New York: NYU Press.

Newlin, K., Knafl, K., & Melkus, G. D. (2002). African-American spirituality: A concept analysis. *Advances in Nursing Science, 25*(2), 57–70.

Nichols, A. (1996). *Epiphany: A theological introduction to Catholicism.* Collegeville, MN: The Liturgical Press.

Orsi, R. A. (2005). *Between heaven and earth: The religious worlds people make and the scholars who study them.* Princeton, NJ: Princeton University Press.

Ott, B., Al-Khadhuri, J., & Al-Junaibi, S. (2003). Preventing ethical dilemmas: Understanding Islamic health care practices. *Pediatric Nursing, 29* (3), 227–230.

Phan, P. C., & Hayes, D. (Eds.). (2004). *Many faces, one church: Cultural diversity and the American Catholic experience.* Lanham, MD: Rowman & Littlefield.

Porter, E. J. (2000). The church family and kin: An older rural black female support group. *Qualitative Health Research, 10*(4), 452–470.

Puncheon, S., & Congdon, J. G. (2003). Spirituality and health in older Thai persons in the United States. *Western Journal of Nursing Research, 25,* 93–108.

Rehm, R. S. (1999). Religious faith in Mexican-American families dealing with chronic childhood illness. *Image, 31*(1), 33–38.

Roberts, K. S. (2002). Providing culturally sensitive care to the childbearing Islamic family. *Advances in Neonatal Care, 2*(4), 222–228.

Sadler, G. R., Dhanjal, S. K., Shah, N. B., Ko, C., Angel, M., & Harshburger, R. (2001). Asian women: Knowledge, attitudes, and behaviors toward breast cancer early detection. *Public Health Nursing, 18,* 357–363.

Sarna, J. D. (2004). *American Judaism: A history.* New Haven, CT: Yale University Press.

Spitler, H. D., Kemper, K. A., & Parker, V. G. (2002). Promoting success for at-risk African-American youth: Perceived barriers and resources in using community-based success criteria. *Family and Community Health, 25,* 37–52.

Swinney, J., Anson-Wonkkka, C., Maki, E., & Corneauu, J. (2001). Community assessment: A church community and the parish nurse. *Public Health Nursing, 18,* 40–44.

Ware, K. (1995). *The orthodox way.* Crestwood, NY: St. Vladimir's Seminary Press.

Wills, D. W. (2005). *Christianity in the United States: A historical survey and interpretation.* South Bend, IN: Notre Dame Press.

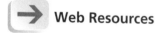 **Web Resources**

http://www.jewfaq.org/torah.htm   About the Torah

http://www.jewfaq.org/holidaya.htm   About Pesach (Passover)

http://www.abc-usa.org   American Baptist Churches

http://www.academicinfo.net/amreligjudaism.html   American Jewish history

http://www.nwmissouri.edu/nwcourses/history155/religion/midtermprojects/connieury   An Overview of American Judaism

http://www.luthhist.org/bibliography/   A Bibliography of Writings on Lutheranism in America

http://www.buddhanet.net   Buddha Dharma Association

http://www.pluralism.org/resources/biblio/islam.php   Buddhism in the United States

http://www.catholic.net   Catholic Net

http://www.wikipedia.org/wiki/Christian_fundamentalism   Christian fundamentalist traditions in the United States

http://www.marybakereddy.org   Christian Science

http://www.mormon,org   Church of Jesus Christ of Latter-day Saints

http://www.encyclopedia.com/html/section/LattrdaCh_History.asp   Church of Jesus Christ of Latter-day Saints

http://www.scientology.org   Church of Scientology

http://www.cnbc.org   Congress of Black Churches

http://www.uscj.org   Conservative Judaism

http://www.pctii.org/cybertab.html   Cyberjournal for Pentecostal-Charismatic Research

http://www.oca.org   Eastern Orthodox Church

http://www.episcopalchurch.org   Episcopal Church USA

http://www.elca.org   Evangelical Lutheran Church in America

http://www.vedanta.org   Hinduism

http://www.pluralism.org/resources/biblio/hinduism.php   Hinduism Bibliography

http://www.geocities.com/RodeoDrive/1415/indexd.html   Hinduism and related resources

http://www.ame-today.com/history/index.shtml   History of the African Methodist Episcopal Church

http://www.ccel.org/b/bangs/history_mec/HMEC09.HTM   History of the Methodist Episcopal Church

http://www.pym.org/exhibit/p045.html   History of the Quakers

http://www.pluralism.org/resources/biblio/islam.php   Islam Bibliography

http://www.islamicedfoundation   Islamic Foundation

http://www.islam-usa.com/e40.html   Islamic Medical Society of America

http://www.usc.edu/dept/MSA/reference/glossary.html   Islamic Terms and Concepts

http://www.news.bbc.co.uk/1/hi/programmes/panorama/2120798.stm   Jehovah's Witnesses

http://www.elca.org   Evangelical Lutheran Church in America

http://www.goatch.org   Greek Orthodox Archdiocese of America

http://www.lcms.org   Lutheran Church-Missouri Synod

http://www.carnegie.org/reporter/04/muslims/index.html   Muslims in America: Identity Develops as a Community Grows

http://www.noi.org   Nation of Islam

http://www.hispanichealth.org   National Alliance for Hispanic Health

http://www.nawho.org   National Asian Women's Health Organization

http://www.naacp.org   National Association for the Advancement of Colored People

http://www.nclar.org   National Council of La Raza

http://www.omhrc.gov   Office of Minority Health

http://www.pcanet.org   Presbyterian Church in America

http://www.pcusa.org   Presbyterian Church USA
http://www.pluralism.org   The Pluralism Project
http://www.diversityRx.org   Resources for Cross Cultural Health Care
http://www.russionaorthodoxchurch.ws/english   Russian Orthodox Church
http://www.uahc.org/jfc/rjnn.shtml   Reform Jewish Nurses Network
http://www.rj.org   Reform Judaism
http://www.quaker.org   Religious Society of Friends
http://www.ccbuscc.org   Roman Catholic Church
http://www.shleimut.org   Shleimut Institute
http://www.searac.org   Southeast Asian Research Action Center

http://www.sbc.org   Southern Baptist Convention
http://www.uahc.org   Union of American Hebrew Congregations
http://www.uua.org   Unitarian Universalist Association
http://www.ucc.org   United Church of Christ
http://www.umc.org   United Methodist Church
http://www.uscj.org   United Synagogue of Conservative Judaism
http://www.vatican.va   The Vatican
http://www.wabashcenter.wabash.edu   The Wabash Center

Community Connections

7

This chapter discusses the connections that the faith community nurse (FCN) will establish with patients, colleagues, institutions, and organizations. The FCN roles of referral agent and advocate will be discussed in-depth. Wuthnow (2004) reminds us that religion is fundamentally social, about relationships among people, with communities and between individuals and organizations, and it is therefore contextual. Its meanings are contextual, given life and given reality through the concrete settings in which it is expressed. Its implications are always conditioned by the contexts in which it occurs (p. 17).

The ability to achieve patient and community outcomes is closely connected to partnerships with others as well as the FCN's ability to manage interdependent and interdisciplinary relationships. Collaboration is considered to be one of the core competencies of advanced practice nursing (American Association of Colleges of Nursing, AACN, 1995; American Nurses Association, ANA, 2004; Davies & Hughes, 1995; National Council on State Boards of Nursing, NCSB, 1993; National Organization of Nurse Practitioner Faculties, NONPF, 1995). Collaboration means "to work together, especially in a joint intellectual effort" (Merriam-Webster, 1983). Hamric, Spross, and Hanson (2000) refer to collaboration as a "dynamic, interpersonal process in which two or more individuals make a commitment to each other to interact authentically and constructively to solve problems and to learn from each other in order to accomplish identified goals, purposes or outcomes. The individuals recognize and articulate the shared values that make this commitment possible" (p. 318). The ability to "make a commitment to interact authentically and constructively" suggests that qualities exist that prospective partners bring to the encounter. The qualities include a common purpose, clinical competence, interpersonal skills, sense of humor, trust, respect, and value of each other's expertise.

Faith Community Nursing: Scope and Standards of Practice (American Nurses Association & Health Ministries Association [ANA-HMA], 2005), *Standard 5—Implementation*, states that the FCN "collaborates with and empowers patients to enhance their spiritual well-being and healthy behaviors, reduce the occurrence of illness, modify health risk behaviors and adapt to chronic changes in health status" (p. 17). *Professional Performance, Standard 11—Collaboration* states: "The FCN collaborates with the patient, spiritual leaders, members of the faith community, and others in the conduct of this specialized nursing practice" (p. 28). Measurement criteria for this standard include collaboration in decision making about clients' health plan, interventions, and desired outcomes; and documentation of the plan and partnering with others to enhance faith-based patient care.

By definition, collaboration identifies relationships that need to be positive and grounded in a problem-solving approach, creating interdependence as a mutually satisfying experience for the parties involved (Smith & Vezina, 2004). Sullivan (1998) adds the concept of power in her definition of collaboration, a "dynamic, transforming process of creating a power-sharing partnership . . . for purposeful attention to needs and problems in order to achieve likely successful outcomes" (p. 6).

Underlying the concept of collaboration is the belief that quality faith community nursing care is achieved by including the contributions of the patient and a team of appropriate professionals. True collaborative practice is a partnership, and it does not have a hierarchy. The contributions of each participant are based on the knowledge or expertise brought to the situation and creative, original visions and strategies are produced.

Archangelo, Fitzgerald, Carroll, and Plum (1996) identify interpersonal attributes that are essential for successful collaboration. They include and are defined as follows:

- *Trust* among all parties establishes a quality-working relationship; it develops over time as the parties become acquainted.
- *Knowledge* is a necessary component for the development of trust. Knowledge and trust remove the need for supervision.
- *Shared responsibility* suggests joint decision making for client care and outcomes as well as practice issues within the organization.
- *Communication* that is not hierarchical but rather two-way ensures the sharing of client information and knowledge. Questioning of the approach to care of either partner cannot be delivered in a manner that is construed as criticism but as a method to enhance knowledge and improve client care.
- *Cooperation* and *coordination* promote the use of the skills of all team members, prevent duplication, and enhance productivity.
- *Optimism* promotes success when the involved parties believe that collaboration is the more effective means of promoting quality of care.

Smith and Vezina (2004) contend that although interpersonal attributes are key in any collaborative relationship, the unique contribution of each member of the team primarily determines a successful outcome. Although several models of collaborative practice exist, they are often distinguished by the following two factors:

1. How is the expertise of each member of the team used to the fullest?
2. Who is responsible for decision making and client care? (p. 458)

Models of collaboration assist in structuring relationships and guiding the process of working partnerships. Strumpf and Whitney (1994) describe three collaborative practice models for nurse practitioners: the parallel model, the sequential model, and the shared model. In the parallel model, the nurse practitioner (NP) manages stable patients, and the physician manages medically complex patients. In the sequential model, the NP performs the intake assessment, and the physician assumes the responsibility for the diagnosis—or the physician screens all patients and refers the less complex ones to the NP. In the shared model, the NP and physician care for all patients on a rotating basis.

Archangelo et al. (1996) identify a fourth model, which they call the collaborative model. Here, the NP is the primary provider who practices autonomously but consults others as needed to provide safe, high quality care. Communication in this model is ongoing and may transition to a point where co-management occurs. This model involves two professionals working together, and an outcome of this model is the learning of new skills for both.

The sequential model and the collaborative model are the two models that can be used by the FCN. In both, the FCN assesses the congregant situation and either manages it autonomously or seeks consultation. The FCN will also assess patient situations and make appropriate and timely referrals.

Smith and Vezina (2004) state that regardless of the model of collaborative practice, the elements of trust and a positive working relationship are key. Collaborative relationships are constantly evolving and are facilitated by interpersonal flexibility and realistic expectations of all of the partners. Over time, mutual expressions of expertise become grounded in a working pattern that is the glue of a successful relationship and reflective of growing skill, trust, and confidence among partners.

Barriers to collaboration include tradition, role, and gender stereotypes, as well as differing agendas, money, and long-held beliefs about "how things should be done" (Hanson &

Spross, 2005). Nurses and other health care providers in the congregation can create barriers for the FCN, if they do not clearly understand the FCN role. And other health ministries may feel excluded or threatened by a new FCN program. Turf issues *do* exist in faith communities, just as they do in community organizations, and hurt feelings create barriers and cause conflict. Everyone needs to feel valued and a part of the larger mission and ministry. Good education and communication are always worth the time and effort to enhance collaborations.

Collaborations with Clients

FCNs provide counseling, expert guidance, and coaching to congregants and their families. Patterson (2003) states that the FCN is available to discuss health concerns, emphasizing an early response to small problems and encouraging healthy lifestyle changes. In doing so, the FCN serves as a mentor, which fosters the development of others to either take the lead or share the pathway of care (Smith & Vezina, 2004). Chase-Ziolek and Iris (2002) conducted a qualitative study on nurses' perspectives on the distinctive aspects of parish nursing. They report that in health counseling situations, parish nurses provided health information, dealt with the feelings associated with the health problem, and focused on manageable goals. Health counseling was perceived as including psychosocial support and spiritual care.

Olson (2000) describes the FCN role of personal health counselor as assisting people to express feelings, identifying the health issues they are facing, identifying possible solutions to address their own health issues, and evaluating their outcomes. These steps follow the standards of care for faith community nursing: assessment, diagnosis, outcome identification, planning, implementation, and evaluation (ANA-HMA, 2005). Personal health counseling can occur as formal or causal interaction in any setting where the patient and FCN meet together. As discussed in Chapter 2, the personal counseling role of the FCN is highly supported by the research literature.

Wuthnow (2004) develops the concept of congregations as caring communities. He states that social interaction in congregations takes place regularly over a long period of time and across a wide variety of activities, and that being part of a congregation necessarily implies a distinction between those who are "insiders" and those who are not. Third, a congregation is characterized by what is called a "thick" set of shared values, beliefs, understandings, traditions, and norms. As caring communities, congregations may function best by encouraging members to help each other, rather than trying to help any and all who may need help in the larger community (p. 65). The concept of congregation as a caring community supports the ministry of faith community nursing.

Collaborations with Colleagues

Consultation is the direct involvement of another practitioner, which denotes the need to confirm findings, diagnosis, or plan of care. The responsibility for care always resides with the primary professional. Consultation can be within the nursing profession or it can be interdisciplinary. In either situation, partnership is necessary for optimal client outcomes (Smith & Vezina, 2004). Because both professional standards and Health Insurance Portability and Accountability Act (HIPAA) requirements demand client confidentiality, the FCN cannot share client information with other professionals without the client's expressed permission.

Clark (2000) describes three elements of collaboration in ministry partnerships: *learning,* which is described as creative interaction between ministry professionals and those who are the focus of their ministry; *boundaries,* which are places where care and influence encounter both respect and limitations; and *dialogue,* a nuanced and creative integration of insights, words, and ministry actions (p. 312). The element of learning involves an openness to see beyond the stereotypical roles of pastor and nurse. The element of boundaries encompasses male/female roles, dominance/subordination issues or power struggles, and turf issues. According to Pope Paul VI (1964), the element of dialogue is both an attitude and a method. As an attitude, dialogue reveals both rootedness and openness; as a method, it can help individuals and groups accomplish a sense of purpose or mission. Dialogue is a form of spiritual communication that is characterized by clarity of language, meekness and peacefulness, trust, and prudence.

In many faith community nursing settings, a health ministry team will provide interdisciplinary team efforts for members of the faith community. According to Howe, Cassel, and Vezina (1998), several dimensions should be considered when working with interdisciplinary teams. The dimensions include the following:

Skills

- Conflict resolution
- Team interaction
- Communication
- Leadership

Attitudes

- Respect for other disciplines
- Respect for client/family input
- Respect for client management and client-focused care
- Awareness of outcome-based practice

Knowledge

- Roles, responsibilities, and scope of practice for each discipline
- Role of the extended team
- Group dynamics
- Application of clinical concepts among disciplines
- Up-to-date knowledge of the health care

Collaboration is the basis for interdisciplinary teams. Smith and Vezina (2004) suggest that team members ask themselves the following questions:

- *Are my own goals consistent with team goals?* This consistency obviously would be a requirement of faith community nursing practice.
- *Do I advocate for solutions for problems that will benefit all team members?* This question may or may not be relevant to faith community nursing practice, depending on the context.
- *Do I work for consensus?* Consensus builds teams and allows everyone to "own" a decision.
- *Do I cooperate with other team members' activities?* This question requires self-reflection and personal honesty.
- *Do I do an equitable share of the group workload?* This question will have differing answers, depending on the model of parish nursing. In a voluntary model where the FCN is providing limited hours of service, equity will not be a team issue.
- *Do I support the team in dealing with larger organizational issues?* Once again, consistency in goals is very important in faith community nursing.
- *Do I actively participate in team meetings and assignments?* Whether the FCN is a part of a health ministry or a clerical team, active participation related to the health of faith community is an expectation of the FCN role.

Smith and Vezina (2004) describe interdisciplinary teaming, with its strong emphasis on relationship-centered care, as a "best practice" for the 21st century. They state that although roles and relationships may be challenged, they also move to a new level where extraordinary achievements can occur.

Hahn, Radde, and Fellers state that effective collaboration in health ministries requires the following simple rules:

- Place God and the client first.
- Respect one another's gifts.
- Respond to the client's preferences and needs.
- Communicate with one another.
- Reserve territoriality for the endangered species.
- Respect one another's differences.
- Communicate about mutual expectations and about areas of potential overlap.
- Plan together.
- Periodically evaluate the effectiveness of working relationships. (2001, p. 60)

Smith (2003) suggests that every member of the health ministry team should have a specific responsibility. She states that the team should meet at least monthly and that the team, not the FCN, should be responsible for program outreach, implementation, and evaluation. The FCN brings clinical expertise and health resources to the team.

Collaborations with Other Faith Communities

Facilitation of collaborations between faith communities to address common health concerns and issues is becoming increasingly important as FCN/health ministries become established in congregations. Collaboration is also a realistic means of sharing human, spatial, and fiscal resources.

Collaborations with Agencies and Institutions

Brudenell (2003) conducted a descriptive study to determine how faith communities form parish nursing programs and what their effect is. Thirteen congregations, representing eight denominations with parish nursing/health ministry programs, participated in the study. Collaboration between faith communities and health organizations were successful using a *limited domain approach* to attain specific health goals. Brudenell was initially surprised when parish nurses and pastors could not identify "partnerships," except with one of the two area medical centers. Rather than partnerships, pastors and parish nurses recognized extensive collaborations. Gunderson (1997) describes two aspects of collaboration, respect for survival and *limited domain collaboration*. In limited-domain collaboration, organizations come together for a specific project and then separate. This type is a useful venue for volunteer-driven organizations, such as faith communities, because it takes less time and commitment than full partnerships.

Ammerman (2004) found that the 83% of connections that congregations had with other organizations involving human services were with local or regional organizations, whereas 17% were with national or international partners. She also found that among congregations with any connections there was little difference in the proportions involved in informal coalitions (62%), involved in cooperative relations with religious nonprofits (66%), or involved in cooperative relations with secular nonprofits (58%). These figures were considerably higher than the proportion of congregations involved in service networks that included governmental units (29%). These figures suggest that congregations are fairly widely connected with specialized nonprofit organizations and, to a lesser degree, with governmental agencies.

The community assessment process, discussed in detail in Chapter 5, provides the FCN with an overview of the health and social service facilities and agencies available in the community and region. To personalize service and make appropriate referrals, the FCN should extend his or her network to key personnel in community agencies.

A key collaboration for the FCN will be with the nearest acute care hospital. Networking with hospital chaplains and home care/discharge planning department nurses will create important information links and referral sources for the FCN.

Schumann and VanDuivendyk (2001) state that as health care professionals, chaplains and parish nurses share the mission of healthy, whole, and integrated communities without walls. Chaplains focus primarily within the hospital setting but may team with community clergy and parish nurses. Parish nurses may work with one or more faith communities and also in another field of nursing. Working toward this mission without walls requires chaplains and parish nurses to minister within the traditional healing community of the hospital and also to involve congregations and communities outside the hospital. To do this, chaplains and parish nurses can collaborate in a number of activities to complement and connect their practice skills, knowledge, and gifts. The authors caution, however, that inherent in any collaboration, are times when complementary connections of ministry patterns, philosophies, and connections become collisions and conflict regarding care roles, boundaries, and priorities. They remind us that collisions of any sort can generate tremendous amounts of energy, whether they involve atoms, automobiles, rain clouds, or people. On the other hand, complementarity of practice skills, knowledge, and gifts creates not only energy but also a synergy that enhances the ideas and abilities of team members.

Schumann and VanDuivendyk (2001) report that collaborative community efforts result in at least four positive outcomes. First, collaboration between congregational ministries and hospital services can strengthen the link between faith and health as congregations move toward healing communities. Second, greater support for health ministry programs is created as congregants share their success stories with others. Third, more comprehensive care is provided as parishes and hospitals work together to coordinate and provide the highest level of holistic care. Fourth, chaplains, parish nurses, and community clergy have the opportunity to learn more about each other and their various roles with this healing mission. And last, each professional can use the skills and abilities of the others while uncovering greater opportunities for collaboration. Collaborative efforts can include referral into each other's specialty areas, as well as consultation across the fields of pastoral care and nursing (p. 67).

Another key agency for the FCN is the health department. Depending upon the state, health departments may have local, county, regional, and/or state offices.

Services and programs vary greatly, depending on state and local health codes, the needs of the community, and available resources. Examples of services that may be provided by local health departments are presented in Box 7-1.

If there is a local health department within a reasonable geographic distance, the FCN should plan to spend a morning or afternoon there. Many health departments provide extensive libraries and support services for health promotion and disease prevention. The FCN needs to be familiar with the services offered (and their costs) to be an effective referral agent for the faith community. If the health department is at a distance, the FCN should become familiar with the resources available from the health department via its Web site.

Home health care is provided by official agencies (health departments), proprietary and voluntary agencies (for-profit home care agencies, visiting nurse associations), combination agencies (public and voluntary), or hospital-based home health agencies. Hospices that provide pal-

BOX 7-1
Examples of Services Provided by Local Health Departments

Addiction
Adult health
Bioterrorism response
Birth and death records
Child health clinics
Dental health clinics
Disaster management
Environmental health
Epidemiology and disease control
Family planning
Food inspection and safety
Health education and information
Health promotion and disease prevention
Home safety programs
Immunizations
Maternal health
Mental health
Mental retardation and developmental
   disabilities
Nursing
School health
Sexually transmitted disease clinics
Tuberculosis

BOX 7-2
Examples of Skilled Nursing Services

Assessing a patient's health status and condition
Providing direct care in administering
   treatments
Teaching the patient and family to carry out the
   physician's orders related to medications, treatments, therapeutic diets, and/or exercise programs
Reporting patient condition changes to the physician and arranging for medical follow-up as
   needed
Assisting the patient and family to identify
   resources that will help the patient toward
   optimal functioning

liative care services may be free-standing or may be a division or a department of a home health agency or acute care facility. In 2002, there were 6,183 Medicare-certified home health agencies and 2,275 hospice agencies, with an average cost per home visit of $138 (Centers for Medicare and Medicaid, 2002). The responsibilities and functions of the disciplines in home health care are dictated by Medicare regulations, professional organizations, and state licensing boards. Medicare certified agencies provide skilled nursing services, physical therapy, occupational therapy, social work services, home health aide services, and speech pathology services. Each patient in a Medicare certified agency is under the care of a physician who certifies (in the plan of care) that the patient has a medical condition.

Only *skilled nursing care* is reimbursable by Medicare and other third party payers. Skilled nursing care is that level of care which can only be provided by a registered nurse. Skilled nursing care is goal-directed, and documentation must indicate client movement toward the goal(s). Examples of skilled nursing services are presented in Box 7-2. As of 2002, all Medicare home care visits are reimbursed on a prospective payment system, which is documented on OASIS (a computer-based documentation system). In prospective payment systems, the home health agency is paid a fixed rate per diagnosis. A financial incentive to the agency is to make fewer visits per client to accomplish goals. Why is this important information for the FCN? One reason is so that the FCN will refer clients appropriately. The FCN also needs to be aware that with tighter controls on who can receive Medicare-paid nursing services, there will be an increased number of elderly clients with unmet nursing needs in the community.

The FCN should make a visit to the local home health agency and hospice to learn about the services offered and to meet the staff. Special attention should be paid to programs and services that will address the needs of the faith community that were identified in the community assessment process. For example, if the faith community is comprised of predominantly young families, the FCN should be sure to investigate maternal-child services. Developing a network of key personnel in agencies personalizes the services the FCN can provide her or his clients, and it provides the FCN with a network of expert consultation.

Both health departments and home care agencies have boards of directors and professional advisory committees. If times permits, volunteering to serve on one of these bodies puts the FCN at the decision-making table, keeps the FCN informed of health-related legislation, and expands the FCN's network of colleagues.

The FCN needs to be aware of mental health services available in the community. Although each state provides mental health services for its residents, the availability and access to these services varies greatly. Mental illness has historically been the stepchild of the American health care system, and health insurers provide them considerably less coverage, both inpatient and outpatient, for psychiatric services than for medical/surgical services. Currently, acute hospitals are converting their inpatient psychiatric beds to medical-surgical beds because of higher reimbursement for medical-surgical conditions. Many counties are completely without inpatient psychiatric beds.

The FCN should make a connection with the local chapter of NAMI (National Alliance for the Mentally Ill). NAMI is a family organization that promotes family support groups, educational programs, public campaigns to reduce stigma, and political advocacy for mental health policy and services at all levels. The FCN should also be aware of crisis intervention services, hot lines, substance abuse treatment and support groups, halfway houses, and domestic violence shelters.

The FCN needs to investigate community resources and services for senior citizens. With the current demographics, the size and needs of the elderly population will greatly increase in the next decade. All families and faith communities will be impacted by the growth and the needs of this sector of the population.

Other community agencies that the FCN should include in his or her network are social service agencies, such as the Department of Welfare, the Social Security Administration, and, if available, food banks. The FCN may need to assist congregants to apply for public assistance, food stamps, Medicaid, unemployment compensation—to name a few.

Collaborations with Organizations

Health-related organizations can provide the FCN with a great deal of information, teaching materials, and professional resources for health programming in the faith community. In urban and suburban areas, health-related organizations maintain offices that provide resources to health care professionals and to consumers. If such offices are available to you, do make use of the resources they provide. If such offices are not geographically available, do visit organizational Web sites and request information and resources. A great deal of free health education materials can be requested via Web sites (with nominal charges for postage). An extensive list of health-related organizational Web addresses is provided at the end of this chapter. The FCN should become familiar with these important resources.

Referrals

As discussed in-depth in Chapter 2, the role of the FCN as referral agent is strongly supported by the research literature. Referral is the process of directing a patient to another source of information, assistance, or service. Clark (2003) states that four considerations enter into a decision to refer a patient to a particular provider, agency, or service:

- Acceptability of the referral to the client.
- Client eligibility for service.
- Situational constraints.
- Availability of resources.

The first and most important consideration in making a referral is the acceptability of the referral to the client. If the client is unwilling to use the resource, the other considerations are not of consequence. Some clients may be unwilling to accept assistance that they perceive as "charity." Other clients may have philosophical or religious differences from those of the referral source. Other barriers to acceptability may include fear of a new provider, prior negative experiences, lack of faith in the referral source, failure to acknowledge a problem requiring referral, and/or concerns about costs.

The second consideration is client eligibility for the service to be provided. Eligibility may be based on age, income level, residency requirements, citizenship, membership in a particular group, or the presence of a specific physical condition.

The presence of situational constraints, or factors in the client situation that would prevent follow-through on the referral, is the third consideration. These constraints might include a lack of transportation, the need for an interpreter, or a lack of funds. The FCN should assess the client situation and take action to eliminate or minimize situational constraints.

The last consideration is the availability (and accessibility) of resources. The FCN who has conducted a community assessment will have the benefit of the resource file developed as a part of this process. The resource file will provide the FCN with information about the types of services that a referral source provides, the criteria for eligibility for services, telephone numbers and addresses, whether a fee is involved and what forms of insurance are honored, and the name of a contact person in the setting. Some agencies require a physician's referral before service can be provided. Dunkle (2000) states that when FCNs identify a need for which a resource does not exist, they are likely to establish one! For example, to help parishioners deal with the effects of chronic illness, an FCN established "healing services."

To be an effective referral agent, the FCN must have excellent assessment skills, be knowledgeable about community resources and how to access them, and understand the culture and values of the faith community. Client assessments may be formal and planned, such as when making home visits, or they may occur unexpectedly in a casual encounter, such as at a post-worship coffee hour. In addition to knowing where and how to refer patients, the FCN needs to have the ability to recognize the factors that promote or hinder people from being receptive to referrals and to assist people to make their own informed decisions regarding the use of community services. Finally, the FCN needs to follow up with patients that have been referred to find out whether the services were effective in meeting the patient's needs.

Ward-Collins (2000) states that values are developed in a three-phase process of choosing, prizing, and acting. *Choosing* is a cognitive process that involves thinking and logic after receiving information. *Prizing* is an affective process that involves an emotional expression of values. She states that once values are received, accepted, and cherished, they become a source of positive self-esteem and willingness to affirm the choice. *Acting* is the behavioral component of valuing. After values are chosen, they are prized and acted upon in a consistent manner. Value systems govern how people conduct themselves, make decisions, and serve as filters for governing how information is taken in or excluded (p. 34).

Advocacy

Another faith community nursing role that is strongly supported by the research literature is that of advocate. Kohnke (1982) defined the classic process of advocacy as including informing, supporting, and affirming. Fundamentally, advocacy entails advising patients of their rights, providing information so patients can make informed decisions, and then supporting those decisions (Mallik, 1997). Advocacy also includes helping patients to clarify their values and make decisions that are compatible with their worldview, thus helping patients to maintain their personal integrity (Liaschenko, 1995). Because illness experiences may cause patients to question values and beliefs, the nurse helps the client to sort out uncertainty by listening, providing information, and by affirming the patient's experience.

The ANA *Code of Ethics* (2001) describes advocacy in broad terms as a commitment to "the health, well being, and safety of the patient across the life span and in all settings. . . . This includes not only those acts that prevent, promote, maintain, and restore health but also those acts that alleviate suffering and promote a peaceful, comfortable and dignified death" (p. 9).

In the advocate role, the FCN works to provide information and resources that are in the best interests of the faith community from a mind-body-spirit wellness perspective. FCNs advocate for patients when they listen to them and affirm and support the informed decisions that the patient makes. At other times, the FCN may have to step in and be the voice, when the patient is unable or unwilling to speak for himself or herself. As with the referral agent role, the nurse advocate must understand the culture and values of the faith community so that he or she can communicate from the same frame of reference. Advocacy also has a mentoring function, and the FCN can assist clients to use the health care system effectively and advantageously.

The idea of patient advocacy is built on the assumption that patients have certain rights, and health care providers have a duty to ensure that those rights are honored (Mallik, 1997). Liaschenko (1995) says that the moral significance of patient advocacy lies in three linked concerns. When a patient's health status suggests a possible loss of quality of life as a result of an illness, he or she deserves a knowledgeable advocate to help restore health or prevent further decline. A second concern comes from the vulnerability of all people to illness and death. The nurse is connected with clients through this shared vulnerability. Societal expectations of health care providers are that they will help those whose health is threatened. The inequality of power between the advocate and patient is a third moral element of advocacy. The advocate's power resides in his or her knowledge, role, health, and affiliation with the institution to which the patient has come for help. Liaschenko states: "The power to act for others in such conditions (illness) is an occasion not only for compassion and nobility of spirit, but also for evil in the form of abuse of power" (p. 3). The advocate is challenged to act on behalf of the patient, not the health care system.

Schroeder and Gadow (2000) view advocacy as a practical partnership between a professional who has expertise to offer and a patient who is experiencing ambiguity inherently associated with significant health concerns. Ward-Collins (2000) states that advocacy emphasizes mutuality, facilitation, protection, and coordination. It involves the active support of autonomy, beneficence, and human dignity, with an understanding and sensitivity to cultural and generational differences.

Hood and Leddy (2003) state that concept of "mutuality means that the nurse and the client together fully describe the client's health situation, agreeing on the direction and nature of change that the client would like to make, explore alternative ways to achieve mutually agreed-upon goals, and work together as the client implements the changes" (p. 511). The advocate makes sure that technical and informational supports are provided and assists the client in accessing health services. The essential elements of mutuality are respect, shared authority, empathy, and a focus on the client's strengths.

BOX 7-3
Comparison of the Nursing Process and the Advocacy Process

NURSING PROCESS	ADVOCACY PROCESS
Assessment/ diagnosis	Information exchange
	Gather data
	Illuminate data
Planning/outcome	Generate alternatives and consequences
	Prioritize actions
Implementation	Decision making
	Support of client
	Assure
	Reassure
Evaluation	Affirmation
	Evaluation
	Reformulation

From Cary, A. H. (2004). Case management. In M. Stanhope and J. Lancaster (Eds.), *Community and public health nursing* (6th ed., p. 459). St. Louis, MO: Mosby.

BOX 7-4
Ethical Principles for Effective Advocacy

1. Act in the patient's best interests.
2. Act in accordance with the patient's wishes and instructions.
3. Keep the patient properly informed.
4. Carry out instructions with diligence and competence.
5. Act impartially and offer frank, independent advice.
6. Maintain patient confidentiality.

From Bateman, N. (2000). *Advocacy skills for health and social care professionals* (p. 63). Philadelphia: Jessica Kingsley.

Snowball (1996) suggests that emphasis on facilitation in the advocacy process requires that the nurse take the responsibility to see that the patient has all of the information necessary to make informed decisions and to support the decisions that are made. Cary (2004) compares the nursing process with the advocacy process (Box 7-3).

Hood and Leddy (2003) identify 12 duties of the nurse serving as advocate. Many of the duties are appropriate to the nurse functioning in an acute care setting. The duties that can be applied to faith community nursing include:

(Interaction with the patient in a manner and quantity that permits)

- Exploration of the patient's personal responses to health or threats to health.
- Evaluation of the environmental circumstances in which the patient exists.
- Identification of strengths and limitations.
- Identification of resources perceived to be needed.
- Clear allocation of responsibilities of patient and nurse, which ensures the patient's assumption of responsibility for health and the nurse's responsibility for the informational and interactional supports needed (p. 514).

Chafey, Rhea, Shannon, and Spencer (1998) suggest that certain traits enhance patient advocacy. They include assertiveness, persistence, ethical awareness, empathy, and nurturance. Bateman (2000) identifies six core skills of advocacy. They include: interviewing, assertiveness and force, negotiation, self-management, legal knowledge and research, and litigation. He places these core skills within the context of six ethical principles for effective advocacy presented in Box 7-4.

Cooper (2001) says that it is easy to advocate for a patient whose values are in concert with those of the nurse. Advocacy is much more challenging when patient values differ from those of the nurse. In such situations, the moral requirement is to recognize that a conflict in values may threaten compassionate care. With this awareness, it is the nurse's responsibility to either provide competent, compassionate care or find another nurse who is willing to do so. The case study presents a situation in which the FCN assists the patient to clarify values before she serves as an advocate and a referral agent.

Although the health educator role is a designated faith community nursing role, it also accomplishes an advocacy function by providing advocating for primary prevention in the form of health promotion.

Summary

This chapter explored community connections and faith community nursing. Definitions of collaboration and strategies for successful collaboration were presented. Collaborations with patients, colleagues, institutions and agencies, and organizations were discussed. The FCN roles of referral agent and advocate were discussed in-depth.

Reflect and Discuss

Your faith community would like to run a health fair with both health promotion activities and health screenings.
1. How might your faith community collaborate with a community-based agency to implement this project?
2. What common goals or outcomes can you identify?
3. What barriers exist that might affect successful collaboration?
4. What are the benefits of a "limited domain" partnership?
5. How might such an event be evaluated?

Case Study

Marion Brown has been the FCN at Prince of Peace Christian Church for 4 years. A strategy that she has found to be helpful to her congregation is to have walk-in office hours on Thursday afternoons. Every few weeks Ellen Mayer stops by to discuss her mother's deteriorating condition with Marion. Ellen has been caring for her mother, an Alzheimer's patient, in her own home for the past 18 months. Previously, Marion had referred the family to home health services and an Alzheimer's disease support group. Currently, Ellen has respite assistance 2 afternoons each week.

This particular week, Ellen is particularly distressed. She shares that her teenage daughters are becoming less accepting of their grandmother's condition and the impact caregiving is having on the family. The teens are reacting by testing limits and staying out of the home as much as possible. Ellen becomes tearful, and the stress of caregiving and dealing with her teens is becoming impossible. She says that it might be time to consider a nursing home placement for her mother. She talks about how good her mother was to her and to her family when she was well, and how guilty she would feel if she put her mother in a nursing home. Although Marion had actually suggested nursing home placement many months ago, she listened carefully to Ellen's comments, reflecting back her words for clarification as needed. Marion discussed the mother-daughter-granddaughter relationship and its rights and responsibilities with Ellen. Together they explored what a nursing home placement for her mother might mean to that relationship. Marion suggested that she and Ellen pray together for the family.

Two weeks later, Ellen shared with Marion that she was ready to begin to make nursing home placement arrangements for her mother. She had prayed on the situation and discussed it with her daughters. At this point, Ellen has decided that although she will feel guilty pursuing the placement, the effect that the in-home caregiving is having on her own daughters is creating even more guilt and concern. Marion tells Ellen that she will assist her in choosing an appropriate facility for her mother and that she will be available to her through the placement process.

References

American Association of Colleges of Nursing. (1995). *The essentials of master's education for advanced practice nursing*. Washington, DC: American Association of Colleges of Nursing.

American Nurses Association (ANA). (2001). *Code of ethics with interpretive statements*. Washington, DC: American Nurses Association.

American Nurses Association (ANA). (2003). *Nursing's social policy statement* (2nd ed.). Washington, DC: American Nurses Association.

American Nurses Association and Health Ministries Association. (2005). *Faith community nursing: Scope and standards of practice*. Silver Springs, MD: American Nurses Association. Washington, DC: American Nurses Publishing.

Ammerman, N. T. (2004). *Pillars of faith: American congregations and their partners serving God and serving the world*. New Brunswick, NJ: Rutgers University Press.

Archangelo, V., Fitzgerald, M., Carroll, D., & Plumb, J. (1996). Collaborative care between nurse practitioners and primary care physicians. *Primary Care, 23*(1), 103–113.

Bateman, N. (2000). *Advocacy skills for health and social care professionals*. Philadelphia: Jessica Kingsley.

Brudenell, I. (2003). Parish nursing: Nurturing body, mind, spirit, and community. *Public Health Nursing, 20*(3), 85–94.

Cary, A. H. (2004). Case management. In M. Stanhope & J. Lancaster (Eds.), *Community and public health nursing* (6th ed.). St. Louis, MO: Mosby.

Centers for Medicare and Medicaid, 2002 data compendium. Available online at: http://www.cms.gov.researchers/pubs/datacompendium/

Chafey, K., Rhea, M., Shannon, A. M., & Spencer, S. (1998). Characterizations of advocacy by practicing nurses. *Journal of Professional Nursing, 14*(1), 43–52.

Chase-Ziolek, M., & Iris, M. (2002). Nurses' perspectives on the distinctive aspects of providing nursing care in a congregational setting. *Journal of Community Health Nursing, 19*(3), 173–186.

Clark, M. B. (2000). Nurses and faith community leaders growing in partnerships. In M. B. Clark & J. K. Olson (Eds.), *Nursing within a faith community: Promoting health in times of transition*. Thousand Oaks, CA: Sage Publications.

Clark, M. J. (2003). *Community health nursing: Caring for populations* (4th ed.). Upper Saddle River, NJ: Prentice Hall.

Cooper, C. (2001). *The art of nursing: A practical introduction*. Philadelphia: WB Saunders.

Davies, B., & Hughes, A. M. (1995). Clarification of advanced nursing practice: Characteristics and competencies. *Clinical Nurse Specialist, 9,* 156–160.

Dunkle, R. M. (2000). In R. Hunt (Ed.), *Readings in community-based nursing*. Philadelphia: Lippincott.

Gunderson, G. (1997). *Deeply woven roots: Improving the quality of life in your community*. Minneapolis, MN: Fortress Press.

Hahn, K., Radde, J. M., & Fellers, J. E. (2001). Spiritual care: Bridging the disciplines in congregational health ministries. *Journal of Health Care Chaplaincy, 11*(2), 49–61.

Hamric, A., Spross, J., & Hanson, C. (2000). *Advanced nursing practice: An integrative approach* (2nd ed.). Philadelphia: WB Saunders.

Hanson, C. M. & Spross, J. A. (2005). Collaboration. In A. B. Hamric, J. A. Spross, & C. M. Hanson, *Advanced practice nursing: An integrative approach* (3rd ed.). St. Louis: Elsevier Saunders.

Hood, L. J., & Leddy, S. K. (2003). *Conceptual bases of professional nursing* (5th ed.). Philadelphia: Lippincott Williams & Wilkins.

Howe, J., Cassel, C., & Vezina, M. (1998). Structuring the GITT didactic experience. In E. Siegler, K. Hyer, T. Fulmer, & M. Mezey (Eds.), *Geriatric interdisciplinary team training* (p. 90). New York: Springer.

Kohnke, M. F. (1982). *Advocacy risk and reality*. St. Louis, MO: Mosby.

Liaschenko, J. (1995). Ethics in the work of acting for patients. *Advances in Nursing Science, 18*(2), 1–12.

Mallik, M. (1997). Advocacy in nursing—a review of the literature. *Journal of Advanced Nursing, 25,* 130–138.

Merriam-Webster. (1983). *Webster's Ninth New Collegiate Dictionary.* Springfield, MA: Merriam-Webster.

National Council on State Boards of Nursing. (1993). *Position paper on the regulation of advanced nursing practice.* Chicago: National Council on State Boards of Nursing.

National Organization of Nurse Practitioner Faculties. (1995). *Advanced nursing practice curriculum guideline and program standards for nurse practitioner education.* Washington, DC: National Organization of Nurse Practitioner Faculties.

Olson, J. K. (2000). Functions of the nurse as health promoter in a faith community. In M. B. Clark & J. K. Olson (Eds.), *Nursing in a faith community: Promoting health in times of transition.* Thousand Oaks, CA: Sage Publications.

Patterson, D. L. (2003). *The essential parish nurse: ABCs for congregational health ministry.* Cleveland, OH: Pilgrim Press.

Paul VI. (1964). *Paths of the church.* Boston: Daughters of St. Paul.

Schroeder, C., & Gadow, G. (2000). An advocacy approach to ethics and community health. In E. Anderson & J. McFarlane (Eds.), *Community as partner: Theory and practice in nursing* (3rd ed., p. 78). Philadelphia: Lippincott Williams & Wilkins.

Schumann, R., & VanDuivendyk, T. (2001). Connections, collisions, and complementarity: The dynamics of health care chaplain, parish nurse and parish clergy collaboration. *Journal of Health Care Chaplaincy, 11*(2), 61–67.

Smith, S. D. (2003). *Parish nursing: A handbook for the new millenium.* New York: The Haworth Press.

Smith, T. D., & Vezina, M. L. (2004). Mediated roles: Working through other people. In L. A. Joel (Ed.), *Advanced practice nursing: Essentials for role development.* Philadelphia: FA Davis.

Snowball, J. (1996). Asking nurses about advocating for patients: "Reactive" and "proactive" accounts. *Journal of Advanced Nursing, 24,* 67–75.

Strumpf, N., & Whitney, F. (1994). Teaching collaborative skills to nurse practitioner students. In E. Siegler & F. Whitney (Eds.), *Nurse-physician collaboration.* New York: Springer.

Sullivan, T. J. (1998). Concept analysis of collaboration: Part 1. In T. J. Sullivan (Ed.), *Collaboration: A health care imperative* (pp. 3–42). New York: McGraw-Hill.

Ward-Collins, D. (2000). "Noncompliant." Isn't there a better way to say it? In R. Hunt (Ed.), *Readings in community-based nursing.* Philadelphia: Lippincott.

Wuthnow, R. (2004). *Saving America: Faith-based services and the future of civil society.* Princeton, NJ: Princeton University Press.

Additional Related Resources

Ammerman, N. T. (1997). *Congregation and community.* New Brunswick, NJ: Rutgers University Press.

Cary, A. (1998). Advocacy or allocation. *Nursing Connections, 11*(1), 1–4.

Chaves, M. (2004). *Congregations in America.* Cambridge, MA: Harvard University Press.

Christoffel, K. K. (2000). Public health advocacy: Process and product. *American Journal of Public Health, 90*(5), 722–723.

Foley, B. J., Minick, M. P., & Kee, C. C. (2002a). How nurses learn advocacy. *Journal of Nursing Scholarship, 34*(2), 181–187.

Foley, B. J., Minick, M. P., & Kee, C. C. (2002b). Nursing advocacy during a military operation. *Western Journal of Nursing Research, 22*(4), 492–498.

Geoffrey, M. (1998). Ritual action and its effect on the role of the nurse as advocate. *Journal of Advanced Nursing, 27*(1), 189.

Green, J. C., & Sherman, A. L. (2002). *Fruitful collaborations: A survey of government-funded faith-based programs in 15 states.* Washington, DC: Hudson Institute.

Hewitt, J. A. (2002). Critical review of the arguments debating the role of the nurse advocate. *Journal of Advanced Nursing, 37*(5), 439.

Mallik, M., & Rafferty, A. M. (2000). Diffusion of the concept of patient advocacy. *Journal of Nursing Scholarship, 32*(4), 399.

Mitchell, G., & Bournes, D. (2000). Nurse as patient advocate? In search of straight thinking. *Nursing Science Quarterly, 13*(3), 204.

Sullivan, T. J. (1998). *Collaboration: A health care imperative.* New York: McGraw-Hill.

Willard, C. (1996). The nurse's role as patient advocate: Obligation or imposition? *Journal of Advanced Nursing, 24,* 60–68.

Wuthnow, R., & Evans, J. H. (2002). *The quiet hand of God: Faith-based activism and the public role of mainline Protestantism.* Berkeley, CA: University of California Press.

→ Web Resources

http://www.Alcoholics-anonymous.org   Alcoholics Anonymous

http://www.alz.org   Alzheimer's Association

http://www.aanma.org   Allergy and Asthma Network

http://www.aap.org   American Academy of Pediatrics

http://www.aacvpr.org   American Association of Cardiovascular & Pulmonary Rehabilitation

http://www.aadenet.org   American Association of Diabetes Educators

http://www.aarp.org   American Association of Retired Persons

http://www.cancer,org   American Cancer Society

http://www.diabetes.org   American Diabetes Association

http://www.eatright   American Dietetic Association

http://www.americanheart.org   American Heart Association

http://www.lungusa.org   American Lung Association

http://www.apha.org   American Public Health Association

http://www.redcross.org   American Red Cross

http://www.arthritisconnection.com   Arthritis Connection

http://www.arthritis.org   Arthritis Foundation

http://www.goaskalice.colombia.ed/Cat8.html   Ask Alice about Relationships

http://www.best4health.com   Best Practice Network

http://www.bazelon.org   Bazelon Center for Mental Health Law

http://www.cancerfacts.com   Cancer Facts

http://www.cancernet.nci.nih.gov   Cancer Net

http://www.cdc.gov   Centers for Disease Control and Prevention

http://www.patientadvocacy.org

http://www.sanhsa.gov   Center for Substance Abuse Prevention and Treatment

http://www.childbirth.org   Childbirth

http://www.chronicillnet.org   Chronic Illness

http://www.smartmarriages.com   Coalition for Marriage, Family, and Couples

http://www.susanlovemd.com   Dr. Susan Love's Breast Cancer Site

http://www.epa.gov   Environmental Protection Agency

http://www.efa.org   Epilepsy Foundation

http://www.florenceproject.org   Florence Project: The Heartbeat of Health Advocacy

http://www.fda.gov   Food and Drug Administration

http://www.healthfinder.gov   Healthfinder

http://www.healthypeople.gov   Healthy People 2010

http://www.nahc.org   National Association of Home Care

http://www.hospicefoundation.org   Hospice Foundation of America

http://www.immunize.org   Immunization Action Coalition

http://www.effo.org   International Osteoporosis Foundation

http://www.jdfcure.org   Juvenile Diabetes Foundation International

http://www.lalacheleague.org   La Leche League

http://www.lupus.org   Lupus Foundation of America

http://www.lymenet.org   Lyme Disease Network

http://www.modimes.org   March of Dimes

http://www.mayohealth.org   Mayo Clinic Health Oasis

http://www.mentalhelp.net   Mental Health Net

http://www.mindbody.harvard.edu   Mind-Body Institute

http://www.mmwrq@cdc.gov   Morbidity & Mortality Weekly Report

http://www.na.org   Narcotics Anonymous

http://www.nami.org   National Alliance for the Mentally Ill

http://www.health.org   National Clearinghouse for Alcohol and Drug Information (NCADI)

http://www.ncadd.org   National Council on Alcoholism and Drug Dependence, Inc.

http://www.nhic-nt.health.org   National Health Information Center (NHIC)

http://www.nhpco.orh   National Hospice and Palliative Care Organization

http://www.niaid.nih.gov/   National Institute of Allergy and Infectious Diseases

http://www.nih.gov/ninr/   National Institute of Nursing Research

http://www.nlm.nih.gov   National Library of Medicine

http://www.nmha.org   National Mental Health Association

http://www.nof.org   National Osteoporosis Foundation

http://www.rosacea.org   National Rosacea Society

http://www.sleepfoundation.org   National Sleep Foundation

http://www.stroke.org   National Stroke Association

http://www.womenshealthnetwork.org   National Women's Health Network

http://www.oncolink.upenn.edu   OncoLink

http://www.pharminfo.com   Pharmaceutical Information Network

http://www.plannedparenthood.org   Planned Parenthood Federation

http://www.pluralism.org   Pluralism Project

http://www.geocities.com/Athens/1501/sheckfil.html   Under Shekina's Wings

http://www.usda   USDA Guidelines

http://www.dhhs.gov   U.S. Department of Health and Human Services

http://www.vnaa.org   Visiting Nurse Association of America

III

Issues in Faith Community Nursing Practice

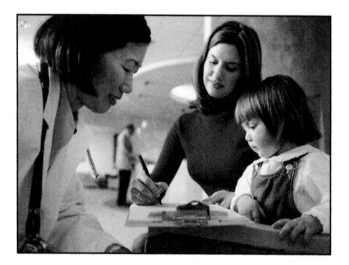

8

Legal Aspects of Faith Community Nursing Practice

T his chapter addresses the legal aspects of faith community nursing practice. At this point in time, no faith community nurse (FCN) has been sued for negligence in practice. However, the FCN is bound to the same legal requirements as nurses practicing in any other settings. Elements of those requirements, including accountability, nurse practice acts and standards of practice, confidentiality and privacy, and documentation, will be addressed as they relate to faith community nursing practice. Specific legal issues relating to faith community nursing will also be addressed.

Accountability and Faith Community Nursing Practice

To be *accountable* is to be answerable for one's professional judgment and actions within a realm of authority (Turnock, 2001). In the congregational setting, the FCN's position description addresses his or her accountability by clearly describing the duties, responsibilities, and expectations of the position. The position description should clearly state *to whom* (in addition to God) the FCN is accountable. It should also describe the types and frequency of reporting methods. For example, the FCN might be expected to provide the pastor, health ministry team, and the congregation with formal quarterly (or semiannual) reports indicating the number and types of nursing services provided during that time period. Several documents address the accountability for practice of the professional nurse. Nurse practice acts (NPAs) describe the educational preparation required for professional nursing and licensure requirements, and they define the legal scope of professional nursing practice. Nurse practice acts are specific to the state or territory where the professional practice is delivered. All FCNs should hold an active RN license (in the state of practice), and this requirement should be included in the position description. All FCNs should be familiar with their state's nurse practice act and with the state board's rules and regulations, because these documents define the scope of nursing practice. Exceeding the limits defined in these documents invites legal action. All state boards of nursing maintain Web sites, where changes to practice acts and to rules and regulations are routinely posted.

Standards of care set minimum criteria for job proficiency, which enable both the nurse and others to judge the quality of care provided. Although standards of care are guidelines, not laws, they are legally significant because they provide the standard a nurse would be held to in a court of law. *Nursing: Scope and Standards of Practice* (ANA, 2004) outlines the expectations of the professional nurse role. The authority for the practice of nursing is based on a social contract that recognizes the professional rights and responsibilities of nursing and includes methods of public accountability. *Nursing's Social Policy Statement* (ANA, 2003) discusses the profession's relationship with society and its obligation to those who receive nursing care. FCNs also practice professional nursing in accordance with *Faith Community Nursing: Scope and Standards of Practice* (American Nurses Association and Health Ministries Association [ANA-HMA],

2005). As discussed in Chapter 1, this document describes the scope and standards of the nursing specialty of faith community nursing practice.

FCNs directly serve individuals and families; they serve the congregation-as-population, the nursing profession, and other colleagues; and, if in a paid capacity, they serve the employer. FCNs are accountable to all of the populations receiving nursing services. According to McDermott (1999), program accountability includes various elements. These elements are as follows:

- Record keeping
- Data collection
- Documentation
- Confidentiality
- Performance evaluation
- Annual reports
- Satisfaction surveys
- Peer-reviewed chart audits
- Quality assurance

Smith (2003) suggests that FCNs increase their program accountability by developing written policies. Policies regarding the definition of a congregant and who is eligible for services clarify who the recipient of service will be. Written policies regarding documentation, confidentiality, scope of practice, medical emergencies in the home, death in the home, safety of the FCN, and policies regarding infectious disease provide both program structure and consistency. Such policies should go through the established channels for congregational approval (and employer approval, if applicable), and they should be reviewed annually.

Legal Bases of Practice

Professional Practice: State Nurse Practice Act

The legal foundation for professional nursing practice is the state nurse practice act (NPA). Although each NPA is unique to its state or territory, most contain similar provisions. NPAs generally include (a) a scope; (b) a purpose and definitions; (c) a description of the compositions of the members of the Board of Nursing; (d) powers and responsibilities of the board members; (e) requirements for initial licensure and license renewal; (f) licensee responsibilities; (g) protected terms, titles, and abbreviations; (h) an approval process to be followed by schools of nursing; (i) a section identifying violations and penalties; (j) a process and grounds for taking disciplinary action; (k) a provision granting the board the authority to seek emergency relief; (l) sections identifying individuals and entities obligated to report practice act violations to the board; (m) exemptions, revenues, fees, and fines; (n) a grandfathering and severability clause; and (o) a provision for repeal of portions of the NPA (Monarch, 2002). Some NPAs have stipulations regarding moral character, good physical and mental health, a minimum age, and/or fluency in English.

In almost every state, the board members are appointed by the governor from a list provided by the state's nurses association. State boards of nursing usually have the authority to create regulations related to the NPA; to delineate the tasks that nurses are permitted to carry out, either independently or in collaboration with a physician; and to establish criteria and administrative processes for disciplinary actions. For example, a nurse who practices while under the influence of alcohol or drugs may have his or her license suspended or revoked pending treatment.

Nurse practice acts discuss the scope of practice in broad terms that do not provide specific guidelines for nursing practice, which is done intentionally so as not to limit nurses to certain activities. It would be literally impossible to enact a new nurse practice act every time a new medical technology is presented. The state boards of nursing are authorized to create, revise, and enforce administrative rules and regulations that explain NPA provisions so that the profession is properly regulated and the public is protected (Monarch, 2002).

The National Council of State Boards of Nursing (NCSBN) is an organization composed of two representatives from each member board. This organization develops and administers the National Council Licensure Examination (NCLEX), maintains licensure and examination statistics, and maintains a national disciplinary data bank. Both the NCSBN and the American Nurses Association (ANA) have published Model Practice Acts (MPAs).

Violations

According to Monarch (2002), many states relegate their violations section of the NPA to one sentence, declaring that violations of the practice act constitute a misdemeanor and are punishable by a fine. The rules and regulations created by the Board of Nursing contain a more specific list of penalties that can be invoked when disciplinary action is taken. The NCSBN encourages member boards to address violations specifically and in detail. Their Model Practice Act states that no person shall:

- Engage in the practice of nursing without a valid license.
- Practice nursing based on illegally or fraudulently obtained diploma, license, or other record.
- Practice nursing while his or her license is suspended, revoked, surrendered, inactive, or lapsed.
- In any way imply that he or she is a nurse unless he or she is duly licensed as an LPN/LVN, RN, or APRN.
- Fraudulently get or supply someone else a license by or for money or for anything of value.
- Knowingly employ unlicensed persons to practice nursing.
- Fail to report conduct that violates the NPA.
- Open a nursing education program without first having the program approved by the Board of Nursing.
- Otherwise violate the NPA or aid or abet anyone else to violate any provisions of the NPA.

Although the Model Practice Act published by the ANA does not identify a list of NPA violations, it does identify 10 sanctions that are available to the Board of Nursing. They include denying, suspending, and revoking a nursing license; imposing fines; requiring attendance at remedial programs; and issuing cease and desist orders.

Keeping Informed About Laws

Public health law consists of all legislation, regulations, and court decisions enacted by federal, state, and local governments to protect the health of the public. Because laws have important implications for faith community nursing practice, nurses need to be informed. Several sources provide information about laws that affect nursing practice: written health codes and local or state department health policies; law schools and legal aid services; and professional associations and public advocacy groups. The references at the end of this chapter provide additional resources for learning about public health laws.

Professional Liability

Austin, Brooks, Glenn, Guido, Keepnews, and Michael (2004) note that, historically, courts have held nurses who work in alternative settings to the same standards as those who work in hospital settings. The authors note that more nurses are being named in lawsuits as a result of the following reasons:

- Clients are more knowledgeable about health care, and their expectations are higher.
- The health care system is more reliant on nurses and nonphysician providers to help contain costs.
- Nurses are more autonomous in their practice.
- The courts are expanding the definition of liability and hold all types of medical professionals to higher standards of accountability.

Liability of the Volunteer Faith Community Nurse

Green (2001) discusses the nurse's liability when functioning in a volunteer capacity. She states that "the current state of the law suggests that if professional nurses render professional nursing services to a person, even though on a free-of-charge and volunteer basis, they could be held professionally liable for negligence. Nurses must be aware that, even with a charitable intent, volunteer nursing activities can involve professional liability" (p. 408). Professional liability coverage provided to nurses by employers provides coverage in the job setting only, so nurses providing services on a volunteer basis need to have liability insurance that will cover them in those circumstances. Good Samaritan Acts protect health care professionals from civil liability only when rendering emergency care outside of a health care facility (Monarch, 2002).

Austin et al. (2004) elaborate that as a nurse, one's responsibilities do not change when that person is donating nursing services, but one's legal status does; it becomes less defined than when a nurse is compensated. In most states, nurse practice acts specify only the legal limits of paid nursing practice. This, however, does not mean that the volunteer nurse is exempt from a lawsuit. A volunteer FCN would, in fact, be held to the standards of the nurse practice act in a court of law. Box 8-1 presents information on minimizing one's liability when volunteering.

Negligence and Malpractice

Patient falls and drug errors, as a result of negligence, are the two most common causes of lawsuits against nurses. Other causes include operating room errors, communication breakdowns, inadequate observation or assessment of patients leading to a delay in diagnosis and treatment and resultant negative outcome(s), and failure to know and follow agency policy, resulting in patient injury (Austin et al., 2004). The only one of these areas of negligence that would pertain to faith community nursing practice is inadequate assessment leading to a negative outcome.

Negligence is the failure to exercise the degree of care that a reasonable person of ordinary prudence would exercise under the same circumstances. A claim of negligence requires that there be a duty owed by one person to another, that the duty be breached, and that the breach results in injury or damage. For example, nurses have a duty to preserve patient privacy, so a failure to do this would constitute negligent behavior on the part of the nurse. To meet the other requirements of negligence, the plaintiff would have to be damaged in some way by the disclosure.

Malpractice is defined as a violation of professional duty or failure to meet a standard of care, or failure to use skills and knowledge that other nurses would use in similar circumstances (Austin et al., 2004, p. 130). Hall and Hall (2001) identified common areas of nursing malpractice that include the following:

- Unsafe environment
- Inadequate assessment
- Failure to follow physician's orders or established protocol
- Medication or treatment errors
- Defective technology or products
- Inadequate infection control
- Poor communication

Because FCNs generally do not engage in nursing actions that involve hands-on nursing care or medication administration, their malpractice liability is less than that of an acute care nurse. However, any time that a nurse provides a client with information about his or her care or treatment, it is considered to be client teaching. Client teaching can be formal or informal. Most NPAs contain wording about health promotion activities, and the faith community nursing scope and standards document addresses the health teaching and health promotion activities of the FCN.

Liability Insurance

All FCNs should carry personal liability insurance and should be covered under the congregation's liability policy as well. To help one assess professional liability insurance needs, find out the degree of protection the FCN is entitled to under the congregational policy and, if applicable, the liability policy of the employing health care facility, one should obtain and review a copy of the policy. Individual liability insurance policies for nurses are readily available and affordable. Box 8-2 describes how to choose liability insurance coverage.

Confidentiality and the Right to Privacy

The *ANA Code of Ethics for Nurses* states that nurses must safeguard the client's right to privacy (2001). Maintaining confidentiality is essential to preserving the trust necessary to be an effective FCN. The ethical principles of *autonomy* and *fidelity* support the concept of confidentiality. Autonomy includes the client's right to maintain control over his or her life and personal information. Fidelity refers to one's faithfulness to agreements.

BOX 8-2
How to Choose Liability Insurance

To find professional liability insurance that fits your needs, compare the coverage of a number of different policies. Make sure the policy provides coverage for in-court and out-of-court malpractice suits and expenses and for defense of a complaint or disciplinary action made to or by a board of nursing. Understanding insurance policy basics will make you a more knowledgeable consumer. If you already have professional liability insurance, the information below may help you better evaluate your coverage.

TYPE OF COVERAGE

Ask your insurance agent whether the policy covers only claims made before the policy expires (claims-made coverage) or whether it covers any negligent act committed during the policy period, regardless of when it is reported (occurrence coverage). Keep in mind that the latter type offers better coverage.

COVERAGE LIMITS

All malpractice insurance policies cover professional liability. Some also cover representation before a board of nursing, general personal liability, medical payments, assault-related bodily injury, and property damage.

The amount of coverage varies, as does the premium. Faith community nurses should carry liability coverage in the amount of at least $1,000,000/3,000,000. This means that the maximum amount that can be paid is 1 million dollars per claim, and the number of claims that can be paid at that amount in 1 year is three. Organizations, such as the ANA, offer group plans at attractive premiums. Remember that professional liability coverage is limited to acts and practice settings specified in the policy. Be sure the policy covers your nursing role as a faith community nurse.

OPTIONS

Check whether the policy would provide coverage for these incidents:
- Negligence on the part of nurses under your supervision
- Misuse of equipment
- Errors in reporting/recording care
- Failure to properly teach clients
- Mistakes made while providing emergency care

DEFINITION OF TERMS

Definitions of terms can vary from policy to policy. If the policy includes restrictive definitions, there will not be coverage for actions outside these guidelines. For the best protection, seek the broadest definitions possible, and ask the insurance company for examples of actions that they have denied.

DURATION OF COVERAGE

Insurance is an annual contract that can be renewed or canceled each year. Most policies specify how they can be canceled—for example, in writing, either by the insured or the insurance company.

EXCLUSIONS

Ask the insurer about exclusions—areas not covered by the policy.

BOX 8-2
How to Choose Liability Insurance (continued)

OTHER INSURANCE CLAUSES

All professional liability insurance policies contain "other insurance" clauses that address payment obligations when a nurse is covered by more than one insurance policy, such as the employer's policy and the nurse's personal liability policy:

- The *pro rata* clause states that two or more policies in effect at the same time will pay any claims in accordance with a proportion established in the individual policies.
- The *in excess* clause states that the primary policy will pay all fees and damages up to its limits, at which point the second policy will pay additional fees or damages up to its limits.
- The *escape clause* relieves an insurance company of all liability for fees or damages, if another insurance policy is in effect at the same time.

Faith community nurses should be covered by the congregation's insurance policy, so be alert to "other insurance" clauses, and avoid purchasing a policy with an escape clause for liability.

ADDITIONAL TIPS

- Insurance applications are legal documents. If false information is given, it may void the policy.
- Be careful that the policy provides coverage for the faith community nurse role. If the faith community nurse is serving as a volunteer, check to be sure that the policy covers donated nursing services.
- After selecting a policy that provides adequate insurance, stay with the same policy and insurer to avoid gaps in coverage that can occur when changing insurers.
- No insurance policy covers nurses for acts outside the scope of practice.
- Be prepared to uphold all obligations specified in the policy; failure to do so may void the policy and cause personal liability for any damages.
- Check out the insurance company by calling the state division of insurance to inquire about the company's financial stability.

Adapted from Austin, S., Brooks, P. S., Glenn, L. M., Guido, G. W., Keepnews, D. M., Michael, J. E., et al. (2004). *Nurse's legal handbook* (5th ed., pp. 146–147). Philadelphia: Lippincott Williams & Wilkins. Used with permission.

Austin et al. (2004) report that state courts have strongly protected a patient's right to have health information kept confidential. In court, the client is protected by the privilege doctrine. In privileged or protected relationships, such as physician and patient, communication occurring between the parties is protected, unless the person who benefits from the protection agrees to disclosure. State law determines which relationships are protected by the privilege doctrine; most states include husband–wife, lawyer–client, and physician–patient relationships. The states of New York, Arkansas, Oregon, and Vermont recognize the nurse–client relationship as protected.

Health Insurance Portability and Accountability Act

The Health Insurance Portability and Accountability Act (HIPAA) of 2003 protects the privacy, confidentiality, and security of medical information. Under HIPAA, only those who have a need to know patient information for the patient's care, and only those authorized by the patient, may have access to the medical record. HIPAA requires safeguards in faxing and electronic transmittal of client medical information. Although FCNs operating in congregational settings are not considered a "covered entity" under HIPAA regulations (because charges are not made for their services), prudence suggests that this standard of privacy be upheld. Oral communications that FCNs have with patients should not be shared with anyone, including the pastor or health ministry team members, without the expressed permission of the patient. A good rule of thumb is simply to ask the patient whether you may share the patient's health information with the pastor and, for example, whether the patient wants to be remembered by name in prayer during services. However, if in your professional judgment, there is a safety risk (such as when a patient verbalizes suicidal intent), you may share information without obtaining the patient's permission. Be sure to document this (Update on HIPAA, 2003).

Documentation and Faith Community Nursing Practice

The Patient Record

The patient record provides legal proof of the nature and quality of care received. Complete, accurate, and timely documentation:

- Reflects the care that the patient was given.
- Provides evidence of the nurse's legal responsibilities for the patient.
- Demonstrates standards, rules, regulations, and laws of nursing practice.
- Reflects consultation with and/or referral to other health care professionals.
- Reflects all patient education and an evaluation of the teaching/learning process.
- Furnishes data for various uses, such as outcomes assessment.
- Reflects case management, research, and quality improvement.

Parker (2004) states that documentation is important in faith community nursing to report to the congregation and to gain program support. Progress reports communicate the quality and quantity of work accomplished by the faith community nursing program as a ministry of the faith community. This type of reporting also communicates available services. Second, reporting enables the FCN and the church staff to evaluate the program, measuring its worth to the congregation and to the community. Reports establish a baseline for future planning and program development.

FCNs screen, assess, counsel, educate, and refer people in various settings. While maintaining confidentiality, the FCN must accurately document health-related findings, referrals, and outcomes of care. *Faith Community Nursing: Scope and Standards Practice* (ANA-HMA, 2005) states that the FCN "synthesizes and stores relevant data in a retrievable format that is both confidential and secure" (p. 11).

Documentation Structure

Several systems exist to give structure to documentation. In the traditional narrative format, the FCN documents ongoing assessment data, nursing interventions, and patient responses in chronologic order. Writing narrative notes is time-consuming and, at times, repetitive. The problem-oriented system uses the SOAP note format: **S** representing subjective client data; **O** for objective findings on observation, assessment, and examination; **A** for assessment of the subjective complaints and objective findings; and **P** for the plan, for both present and future care. Another method, called *focus charting,* makes the patient care problems the focus of concern. It may be a nursing diagnosis, a sign or symptom, a client behavior, a special need, or a change in the patient's condition. The focus is identified by reviewing the assessment data and then precisely documenting the focus. Yet other charting

---

BOX 8-3
Documentation Tips

HOW TO DOCUMENT
- Use the appropriate form, and document in ink.
- Record the patient's name on every page of the record.
- Document the care given in a timely manner.
- Include patient statements in quotations when significant.
- Be specific. Avoid general terms and vague expressions.
- Use standard abbreviations only.
- Use medical terminology correctly.
- Document symptoms using the patient's own words.
- Document objectively.

WHAT TO DOCUMENT
- Document all nursing actions taken in response to the patient's problem(s).
- Document patient responses to treatment or education.
- Document any protective measures taken.
- Document observations.
- Document all patient education and an evaluation of the teaching–learning process.
- Document titles of health literature given to the patient.
- Document referrals and follow-ups on outcomes of referrals.
- Write on every line. Place a line through empty space.
- Sign every entry.

Adapted from Austin, S., Brooks, P. S., Glenn, L. M., Guido, G. W., Keepnews, D. M., Michael, J. E., et al. (2004). *Nurse's legal handbook* (5th ed., p. 239). Philadelphia: Lippincott Williams & Wilkins. Used with permission.

---

method, PIE charting, groups information into three categories: **P**roblem, **I**ntervention, and **E**valuation. PIE charting integrates the plan into the nurse's notes, so a separate plan of care is not needed. The FCN keeps an assessment flow sheet and progress notes. FCNs should choose a documentation system with which they are comfortable. Documentation tips are provided in Box 8-3.

Documentation Storage

Congregational client records should be stored in a locked file cabinet or in a secure computer file. In most cases, if the FCN is employed by a health care agency, the agency legally owns the medical records. If the FCN is a direct employee of the congregation or a volunteer, the records belong to the congregation. Inactive client records must be stored for at least 10 years. Records on children must be kept until the child reaches the age of 21, and any records involved in litigation should be kept for 21 years (Update on HIPAA, 2004). Under HIPAA regulations, all clients have access to their records. The FCN should ask for a dated, signed statement showing that a copy of the record was shared with the client, and it is advisable to initial each page as it is copied, so that copies cannot be easily altered (Update on HIPAA).

Documentation in Practice

Parker (2004) studied volunteer FCNs' perceptions of their responsibility to document their activities as health care providers. Eighty-one FCNs participated in the study by completing questionnaires. Parker found that 88% indicated that they documented the services provided; 71% noted observations made in assessments; and 78% listed referrals to other health care professionals. Only 48% documented their follow-up on referrals. Surprisingly, only 50% provided a written report to the pastor, church staff, or church board. Thirty-four percent indicated that they *never* provide a written report to the church.

Parker voices concern over his findings and states that improvement is needed to be compliant with both state practice acts and the HMA-ANA standards of practice for faith community nursing practice. His study showed that the least frequent documentation was related to follow-up and outcomes of referrals to other health care providers. He cautions that FCNs need to recognize the importance of documentation regarding client follow-up in today's liability-conscious world (2004).

Green (2001) speaks to this issue as well. She also advises that when nurses are participating in screening activities, parameters should be set for referring persons with abnormal findings to a physician or to an emergency department. Nurses could be held potentially liable, if they do not provide appropriate follow-up and referral and have it documented.

Boss (2004) reports that the application of the *Faith Community Nursing: Scope and Standards of Practice* (HMA-ANA, 2005) varies from congregation to congregation, particularly in the volunteer model. She questions whether volunteer FCNs are violating professional boundaries by inconsistent behaviors, sacrificing principles, and letting the end justify the means. She strongly admonishes that the FCN is not retired from professional nursing and cannot pick and choose preferred nursing activities at the expense of legally required activities.

Legal Issues Related to Faith Community Nursing Practice

Patient's Bill of Rights

The concept of a formal document enumerating the rights of patients has been around since the late 1950s. Over the years, nursing, hospital, hospice, and legal organizations have crafted documents called "Patient's Bill of Rights." In 1973, Minnesota became the first state to enact a patient's bill of rights into law. Since that time, several other states have enacted patient's bill of rights legislation. Bills of rights that have become laws carry the greatest authority because they give the patient specific legal recourse. Bills of rights issued by organizations and institutions are not legally binding.

Presently, there is no national patient's bill of rights. National bills of patient rights have been proposed but have not been passed by Congress. Unfortunately, they have been a part of other health care bills that were not passed by both houses.

Informed Consent

Most nurses are familiar with the patient right of *informed consent*. Informed consent basically means that the patient or someone acting on the patient's behalf has enough information to know what the patient is risking if he or she decides to undergo a proposed treatment or surgery, what the expected outcome of the proposed treatment or surgery will be, and what the anticipated results of nonaction would be. Informed consent includes telling the patient about the available alternatives to the proposed treatment and the risks and dangers associated with each alternative. The patient must also be informed of the name and credentials of the person who will perform the procedure and, if others will assist, their names and qualifications. Patients have the right to refuse to consent or to change their minds after giving consent.

In the faith community nursing setting, informed consent is required prior to screening procedures. FCNs who provide flu immunizations are also required to provide the patient with information about the vaccine, allergies that contraindicate its use and possible side effects, to obtain the patient's informed consent.

Usually, the person giving consent for the care of a child under the age of 18 (minor) is a parent or other designated adult, but state laws do vary. Parental consent is required for most medical procedures in most states; however, under federal law, adolescents can be tested and treated for HIV without parental involvement. Some states permit minors to consent to contraceptive services, and parental consent is not always needed for a teen to seek prenatal care or for diagnosis and treatment of a sexually transmitted disease. Every state will allow an *emancipated minor (a minor who has legal independence from his or her parents),* to consent to his or her own medical care and treatment. Additionally, teenagers who are pregnant or have a child, are self-supporting, or are living apart from their parents, are considered independent in some states (Brooke, 2005).

Freedom of Religion

The courts usually uphold a patient's right to refuse medical treatment because of the constitutionally protected right to religious freedom. Jehovah's Witnesses oppose blood transfusions, based on their interpretation of a biblical passage that forbids "drinking" blood. Other religious freedom court cases involve Christian Scientists who oppose many medical interventions, including the use of medicines (Austin et al., 2004).

In most instances, the severity of illness dictates whether courts will overrule parental decisions. In life-threatening situations, the court is more likely to overrule a parent's religious objections to treatment (Austin et al., 2004).

Child Abuse, Domestic Violence, and Elder Abuse

Child abuse, domestic violence, and elder abuse are societal ills that cross all socioeconomic levels and all ethnic groups. In 1973, Congress passed the Child Abuse Prevention and Treatment Act. The act requires states to meet certain uniform standards to be eligible for federal assistance in child abuse programming, prevention, and treatment. The act also established a national center on child abuse and child neglect. The three most common features of state laws about child abuse are:

- Empowering of social agency welfare or law enforcement bureau to receive and investigate reports of actual or suspected abuse.
- Granting of legal immunity from liability, for defamation or invasion of privacy, to a person reporting an incident of actual or suspected abuse.
- Nullification of confidentiality, privacy, and privilege mandates that would otherwise be required of the nurse–client relationship.

All nurses are legally required to report suspected child abuse, and, in many states, failure to report actual or suspected child abuse is a crime. Nearly every state has laws mandating that suspected elder abuse be reported to authorities. However, not all states define elder abuse per se. As the elder population of America continues to grow in numbers, incidences of elder abuse will continue to increase. Laws regarding domestic violence are less clear. FCNs, however, should be alert to signs and symptoms of domestic violence and should be aware of community supports for shelter, counseling, emergency medical, and law enforcement.

Chapter 17 provides information about vulnerable populations, and the issues of abuse and domestic violence are further addressed.

Rights of Persons with Disabilities

The Americans with Disabilities Act (ADA) was signed into law in 1990 to protect the civil liberties of the many Americans living with disabilities. The ADA essentially prohibits discrimination on the basis of disability in employment, state, and local government, public accommodations, commercial facilities, transportation, and telecommunication. The definition of a disabled person used in application of the ADA is "a person who has a physical or mental impairment that substantially limits one or more major life activities, a person who has a history or record of such impairment, or a person who is perceived by others as having such impairment (U.S. Department of Justice, 2002, p. 2). The ADA sets the standard for several subsequent laws that expand protection for persons with disabilities. A guide to disability rights laws is available at http://www.usdoj.gov/crt/ada/cguide.htm. Chapter 17 provides additional information and resources about persons with disabilities.

Right to Die

Most states have enacted right-to-die laws, which recognize a patient's right to choose death by refusing extraordinary treatment, when there is no hope of recovery. Whenever a competent person expresses specific wishes, the health care providers should attempt to follow them. Written evidence of the patient's wishes provides the best indication of what treatment the client would consent to, if he or she were able to communicate. This information may be provided through

- A living will—an *advance directive* document that specifies a person's wishes with regard to medical care, if he or she were to become terminally ill, incompetent, or unable to communicate. All states have living will laws that outline the documentation requirements for living wills.
- Durable power of attorney for health care—an individual designates a person who will make medical decisions when the patient is unable to do so. Each state with a durable power of attorney for health care law has specific requirements for executing the document.

Education about advance directives may be requested of FCNs. The FCN should review state requirements for advance directives and confer with legal counsel to provide accurate information. Advance directives have implications for patients who wish to die at home and for those in hospice care.

Summary

The chapter addresses the legal aspects of faith community nursing. The key point of this chapter is that the FCN, whether paid or volunteer, is held to the same standards of care that a registered professional nurse is held to in traditional hospital nursing settings. Although the FCN has a lower liability risk (because FCNs generally do not perform hands-on nursing actions) than acute care nurses, faith community nursing practice in accord with the legal mandates of the state practice act and professional standards is required. These legal mandates relate to accountability, scope of practice, patient's rights, and documentation.

The chapter also discusses confidentiality and suggests that FCNs adhere to the HIPAA. Professional liability, documentation, and legal issues pertaining to faith community nursing practice were addressed.

Reflect and Discuss

1. What is the FCN's first action?
2. What is the legal basis for this action?
3. What responsibilities does the FCN have regarding confidentiality in this situation?
4. What documentation (if any) should be done of this situation and why?
5. What follow-up is the FCN expected to do in this situation?

Case Study

Alice Kent has been the FCN at a suburban Christian church for 2 years. She recently made a home visit to a new mother, Mrs. Kay, to assess the health and needs of the new mother and infant. Alice performed a health assessment on the newborn and found him to be well nourished, hydrated, and clean. She complimented Mrs. Kay on her mothering abilities. At that point, Mrs. Kay became tearful and told Alice that she feels overwhelmed by motherhood and doesn't think she will ever learn to be good at it. Alice encouraged Mrs. Kay to express her feelings, and together they prayed for God's help and support.

One week later, Alice received a tearful telephone call from Mrs. Kay, who relates that she has just taken 25 tablets of acetaminophen.

References

American Nurses Association. (2001). *Code of ethics for nurses with interpretative statements.* Washington, DC: Author.

American Nurses Association. (1996). *Model practice act.* Washington, DC: Author.

American Nurses Association. (2004). *Nursing: Scope and standards of practice.* Washington, DC: Author.

American Nurses Association. (2003). *Nursing's social policy statement.* Washington, DC: Author.

American Nurses Association and Health Ministries Association. (2005). *Faith community nursing: Scope and standards of practice.* Silver Spring MD: American Nurses Association.

Austin, S., Brooks, P. S., Glenn, L. M., Guido, G. W., Keepnews, D. M., Michael, J. E., et al. (2004). *Nurse's legal handbook* (5th ed.). Philadelphia: Lippincott Williams & Wilkins.

Boss, J. G. (2004). Volunteering as a parish nurse—a response. *Parish Nurse Perspectives, 3*(1), 10.

Brooke, P. S. (2005). Legal context for community/public health nursing practice. In F. A. Mauer & C. M. Smith (Eds.), *Community and public health nursing practice* (3rd ed.). St. Louis, MO: Elsevier Saunders.

Green, M. L. (2001). The nurse in the community. In N. J. Brent (Ed.), *Nurses and the law* (2nd ed.). Philadelphia: WB Saunders.

Hall, J. K., & Hall, D. (2001). Negligence specific to nursing. In M. E. O'Keefe (Ed.), *Nursing practice and the law: Avoiding malpractice and other legal risks* (pp. 132–149). Philadelphia: FA Davis.

McDermott, M. A. (1999). Accountability and rationale. In P. A. Solari-Twadell & M. A. McDermott (Eds.), *Parish nursing: Promoting whole health within faith communities* (pp. 227–232). Thousand Oaks, CA: Sage.

Monarch, K. (2002). *Nursing & the law: Trends and issues.* Washington, DC: American Nurses Association.

National Council of State Boards of Nursing, Inc. (1994). *Model nursing practice act.* Chicago: National Council of State Boards of Nursing.

Parker, W. (2004). How well do parish nurses document? *Journal of Christian Nursing, 21*(2), 13–14.

Smith, S. D. (2003). *Parish nursing: A handbook for the new millennium.* New York: Haworth Press.

Turnock, B. J. (2001). *Public health: What it is and how it works* (2nd ed.). Gaithersburg, MD: Aspen.

Update on HIPAA. (2004, Winter). *Perspectives on Parish Nursing, 3*(1), 6.

Update on HIPAA. (2003, Fall). *Perspectives on Parish Nursing, 2*(4), 6.

U.S. Department of Justice. (2002). *A guide to disability rights laws.* [On-line]. Available: http://www.usdoj.gov/crt/ada/cguide.htm.

Web Resources

http://www.taana.org   American Association of Nurse
  Attorneys
http://www.ahla.org   American Health Lawyers
  Association
http://www.aslme.org   American Society for Law,
  Medicine, and Ethics
http://www.usdoj.gov/crt/ada/adahom1.htm   American
  with Disabilities Act
http://www.childhelpusa.org   Childhelp USA
http://www.apa.org/pubinfo/rights/right.html   Mental
  Health Patient's Bill of Rights
http://www.ncadv.org   National Coalition Against
  Domestic Violence
http://www.nca-online.org   National Children's
  Alliance
http://www.ncd.gov   National Council on Disability
http://www.ncfr.org   National Council on Family
  Relations

http://www.nationalcasa.org   National Court
  Appointed Special Advocate Association
http://www.ndvd.org   National Domestic Violence
  Hotline
http://www.nfcacares.org   National Family Caregivers
  Association
http://www.healthlaw.orh   National Health Law
  Program
http://www.npdb-hipdb.com   National Practitioner
  Data Base; Healthcare Integrity and Protection
  Data Bank
http://www.resourcesharingproject.org   National
  Sexual Assault Coalition Resource Sharing Project
http://www.hhs.gov/news/press/1999pres./990412.html
  Patient's Bill of Rights in Medicare and Medicaid
http://www.rainm.org   Rape, Abuse, and Incest
  National Network
http://www.stop-violence.org   STOP Violence
  Coalition, Inc.

9

Ethical Issues and Faith Community Nursing Practice

Faith community nursing is the only nursing specialty that is viewed as both a practice and a ministry. A ministry within a faith community, it is bound by and to the teachings, beliefs, and values of the faith community it serves. Ethical decisions within faith community nursing are guided by the American Nurses Association (ANA) *Code of Ethics for Nurses* (2001) (the professional nursing element), the teaching, beliefs, and values of the faith community (the theological element), and the lifelong development of beliefs and values of the individuals faced with the decision (the personal element).

Ethical Codes

Professional ethical codes are guidelines for the appropriate conduct of moral decision making. They are intended to serve as standards of conduct for what it means to practice ethically in the specified discipline. For nursing, the American Nurses Association *Code of Ethics for Nurses with Interpretative Statements* (2001) provides ethical guidelines for nursing practice, research, and education. It makes explicit the primary goals, values, and obligations of the profession. The preface states that the *Code of Ethics for Nurses* serves the following purposes:

- A succinct statement of the ethical obligations and duties of every individual who enters the nursing profession.
- The profession's nonnegotiable ethical standard.
- An expression of nursing's own understanding of its commitment to society. (p. 5)

The Code of Ethics consists of two components: nine provisions and accompanying interpretative statements. The first three provisions describe the most fundamental values and commitments of the nurse. The second three provisions address boundaries of duty and loyalty. The last three provisions address aspects of duties beyond individual client encounters. The interpretative statements provide greater specificity for practice and are responsive to the contemporary context of the profession.

The *Public Health Code of Ethics* (Public Health Leadership Society, 2001) consists of a preamble, 12 principles and related commentary about the ethical practice of public health, and 11 values and beliefs that focus on health, community, and action.

This code is valuable to the faith community nurse (FCN) because it focuses on keeping aggregates healthy—the same focus as health ministry. The preamble of the Public Health Code of Ethics asserts that keeping people healthy is the collective and societal nature of public health. The Code addresses the ethical tenets of preventing harm; doing no harm; promoting good; respecting individual and community rights; respecting autonomy, diversity, and confidentiality; ensuring professional competency; accountability; and promoting advocacy for disenfranchised people.

The Canadian Nurses Association's (CNA) *Code of Ethics for Registered Nurses* (2002) describes the ethical behavior expected of registered nurses in Canada. The code provides guidance for ethical decision making, a process for self-reflection and self-evaluation, and a basis for feedback, peer review, and advocacy for quality practice environments. The code of ethics is structured around eight primary values: safe, competent, and ethical care; health and well-being; choice; dignity; confidentiality; justice; accountability; and quality practice environments.

Faith Community Nursing: Scope and Standards of Practice

As discussed in Chapter 8, the ANA document *Faith Community Nursing: Scope and Standards of Practice* (American Nurses Association & Health Ministries Association [ANA-HMA], 2005) delineates the expectations practice for this nursing specialty. Professional Performance Standard 12 of the *Faith Community Nursing: Scope and Standards of Practice* (ANA-HMA, 2005, p. 29) speaks explicitly to ethics. It states: "The faith community nurse integrates ethical provisions in all areas of practice." The measurement criteria for this standard states that the faith community nurse:

- Uses *Code of Ethics for Nurses with Interpretative Statements* (2001) to guide practice.
- Acknowledges and respects tenets of faith and spiritual belief system of a patient.
- Delivers care in a manner that preserves and protects patient autonomy, dignity, rights, and spiritual beliefs and practices.
- Maintains patient confidentiality within religious, legal, and regulatory parameters.
- Serves as a patient advocate assisting patients in developing skills for self-advocacy in support of their spiritual beliefs and practices.
- Maintains a therapeutic and professional patient-nurse relationship with appropriate professional role boundaries.
- Demonstrates a commitment to practicing self-care, growing spirituality, managing stress, and remaining connected both with a centered self and with others.
- Contributes to resolving ethical issues of patients, colleagues, or systems, as evidenced in such activities as participating on ethics committees.
- Reports illegal, incompetent, or impaired practices.
- Participates on multidisciplinary and interdisciplinary teams that address ethical risks, benefits, and outcomes. (ANA-HMA, 2005, p. 29)

The Context of Ethical Practice in a Faith Community

FCNs face increasingly complex ethical concerns as changes in economics, technology, law, and morality interact within the context of health care. Although a service to people, health care and health insurance in today's world have become a profitable business. Corporate values and financial motivation conflict with the values of health professionals, and they impact the quality of care provided to clients. Beliefs about the nature and development of human life and health care are being challenged in ways unimaginable a few years ago. Genetic and technological innovations produce possibilities for creating and, to some degree, controlling new life, whereas sanctity and quality of life compete with each other at the end of life.

Fowler (1999) states that the fundamental ethical issues that FCNs face are much the same as those faced by nurses in other settings. Issues of respect for the congregant's wishes, of capacity to give consent, of privacy and confidentiality, end-of-life decisions, of truthfulness and promise keeping, of advocacy and intercession, and of equitableness and discrimination confront all nurses in all settings. However, faith community nursing practice gives new meaning and emphasis to ethical practice. The setting itself, a faith community with a commitment to pray for each other, and a shared faith journey are norms from which moral actions follow. Hence, the nature of the faith community may modify the way in which the FCN exercises his or her ethical responsibilities. The discernment of good and evil, right and wrong is tied to a methodology that is different from the secular world. Scripture, prayer, creeds, and confessions are essential elements to that discernment.

Fowler (1999) continues by saying that faith community nursing joins the concepts of *vocation* and *covenant community* together with a specialized clinical nursing practice. "Its identity is vocational, its intent is ministry, its instrument is nursing and its involvement is covenantal" (p. 187). The vocational aspect is a call to a special work for which one has been given gifts and in which one finds self-identity. The intent is ministry that serves a spiritual function to bring about whole person health or shalom. The FCN's instrument is nursing, and his or her nursing practice is covenantal in that the nurse is a member of a community in which all members are bound to one another by their God. One's view of faith community nursing is informed and shaped by the community of worship and fellowship, the sacred Scriptures, creeds and confessions, and the canons of faith and prayer.

Douglas (2001) states that ethics is central to nursing knowledge and that morally responsible individual and organizational comportment requires reasoning that is grounded not only in ethical theories and moral principles, but also in moral reasoning, caring, and evolving conceptions of organizational ethics. The author again makes a point of the relationship between the individual (FCN) and the organization (faith community).

Definitions

Ethics is the division of philosophy concerned with the systematic study of morality, the traditions of belief about what is right and wrong. Ethics is concerned with standards of moral conduct and moral judgments. A moral dilemma is an ethical problem caused by a conflict of rights, values, and responsibilities. *Bioethics* is the application of ethical theories and moral principles to life and work. Nursing and medical ethics are dimensions of bioethics. Bioethics evolves from and is influenced by philosophy, theology, and psychology.

White (2003) states that, strictly speaking, an *ethical dilemma* occurs when, to serve one value or principle, another equally important value or principle will be violated. Shelley (2003) describes an ethical dilemma as being essentially a situation with no good alternative—in which it is impossible to do the right thing—and only the *least-worst* alternative. An example would be continuing painful treatment—or not, for a patient with an aggressive and terminal cancer.

Theories

Although agreement does not always occur on the usefulness of applying ethical theories and moral principles in practice, an overview is presented as a general guide to making ethical judgments. The ethic of care and Judeo-Christian ethical theories are discussed in-depth because they are highly relevant to the practice of faith community nursing.

Utilitarianism

Utilitarianism is a well-known teleological theory that bases decision making on doing the greatest good (or least harm) to the greatest number of people. This theory appears to justify imposing suffering or harm on a few for the benefit of the majority. Using teleological theories, ethical decisions are made through a process called *risk-benefit analysis*—determining whether the benefits are worth the risk(s) involved. In this theoretical framework, it is assumed that good and harm can be quantified and evaluated. However, many aspects of health-related ethical decisions are difficult to measure in quantitative terms.

Deontology

Deontological, ethical theories emphasize moral obligation or commitment. They emphasize moral laws and duty and argue that people are not morally obligated to seek the best outcome for their action(s), but rather they are obligated to perform those actions that are in accordance with moral duties and rules. Although considered a preferable theoretical model for use in health care, dilemmas can occur when duties and rules conflict with one another.

Virtue Ethics

Virtue ethics or *character ethics* is an ethical theory that presents the idea that the actions of individuals are based on innate moral virtues. It dates back to the time of Plato and Aristotle. Virtue ethics is not concerned with action, and rather it asks the question, "What kind of person should I be?" The goal of virtue ethics is to flourish as a person (Silva, Fletcher, & Sorrell, 2004). According to Aristotle, virtues are acquired character traits that cause humans to act in accordance with their natural good. Western moralism emerged with the idea of cardinal virtues: wisdom, courage, temperance, justice, generosity, faith, hope, and charity. Burkhardt and Nathaniel (2002) add honesty, compassion, caring, responsibility, integrity, discernment, trustworthiness, and prudence to this list. They state that the concept of virtue ethics presents a challenge to deontological and utilitarian theories, both of which look to what action we ought to do. Virtue ethics posits that the basic function of morality is the moral character of a person.

Fowler (1999) reports that, historically, the nursing profession relied almost entirely upon virtue ethics to guide its practice. It was presumed that, if a nurse possessed the proper moral character, that nurse would inevitably do what was right. Nightingale placed great emphasis on the moral character of her nurses, and this emphasis was continued in the American version of Nightingale training schools (Kalisch & Kalisch, 2004). Fowler suggests, however, that it is not an "all or nothing" situation; both virtue ethics and the ethics of norms and obligation are needed.

Ethic of Care

Emery (2003) states that the *ethic of care* asserts that an action is right, if it involves an empathic understanding of the person and the complex situation. Douglas (2001) states that although, for a long time, nursing ethics has been imbedded in bioethics and biomedical ethics, an ethics of care is emerging. Caring is concerned with reciprocal human relationships and connections, preserving personhood, alleviating vulnerability, and is a moral ideal in itself. The concept of caring is highly congruent with the ministry of faith community nursing.

Seminal work on caring was done by nurse scholars in the late 1980s and early 1990s. Leininger (1984) wrote about caring as the essence of nursing, Watson (1985) wrote about caring as a moral imperative, Benner and Wrubel (1989) wrote about the primacy of caring, and Bishop and Scudder (1991) wrote about the practice of caring. These conceptualizations and the resulting nursing theories provide a framework for nursing practice that is more than and different from the medical-technological model. The discussion of the centrality of caring in nursing continues today. A current example is Eriksson's work on caring science theory, which she describes as ethical in its essence (2002).

Benner also addresses the idea of the primacy of caring in nursing practice. She states that outcomes are not the only issues of care, but that maintaining ties, human connectedness and human concerns, responding to creation and to life as a gift are understood as constituting what it is to be a person. She describes ministering in specific ways, to specific others, as being a profoundly sacred and hopeful practice (1999). Benner's ideas about nursing are highly congruent with faith community nursing practice.

Cooper (2001) reports that the ethic of care has been used as an ethical approach by many nurses. In this framework, the right action is determined by the needs that arise in a caring relationship not by ethical imperatives or focus on outcomes. Engaging with clients, promoting the welfare of clients and families, and meeting their needs are paramount. The nurse's response is based on client circumstances that are revealed in the nurse-client interaction. Within the context of the ethic of care, Cooper highlights the ethical principles of autonomy, truthfulness, beneficence, confidentiality, fidelity, and justice. She states that information is essential to autonomy.

Cooper (2001) also speaks to the importance of personal values in the provision of ethical caring because they are the starting point for ethical behavior and personal integrity. Yeo and Moorhouse (1996) state that when someone has integrity, he or she acts from a position of ethical self-determination or autonomy. The need to rely on others for direction about the right thing to do does not exist. The person with integrity assumes that control over and accountability for one's actions is faithful to promises made and advocates for the client, providing a safe climate that supports healing. Ethical dilemmas involve differences in perspectives and values not differences in facts. A feature of ethical practice is the ability to recognize and to respect perspectives and values other than your own. Cooper encourages understanding values through dialogue.

Findings from four phenomenological studies about the experiences of ethical problems suggest that giving quality care means that nurses must recognize their own humanity with clients. When nurses see their clients through the eyes of compassion, they realize that clients, too, desire to live according to their best ethical and spiritual values, even when some clients appear to behave in contrary ways. Compassion will help both nurses and their clients live up to these values (Cameron, 2003).

Uustal (2003) describes the ethic of care from a Christian perspective. She states emphatically that the nurse is the ethic of care and that nursing as a ministry is a response to one's faith. She states that Christian nurses:

- Recognize that nursing is a calling from God.
- Believe that God has given them a special gift to serve others.
- View nursing as a ministry with a commitment to service as well as a covenantal relationship with the client, which involves beneficence-in-trust.
- View compassionate caring as an act of faith.
- Experience the ethic care from God, who promises us, "Those who wait for the Lord shall renew their strength, they shall mount up with wings like eagles, they shall run and not be weary, they shall walk and not faint" (Is. 40:31). (pp. 14–17)

Uustal describes the ethic of care "in a nutshell" to be show up, shut up (be fully present, seek the client's story, suspend judgment, and stick with them), and assure the client that you will help. She encourages nurses to practice the ethic of care in all of their relationships.

Theological Ethics

Another type of ethical theory with application to faith community nursing practice is theological ethics. In theological ethical theories, the moral principles are based in religious traditions. Different faith traditions have different value systems and theologies. FCNs need to be knowledgeable about the values, theology, and ethics of the faith community being served. Scriptural theology addresses questions that are addressed by Scripture. Historical theology deals with what the church or faith community has believed and held to be the rule across centuries, with regard to specific issues, such as usury, celibacy of priests, nonmarital sexual relations, and infanticide, and how these positions have developed. Constructive theology uses both approaches to address issues.

Judeo-Christian Ethic

The Judeo-Christian ethic is based on God's holy, unchanging character. The standard of right and wrong is taught in Scripture and based on the holy, just, and loving character of God (Uustal, 2003). Judeo-Christian principles of social thought have as their basis the writings of the Old and New Testaments. They outline themes or principles of justice for contemporary society, living with respect and love of God, and the principle of loving and caring for one another. The manner in which faith communities interpret and actualize these principles may be different, but the basics remain the same. The FCN must recognize these principles and how they are applied in the faith community he or she serves.

The seven principles or themes are as follows:

1. *Life and Dignity of the Human Person.* As children of God created in God's image, human persons have a preeminent place in creation. Human dignity is the result of human existence. Human dignity is not earned by achievements or bestowed by any authorities other than God. Human dignity is not dependent on race, creed, color, economic class, political power, social status, culture, personal abilities, gender, sexual orientation, or any other dimensions by which people discriminate social groupings. Human dignity can be recognized and protected only in community with others.
2. *Call to Family, Community, and Participation.* Human beings are not only sacred, but also social. This principle gives direction to issues related to family, marriage, education, and health care systems and resources.
3. *Rights and Responsibilities.* All human persons enjoy inalienable rights. These rights have been codified by the United Nations into a covenant of civil and political rights and a covenant of economic, social, and cultural rights. These rights belong to the person because of his or her being a person; they are not earned by achievement, wealth, or any other measure. These rights are realized in community and are essential for the promotion of justice, human development, and solidarity. With human rights come the responsibilities to honor and protect the rights of all others and to build on the kind of society that protects and nourishes the rights of all.
4. *Concern for the Poor and Vulnerable.* All persons are required to reach out to those whose dignity is most often ignored, overlooked, at risk, or disdained and those who experience the failings and shortcomings of social systems. Their experiences, insights, and concerns offer important evidence in the search for more just systems of social life to which God is calling the human community.
5. *The Dignity of Work and the Rights of Workers.* Work can and must be an individual's humanity and dignity. Work is the way that humans share in the activity of God and express their sacred dignity as human persons and as children of God. Concerns here

involve the right to earn a living wage, working conditions, and benefits and protection from undue risks.

6. *Solidarity.* We belong to one human family, and, as such, we have mutual obligations to promote the rights and development of all people across communities, nations, and the world.

7. *Care for God's Creation.* People are to respect and share the resources of the earth as a part of the community of creation. (http://www.coc.rsv/catholic.html)

Kilner (1992) describes a biblical ethic for health care that, according to Shelly and Miller (1999), blends the best of other ethical theories. Kilner identifies his approach as God-centered, reality-bounded, and love-impelled. A God-centered ethic begins with who God is, what his purposes for people are, and what his image in people looks like. Because man's reasoning is both sinful and limited, both the guidance of the Holy Spirit and moral strength to do what is right are required to help people discern complex issues.

Kilner states that the reality boundaries define good and evil and give moral guidance to our lives. He identifies four ethical guides that are pertinent to health care: (a) promoting life, (b) acting justly, (c) respecting freedom, and (d) telling the truth. Finally, a biblical ethic is love-impelled, building others up, and helping them to experience as much good as possible. Neighbor-love is expressed in community and takes into account how one's actions will affect others. Kilner's ethical guidelines provide direction for the FCN and are supportive of health ministry activities.

Bioethics

Engelhardt (2000) posits that secular bioethics emerged to remedy difficulties posed by Christian bioethics. "As Christian bioethics has the difficulty of being (1) plural, since there is not one Christianity, but many, and therefore many Christian bioethics, and (2) particular, since Christian bioethics as Christian is not open to all but only those who accept its premises, embrace its faith, and are transformed by its Grace. Secular bioethics promised to overcome the difficulties of a Christian bioethics by providing a single universal moral account accessible to all and therefore appropriate for a secular society" (p. 2). This single, universal standard is respect for the autonomy of the individual, letting each one choose his or her own path. Engelhardt contends that Christian bioethics has far greater depth. He states: "A religious bioethics in the sense of a bioethics grounded in the recognition or experience of a transcendent God and in one's obligations to that God offers the possibility of a deep anchor for a content-full morality" (p. 3). Fowler (1999) points out that in faith community nursing practice, discernment of right and wrong, good and evil is tied to the faith tradition's theology, because this will shape and inform client counseling and decision making.

Ethical Principles

Nurses have specific obligations that exist because of the practices and goals of the profession. These obligations have been interpreted as the principles of bioethics: respect for autonomy, nonmaleficence, beneficence, distributive justice, confidentiality, veracity, and fidelity. Although these principles have no inherent rank, context and value systems may create rankings. Rules derived from these principles include the rules of informed consent, privacy, sanctity of life, and quality of life. Douglas (2001) states that ethical principles serve as a foundation for moral conduct, and although less abstract and more content specific than ethical theories, they are at a higher level of abstraction than rules or policies. See Box 9-1 for definitions of these principles.

BOX 9-1
Ethical Principles

Autonomy. Based on human dignity and respect for individuals. Autonomy requires that individuals be permitted to choose those actions and goals that fulfill their life plans, unless those choices result in harm to another. Autonomy is threatened by interfering too much (excessive control or paternalism) or by not interfering enough (abandonment).

Nonmaleficence. "To do no harm." It requires that nurses act according to the profession's standards of care.

Beneficence. Complements nonmaleficence by requiring that people "do good," to act in ways that benefit the patient, and to prevent or remove harm or evil. Beneficent acts are moral and legal professional requirements.

Distributive Justice. Requires that there be a fair distribution of the benefits and burdens in a society based on the needs and contributions of its members.

Veracity. Refers to the practice of telling the truth.

Confidentiality. Requires nondisclosure of private information with which one is entrusted. This principle is clearly addressed in nursing ethical codes and by legislation (HIPAA, 2003).

Fidelity. Concept of faithfulness and practice of keeping promises. For nurses this means being faithful to the scope and standards and code of ethics of the nursing profession.

From Beauchamp, T. L., & Childress J. F. (2001). *Principles of biomedical ethics* (5th ed.). New York: Oxford University Press; Burkhardt, M. A., & Nathaniel, A. K. (2002). *Ethics and issues in contemporary nursing* (2nd ed.). Clifton Park, NY: Delmar; and Munson, R. (2004). *Intervention and reflection: Basic issues in medical ethics* (7th ed.). Clifton Park, NY: Delmar. (Used with permission.)

Nurses often identify ethical principles and strive to honor them in making ethical decisions. The use of the principles in ethical decision making is called *principalism.* The nurse deductively uses general ethical principles to logically determine the best resolution of an issue, which is effective only as long as ethical principles are not in conflict with each other. Another issue that arises in using the principles is the need to achieve a balance between paternalism and abandonment of the patient/client, while continuing to preserve patient/client autonomy. Even passive decisions, such as remaining silent or not taking a stand on an issue, are based on moral judgments.

Ethical Decision Making

Each of the roles of the FCN will require ethical decision making. Often the FCN will be the person who is sought out by a congregant for help in resolving an ethical dilemma. Some of these dilemmas will be related to health care issues, and some will not. An important first step in the process of assisting others in resolving ethical dilemmas is values clarification. Emery (2003) states that first, FCNs should identify their core values, those that do not change over time. The clearer that one is about what one believes and values, the more likely that that person will respond in a consistent way on his or her convictions. Once those values have been communicated to others, one will be held accountable to that standard of conduct. Emery advises that nurses align their lives with their values—"walk the talk."

Ethical decision-making frameworks use problem-solving processes and serve as guides to making sound decisions that can be morally justified. Frameworks provide structure and objectivity to the decision-making process; they do not, however, provide the answers to dilemmas. Human beings are fallible, and it is impossible to gather all of the facts or to be completely without

BOX 9-2
Approaching Ethical Decisions

When faced with an ethical dilemma, consider the following questions:

- What health issues are involved?
- What ethical issues are involved?
- What further information is necessary before a judgment can be made?
- Who will be affected by this decision?
- What are the values and opinions of the people involved?
- Must a decision be made? If so, who should make it?
- What alternatives are available?
- For each alternative, what are the ethical justifications?
- For each alternative, what are the possible outcomes?

From Austin et al. (2004). *Nurse's legal handbook* (5th ed., p. 300). Philadelphia: Lippincott Williams & Wilkins. Used with permission.

bias. Psychological, emotional, and spiritual factors will all have an effect on decision making. Moral reasoning is the psychological interpretative process of helping one to connect one's moral values with one's ethical choices. Using moral reasoning, one examines and analyzes an ethical dilemma and chooses a course of action congruent with one's values and beliefs (Douglas, 2001). Box 9-2 provides questions to consider when approaching ethical decisions.

Silva, Fletcher, and Sorrell (2004) present a generic ethical decision-making framework that includes the following seven steps:

1. Identify the ethical issues and dilemmas.
2. Place them within a meaningful context.
3. Obtain all of the relevant facts.
4. Reformulate ethical issues and dilemmas, if needed.
5. Consider appropriate approaches to actions or options (utilitarianism, deontology, principalism, virtue ethics, ethics of care, feminist ethics).
6. Make decisions and take action.
7. Evaluate the decision and the action. (p. 133)

These seven steps will be used in the case study.

Cooper (2001) suggests that factors to consider in ethical decision making include medical indications, client preferences (respect for autonomy), quality of life, and contextual features, such as the effects of the decision on the family. She identifies competing obligations and technology as challenges to ethical practice.

Austin et al. (2004) suggest using the nursing process as a framework for ethical decision making because it is continuous, systematic, and rational. In the assessment phase, the nurse gathers data—facts, opinions, and perceptions about the ethical problem. The FCN would talk with the client and family, with other members of the health care team, and with the client's permission, members of the clergy, and/or health ministry team. The FCN would identify the people involved in the problem and assess their roles and responsibilities, authority, and decision-making abilities. Validation of information is critical. Never base ethical decisions on hearsay, rumors, or first impressions. The FCN would also identify available resources, which may include a health ministry ethics committee. In the assessment phase, the FCN would help decision makers to participate in values clarification.

In the diagnosis phase of the nursing process, the FCN would clearly describe and define the ethical dilemma. In the planning phase, the following activities would occur:

- Identification of the types of moral dilemmas involved—beneficence, autonomy, justice, fidelity, nonmaleficence, confidentiality, and/or veracity.
- Examination of the rights, duties, and values that are in conflict.

- Identification of possible courses of action and the risks and benefits of each.
- Praying with the client and family about the decision-making process and the ethical dilemma.
- Prioritization of the ethical goals and objectives desired by the persons involved.
- Determination of the ethical obligations of those involved and the ethical principles that shape their actions.

In the implementation stage, the FCN would work with all persons involved to develop an ethical goal that maximizes the greatest good and determine the ethical action that will produce the results closest to the ethical ideal. The action is then carried out. In the evaluation phase of the nursing process, the outcome is evaluated against the goal. If the results fall short of the goals, determine what new moral dilemmas have been created and reassess.

Weston (1997) believes that individuals tend to polarize ethical values into only two possibilities—pro and con. He also states that individuals believe that their perspective is the *right* perspective. The challenge is to consider those points worthy of moral consideration and justification—that is, "what *each* side is *right* about" (p. 54). Weston calls this "right versus right," which is in sharp contrast to pro versus con.

When right versus right does not provide a solution, he recommends integration and compromise. In integration, the common ground among positions and not the points of contention are sought and respected. Through finding out what is right about each position, ethical conflicts are elevated to a higher level of creativity and respect for persons.

Ethical Issues in Health Care

Advances in medical science have outpaced society's ability to solve the ethical problems associated with new health care technologies. In nursing practice, ethical decision making is complicated by sociocultural factors, legal controversies, and consumer involvement in health care. Secular ethics places great emphasis on the principle of autonomy—the right of the individual to choose one's path. However, because faith communities hold values and ethics that are congruent with their theological traditions, reliance on the principle of autonomy may be an insufficient (or inappropriate) guide for the FCN. When the FCN is a member of the faith community served, he or she is familiar with and ascribes to their values, theological, and faith traditions. When the FCN is not a member of the congregation, it is his or her responsibility to learn the values, theological, and faith traditions of the congregation, and to respect them in providing nursing services. Ethical decisions related to right and wrong will be made within that context, and, in almost all faith communities, ethical decision making will include prayer.

Another role of the FCN is one of health educator. New technologies in health care are complex. Before anyone can make an informed health care decision or take an ethical stand on an issue, understanding the issue is critical. Often the FCN will be sought out to provide or interpret complex and technical medical information. Therefore, that the FCN be well informed about developing medical technologies is an ethical imperative.

Right to Die

One of the most difficult ethical decisions in health care is whether to initiate or to withhold life-sustaining treatment for clients who are irreversibly comatose or vegetative or suffering with end-stage terminal illness. *Surrogate decision makers*—people who are designated to act when a person is no longer capable of deciding his or her own fate—face tremendous moral and emotional pressures. At times, the client's expressed wishes to withhold life-sustaining treatment are ignored or overridden by others. For example, if a surrogate decision maker chooses to approve heroic measures to preserve life, when a terminally ill person has requested that no heroic measures be undertaken, the client's expressed wish is ignored.

No clear consensus is known on what constitutes death. Some people define death as the loss of all vital functions, whereas others define death by neurological criteria. Some positions maintain a strong ethical belief in the absolute sanctity of life, whereas others believe that it is ethically wrong to prolong a life devoid of dignity. Definitions vary both between and within faith communities. Chapter 6 addresses viewpoints on death from diverse faith traditions.

Clients do have the right to refuse treatment. This right is grounded in the ethical principle of respect for the autonomy of the individual. It also provides the basis for the concept of informed consent. Clients who refuse life-sustaining treatment still have the right to supportive measures, such as comfort, hygiene, and pain control.

FCNs will be sought out by families faced with making difficult health-related decisions. These families can be assisted by encouraging questions, providing medical information in simple, clear language, and clarifying or correcting misunderstood information. FCNs should also be informed and should educate others about *living wills* and *Durable Power of Attorney* designation. FCNs will be sought out to help congregants understand these issues, in light of their faith tradition and state laws.

Organ Transplantation

Some organ transplantation procedures pose few ethical issues. Blood transfusions and cornea or bone marrow transplants are widely accepted and ethically untainted procedures— although not universally accepted by all faith traditions.

Procurement of essential organs (hearts, kidneys, livers, lungs) is ethical only if steps are taken to ensure that the donor's life and functional integrity are not compromised. When a living person donates an organ, the key issue is informed consent, which includes full awareness of the risks and benefits that may result from the procedure. Recovering organs from a deceased donor poses a different set of ethical issues. Essential organs can only be recovered from brain dead "beating heart" cadavers. A person is pronounced brain dead only when all functional brain activity has ceased. This definition of death is not universally accepted by health care workers, ethicists, or lay people.

The Uniform Anatomical Gift Act allows a person to donate specific or all organs for organ transplantation. All states have enacted required request acts. These acts require hospitals to ask families of potential donors to permit organ donation. The required request laws are intended to increase the availability of organs. Family members are under no obligation to grant permission.

Because the number of potential transplant recipients far exceeds the number of available donors, the selection of organ recipients depends on value judgments. Organ donation is coordinated regionally, with persons having the greatest need and best survival potential assigned the highest priority.

Organ donation and transplantation is not acceptable to all faith traditions. Chapter 6 addresses this issue, as it relates to diverse faith traditions.

Abortion

Abortion has become the focus of a long and bitter political struggle. Pro-life opponents of legal abortion argue that human life begins at conception and therefore abortion is murder. Since 1869, the Roman Catholic Church has condemned all abortions as a form of murder (except in a situation where it is the only recourse in saving the life of a mother). The pro-choice position asserts that an embryo or a young fetus represents the potential for human life but should not be considered a human being. This view sees abortion as a type of surgery necessary for the physical or psychological well-being of certain women. It contends that abortions have always existed in society whether legalized or not. It also argues that elective abortions decrease the number of unwanted children and forced marriages. The ethical principle of autonomy is an important aspect of the abortion debate. This principle upholds a woman's right to control her own body; however, autonomy does not address the fetus. Where one stands on the spectrum of the pro-life/pro-choice continuum is often dependent upon situational context, and decisions are never easy.

Prenatal tests, such as amniocentesis, ultrasound, alpha-fetoprotein screening, and chorionic villus sampling, have made it possible to detect inherited disorders and congenital abnormalities well before birth. In some cases, this early diagnosis allows surgical repairs to be made in-utero. However, cases do exist in which repair or cure is not medically possible. In these situations, the family is faced with making a very difficult decision about whether or not to continue the pregnancy.

Many faith traditions oppose legal abortions, and the topic is highly sensitive. FCNs need to be well versed on the position that the faith community holds on this issue. Denominational Web sites provide faith community policy positions about sensitive ethical issues. If there is not a link to "bioethics" or "social policy," use the search feature to find bioethics policies. Web sites serve as a resource to FCNs, especially to those FCNs who may be serving a faith community in which she or he is not a member. Box 9-3 provides Web addresses.

Reproductive Technologies

In Vitro Fertilization

In vitro fertilization (IVF) refers to the process of recovering ova from a woman's ovaries, placing them in a petri dish filled with a sterile growth medium and covering them with motile spermatozoa for fertilization. Three to five fertilized ova are implanted into the woman's uterus 10 to 14 days after fertilization, and the remaining fertilized ova are frozen for future use or discarded. IVF can be homologous (sperm from the partner) or donated sperm (heterologous). IVF is a complex and expensive procedure that has been called both a medical miracle and a moral dilemma.

Surrogate Mothers

A *surrogate mother* is a woman who gives birth after carrying the fertilized ovum of another woman, or after being artificially inseminated with sperm from the biological father. In this case, the infant is then legally adopted by the wife of the biological father. Surrogate motherhood offers hope to couples in which the woman is the infertile partner. All of the parties in the surrogate motherhood picture are highly vulnerable to exploitation. Some people will view this reproductive option as a form of baby-selling.

Genetics

Gene therapy, or the placement of beneficial genes into cells of patients, opens the door to revolutionary new treatments. *Eugenics,* or good genes, will be capable of preventing genetic disease as well as producing designer babies. White (2003) wonders whether those who request such genetic perfection and those who provide it are "playing God." Access issues related to genetic technologies will also present ethical dilemmas.

BOX 9-3
Web Resources for Faith Traditions

African Methodist Episcopal   www.amecnet.org
American Baptist Church   www.abc-usa.org/resources/resol/
Buddhist Bioethics   www.changesurfer.com/Bud/BudBioethics.html.
Christian Science   www.marybakereddylibrary.org
Center for Applied Christian Ethics   www.wheaton.edu/CACE/
Christian Bioethics (journal)   www.szp.swets.nl/szp/journal/cb.htm
Conservative Judaism,   www.uscj.org
    www.uscj.org/embryonic_stem_cell_5809.html
Eastern Orthodox Church   www.oca.org/pages/orth_chri/q_and-a_old/stem-cells.html
    www.oca.org/pages/ocaadm/documents/pastoral-letters/2002-cloning.html
Episcopal Church   www.ecusa.anglican.org
Evangelical Lutheran Church in America
    www.elca.org/faithandscience
    www.elca.org/dcs/studies
Greek Orthodox Church   www.goarch.org/en/ourfaith/ethics
Islamic Organization for Medical Sciences   www.islamset.com/index.html
Islamic Perspectives in Medical Ethics   www.islam-usa.com
Jehovah's Witnesses   www.watchtower.org/medical_care_and_blood.htm
Journal of Buddhist Ethics   www.jbe.gold.ac.uk/2/dkhughes.html
Latter-day Saints   www.lds.org
National Catholic Bioethics Center   www.ncbcenter.org
National Institute of Judaism and Medicine   www.nijm.org
Orthodox Judaism   www.ou.org
Quakers   www.quaker.org
Presbyterian Church USA   www.pcusa.org
Reformed Judaism   www.rj.org
Roman Catholic Church   www.catholi.org
    www.americancatholic.org
Seventh-Day Adventist   www.adventist.org
Southern Baptist Convention   www.sbc.net/aboutus/pssantity.asp
Unitarian Universalist   www.uua.org/news/010827.html
United Church of Christ   www.ucc.org
United Methodist Church   www.umc.org
U.S. Conference of Catholic Bishops   www.nccbuscc.org

CLONING

Both *reproductive cloning* and *therapeutic cloning* begin with the same process called *somatic cell nuclear transfer* (SCNT). *Therapeutic cloning* is the most popular term used to describe the cloning of human embryos with the intent to harvest their stem cells.

The result of removing stem cells from embryos is death. This creates the ethical debate about stem cell research and the moral status of human embryos (O'Mathuna, 2003). In *reproductive cloning*, the embryos are implanted into the mother with the intent of producing live offspring. Although there is almost unanimous agreement worldwide that human reproductive cloning is wrong, the state of stem cell research is at a moral impasse. Currently in the United States, there is a moratorium (until 2006) on therapeutic cloning while adult stem cell research is aggressively pursued (President's Council on Bioethics, 2002).

Keller (2004) reports that the Union of Concerned Scientists published a statement in February 2004, condemning the Bush administration's stance on scientific research policies, including its restrictions on stem cell research. More than 4,000 scientists, including 48 Nobel prize winners, have signed this document.

Most ethical discussions regarding the use of embryonic stem cells for science revolve around the moral status of the fetus. Dorff (2002) provides a Jewish perspective and states that genetic materials outside of the uterus have no status in Jewish law and that, if materials for stem cell research are procured in permissible ways, the technology is morally neutral. Farley (2002) describes two Roman Catholic viewpoints. The first says that human embryos must be protected on a par with humans. The other view is that early embryos are not differentiated, so some respect is required, but less than that accorded to a fully developed human.

The Pew Forum on Religion & Public Life and the Pew Research Center for the People & the Press conducted a nationwide telephone survey of a random sample of 1,512 adults in August 2004. Overall, 52% of respondents believed that it was more important to conduct stem cell research than not to destroy embryos in the creation of stem cells. Among religious groups, nearly two thirds of white, nonevangelical Christians (65%) now place greater importance on conducting stem cell research than on not destroying embryos.

Additional information and recommendations related to assisted reproduction is available in the President's Council on Bioethics Report titled, *Reproduction and Responsibility: The Regulation of New Biotechnologies* (2004). This report is available online at http://www.bioethics.gov/reports/reproductionandresponsbilibility/index.html.

Some or all forms of reproductive technologies are unacceptable to some faith traditions. The FCN needs to be aware of the values and theological positions of his or her faith community.

Summary

This chapter has provided content about the context of faith community nursing and ethical theories, with an in-depth focus on Judeo-Christian theories and the ethic of care. Moral principles and professional codes of ethics were presented and discussed. Ethical decision-making frameworks were provided, discussed, and applied to a case study. And, finally, an overview of contemporary ethical issues in health care was provided.

FCNs are encouraged to clarify their own personal values. FCNs need to be cognizant of the values, theological positions, and faith traditions of the faith communities that they serve. This statement is mentioned with the caveat that there will be differences of opinion within faith communities as well as between faith communities. When working with congregants, exploration of values and beliefs is an important starting point in a dialogue. Faith community nursing is both a ministry and covenantal relationship with a faith community. Because "right" and "wrong" are defined differently in different contexts, ethical positions and decisions will be made and defended within the context of the faith tradition.

FCNs are strongly advised to read and learn about emerging medical technologies to serve as a resource person and educator of the faith community. All ethical decision-making frameworks begin with establishing a situational context for making a decision, and having up-to-date and accurate information is critical to this process.

Reflect and Discuss

Refer to the case study presented below and consider the following questions:

1. How might this situation differ in a different faith tradition? Consider the case study from Roman Catholic, Jewish, and Islamic perspectives.
2. Under what conditions would the use of an aborted fetus as a source for human embryonic stem cells NOT pose an ethical dilemma?
3. Are there ethical similarities between organ transplantation and stem cell implantation?
4. What resources are available to the FCN to learn about new medical technologies?
5. What resources provide ethical decision-making resources to the FCN?

Case Study

Anne Marie Harris has been the faith community nurse at Calvary Fellowship for 2 years. It is a small, conservative Christian congregation in a suburban community. Members of this congregation know each other well and are comfortable praying for each other by name in group worship settings. For many months, the congregation has been praying for a cure for Cindy, a 3-year-old child who has a complex endocrine disorder.

One afternoon Anne Marie receives a telephone call from Cindy's mother Kendra. She requests that Ann Marie make a home visit to her as soon as she can. Anne Marie immediately addresses the health status of the child, and Kendra assures her that no adverse changes have occurred, but that she needs a home visit to discuss something privately with Anne Marie. An appointment for a home visit is then made for the following morning.

On arrival, Anne Marie assesses Cindy and finds her to be pale and afebrile. After the physical assessment is complete, Cindy begins to play quietly with her dolls and stuffed animals. Anne Marie joins Kendra in the kitchen for a cup of tea, and Kendra hesitantly begins to share that there may be a cure for Cindy's condition. She shares that she and her husband were referred to a physician at a university-affiliated medical center. This doctor has had some success with curing Cindy's condition with embryonic stem cell implantations. Kendra and her husband are cautiously excited about the possibilities that this treatment might provide for their daughter. Kendra states that this opportunity is surely a result of the prayer of her faith community. But, she wonders, would the faith community approve of this treatment for her child? She states that she just wouldn't know what to do, if the congregation disapproved. She asks Anne Marie what biblical directions might support a decision to use this treatment. They then prayed together for God's assistance and for Cindy's health.

Use the following ethical decision-making steps to address the situation described in the case study. You are approaching this process in the role of the faith community nurse.

1. Identify the ethical issues and dilemmas in this case study.
2. Place them in a meaningful context.
3. Obtain all the relevant facts.

4. Reformulate ethical issues and dilemmas, if needed.
5. Consider appropriate approaches to actions or options using Judeo-Christian ethical theory.
6. Make a decision and take a stand.
7. What are expected outcomes of this decision?

References

American Nurses Association. (2001). *Code of ethics for nurses with interpretative statements.* Washington, DC: Author.

American Nurses Association & Health Ministries Association. (2005). *Faith Community Nursing: Scope and Standards of Practice.* Silver Springs, MD: ANA.

Austin, S., Brooke, P. S., Glenn, L. M., Guido, G. W., Keepnews, D. M., & Michael, J. E., et al. (2004). *Nurse's legal handbook* (5th ed.). Philadelphia: Lippincott Williams & Wilkins.

Beauchamp, T. L., & Childress, J. F. (2001). *Principles of biomedical ethics* (5th ed.). New York: Oxford University Press.

Benner, P. (1999). Caring as a context for practice. In P. A. Solari-Twadell & M. A. McDermott (Eds.), *Parish nursing: Promoting whole person health within faith communities* (pp. 171–180). Thousand Oaks, CA: Sage Publications.

Benner, P., & Wrubel, J. (1989). *The primacy of caring: Stress and coping in health and illness.* Menlo Park, CA: Addison-Wesley Publishing Company.

Bishop, A. H., & Scudder, J. R. (1991). *Nursing: The practice of caring.* New York: NLN.

Burkhardt, M. A., & Nathaniel, A. K. (2002). *Ethics and issues in contemporary nursing* (2nd ed.). Clifton Park, NY: Delmar Learning.

Cameron, M. E. (2003). Legal and ethical issues: Our best ethical and spiritual values. *Journal of Professional Nursing, 19*(3), 117–118.

Canadian Nurses Association. (2002). *Code of ethics for registered nurses.* Ottawa: Author.

Cooper, C. (2001). *The art of nursing.* Philadelphia: WB Saunders.

Dorff, E. N. (2002). Stem cell research—a Jewish perspective. In S. Holland, K. Lebacqz, & L. Zoloth (Eds.), *The human embryonic stem cell debate.* Cambridge, MA: MIT Press.

Douglas, M. R. (2001). Ethics in nursing practice. In N. J. Brent (Ed.), *Nurses and the law: A guide to principles and application* (2nd ed., pp. 31–52). Philadelphia: WB Saunders.

Emery, P. (2003). Moral integrity: Faithful living in a fallen world. *Journal of Christian Nursing, 20*(4), 8–12.

Engelhardt, H. T. (2000). *The foundations of Christian bioethics.* Lisse, Netherlands: Swets & Zeitlinger.

Eriksson, K. (2002). Caring science in a new way. *Nursing Science Quarterly, 15*(1), 61–65.

Farley, M. A. (2002). Roman Catholic views on research involving human embryonic stem cells. In S. Holland, K. Lebacqz, & L. Zoloth (Eds.), *The human embryonic stem cell debate.* Cambridge, MA: MIT Press.

Fowler, M. (1999). Ethics as a context for practice. In P. A. Solari-Twadell & M. A. McDermott (Eds.), *Parish nursing: Promoting whole person health within faith communities* (pp. 1181–1194). Thousand Oaks, CA: Sage Publications.

Kalisch, P. A., & Kalisch, B. J. (2004). *American nursing: A history* (4th ed.). Philadelphia: Lippincott Williams & Wilkins.

Keller, J. C. (October 2004). Politicians weigh scientific progress against policy. *Science & Theology News, 5*(2), 8.

Kilner, J. F. (1992). *Life on the line: Ethics, aging, ending patients' lives and allocating vital resources.* Grand Rapids, MI: William B. Eerdmans Publishing Co.

Leininger, M. (Ed.). (1984). *Care: The essence of nursing and health.* Thorofare, NJ: Slack.

O'Mathuna, D. P. (2003). Human cloning: Investigating the issues. *Journal of Christian Nursing, 20*(4), 20–24.

The President's Council on Bioethics. (2002). *Human cloning and human dignity: An ethical inquiry.* Available online at: http://www.bioethics.gov/reports/cloningreport/index.html.

The President's Council on Bioethics. (2004). *Reproduction and responsibility: The regulation of new biotechnologies.* Available online at: http://www.bioethics.gov./reports/reproductionandresponsibility/index.html.

Public Health Leadership Society. (2001). *Public health code of ethics.* New Orleans, LA: Public Health Institute.

Shelley, J. A. (2003). No easy answers (Editorial). *Journal of Christian Nursing, 21*(4), 3.

Shelly, J. A., & Miller, A. B. (1999). *Called to care: A Christian theology of nursing.* Downers Grove, IL: InterVarsity Press.

Silva, M.C., Fletcher, J. J., & Sorrell, J. M. (2004). Ethics in community-oriented nursing. In M. Stanhope, M. and J. Lancaster, *Community & public health nursing* (6th ed., pp. 130–147). St. Louis: Mosby.

Uustal, D. B. (2003). The ethic of care: A Christian perspective. *Journal of Christian Nursing, 20*(4), 13–17.

Watson, J. (1985). *Nursing: Human science and human care.* Norwalk, CT: Appleton Century Crofts.

Weston, A. (1997). *A practical companion to ethics*. New York: Oxford University Press.

White, B. J. (2003). Playing God: Moral tensions in health care. *Journal of Christian Nursing, 20*(4), 4–7.

Yeo, M., & Moorhouse, A. (1996). *Nursing ethics* (2nd ed.). Ontario, Canada: Broadview Press.

Additional Resources

Benjamin, M. (2001). Between subway and spaceship: Practical ethics at the outset of the twenty-first century. *Hastings Center Report, 31*(4), 24.

Berwick, D., Hiatt, H., Janeway, P., & Smith, R. (1997). An ethical code for everybody in health care. *British Medical Journal, 315*, 1633–1634.

Callahan, D., & Jennings, B. (2002). Ethics and public health: Forging a strong relationship. *American Journal of Public Health, 92*(2), 169.

Cameron, M. E. (2002). Older persons' experience of ethical problems involving their health. *Nursing Ethics, 9*, 547–566.

Center of Concern. (2004). Catholic Social Teaching Principles. Available online at: http://www.coc.org/rvs/catholic.html.

Dyck, A. J. (2002). *Life's worth: The case against assisted suicide*. Grand Rapids, MI: William B. Eerdmans Publishing Co.

Emery, P. (2003). Moral integrity: Faithful living in a fallen world. *Journal of Christian Nursing, 21*(4), 8–10.

Espejo, R. (Ed.). (2003). *Biomedical ethics: Opposing viewpoints*. Farmington Mills, MI: Greenhaven Press.

Evans, J. (2000). A sociological account of the growth of principalism. *Hastings Center Report, 30*(5), 31.

Hall, J. K. (2002). *Law and ethics for clinicians*. Amarillo, TX: Jackhal Books.

Hanford, J. (2002). *Bioethics from a faith perspective: Ethics in health care for the twenty-first century*. Binghamton, NY: Haworth Press.

Hinderer, D. E., & Hinderer, S. R. (2001). *A multidisciplinary approach to health care ethics*. Mountain View, CA: Mayfield.

Horner, S. D. (2004). Ethics and genetics: Implications for CNS practice. *Clinical Nurse Specialist, 18*(5), 228–231.

Hui, E. C. (2002). *At the beginning of life: Dilemmas in theological bioethics*. Downers Grove, IL: InterVarsity Press.

Kass, N. (2001). An ethics framework for public health. *American Journal of Public Health, 91*(11), 1776.

Kilner, J. F., Cunningham, P. C., & Hager, W. D. (2000). *The reproductive revolution: A Christian appraisal of sexuality, reproductive technologies and the family*. Grand Rapids, MI: William B. Eerdmans Publishing Co.

Kilner, J. F., Hook, C. C., & Uustal, D. (Eds.). (2002). *Cutting edge bioethics: A Christian exploration of technologies and trends*. Grand Rapids, MI: William B. Eerdmans Publishing Co.

Milton, C. L. (2003). The American Nurses Association *code of ethics*: A reflection on the ethics of respect and human dignity with nurse as expert. *Nursing Science Quarterly, 16*(4), 301–304.

Munson, R. (2004). *Intervention and reflection: Basic issues in medical ethics* (7th ed.). Clifton Park, NY: Delmar.

Shapiro, H. T. (1999). Reflections on the interface of bioethics, public policy, and science. *Kennedy Institute of Ethics Journal, 9*(3), 209–224.

Smith, R., Hiatt, H., & Berwick, D. (1999). A shared statement of ethical principles for those who shape and give health care: A working draft from the Tavistock group. *Annals of Internal Medicine, 130*, 143–147.

Stassen, G. H., & Gushee, D. P. (2003). *Kingdom ethics: Following Jesus in contemporary context*. Downers Grove, IL: InterVarsity Press.

Ubel, P. A. (1999). The challenge of measuring community values in ways appropriate for setting health care priorities. *Kennedy Institute of Ethics Journal, 9*(3), 263–284.

Veatch, R. M. (2000). *The basics of bioethics*. Upper Saddle River, NJ: Prentice Hall.

Volbrecht, R. M. (2002). *Nursing ethics: Communities in dialogue*. Upper Saddle River, NJ: Prentice Hall.

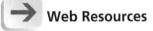 ## Web Resources

http://www.acponline.org/ethics   American College of Physicians, Center for Ethics and Professionalism

http://www.mitpress.mit.edu   *American Journal of Bioethics*

http://www.ama-assn.org/ama/pub/category/2558.html   AMA Institute for Ethics

http://www.asbh.org   American Society for Bioethics and Humanities

http://www.aslme.org   American Society of Law, Medicine, & Ethics

http://www.primr.org/arena.html   Applied Research Ethics National Association (ARENA)

http://www.hopkinsmedicine.org/bioethics   Berman Bioethics Institute at Johns Hopkins

http://www.bioethics.com   Bioethics.com

http://www.nymc.edu/FHP/institutes/Bioethics/mission.asp   Bioethics Institute of New York Medical College

http://www.bioethics.ca   Canadian Bioethics Society

http://www.medicalethics.ca   Canadian Resources for Medical Ethics

http://www.cathmed.org   Catholic Medical Association

http://www.bioethicscolumbia.org   Center for Bioethics, Columbia University

http://www.pitt.edu   Center for Bioethics and Health Law at University of Pittsburgh

http://www.cbhd.org   Center for Bioethics and Human Dignity

http://www.bioethics.upenn.edu   Center for Bioethics at University of Pennsylvania

http://www.bcm.tmc.edu/ethics   Center for Medical Ethics and Health Policy

http://www.mcu.edu   Center for the Study of Bioethics

http://www.csmeh.mc.duke.edu/home.html   DUMC Center for the Study of Medical Ethics and Humanities

http://www.eppc.org   Ethics and Public Policy Center

http://www.ethics.org   Ethics Resource Center

http://www.thehastingscenter.org   Hastings Center

http://www.utmb.edu/imh   Institute for Medical Humanities at UTMB

http://www.bioethics-international.org   International Association of Bioethics

http://www.jme.bmjjournal.com   *Journal of Medical Ethics*

http://www.georgetown.edu/research/nrcbl/   Kennedy Institute of Ethics

http://www.llu.edu/llu/biioethics   Loma Linda University Center for Christian Bioethics

http://www.ethics.bsd.uchicago.edu   McClean Center for Clinical Medical Ethics

http://www.islammedicine.org/ethics   Medical Ethics in Islam

http://www.midbio.org   Midwest Center for Practical Bioethics

http://www.va.gov/vaethics   National Center for Ethics in Health Care

http://www.ncehr.medical.org   National Council on Ethics in Human Research

http://www.nhgri.nih.gov   National Human Genome Research Institute

http://www.nursingethicsnetwork.org   Nursing Ethics Network

http://www.parkridgecenter.org   Park Ridge Center for Health, Faith, and Ethics

http://www.metanexus.net   Philadelphia Center for Religion and Science

http://www.pccef.org   Physicians for Compassionate Care

http://www.bioethics/gov   President's Council on Bioethics

http://www.pbs.org/wnet/religionansethics   Religion & Ethics News Weekly/PBS

http://www.bioethics.net   *The American Journal of Bioethics*

10

Complementary and Alternative Modalities

According to Eisenberg, Davis, Ettner, Appel, et al. (1998), Americans spend more than $22.1 million on complementary therapies during a 1-year period, and this amount is paid for by the consumer alone. Over 70% of the world's population use non-Western health care practices (Kreitzer & Jensen, 2000). Health care consumers have reported that they do not want the treatment for a health problem to make them sicker than the actual health problem itself. Eighty-two percent of patients who use an alternative modality reported the side effects of medications as a reason for seeking complementary therapies (Mitzdorf et al., 1999). Public interest in complementary therapies has also been related to an increased interest in spirituality. In a large national survey, Ray (1997) conducted a large national survey that found that 25% of the population ascribe to a certain set of values that include a holistic philosophy of health and valued spirituality. Astin (1998) found that those who adhere to this value system are large users of complementary healing modalities.

Complementary and alternative modalities (CAM) enhance conventional medicine. According to Kreitzer and Jensen (2000), there are more than 1,800 modalities that have been identified as complementary. Many health care consumers have had some experience with alternative modalities, such as acupuncture and homeopathy; however, many other alternative therapies exist that may be unfamiliar to those who practice only traditional Western medicine. Symptoms, such as pain, are a manifestation of a more serious underlying physiologic problem. These modalities, and the practitioners who participate in their use, are more interested in the underlying cause of the disease and less interested in the manifestations (symptoms) of the disease. Therefore, common to see are several treatment modalities applied to many disease conditions that are unrelated. This stems from the philosophy that many illnesses manifest themselves from a common cause. Last, and most important, is the role of the mind-body connection in alternative modalities. One cannot separate the client from his or her social life, family, and work life (Novey, 2000).

With an increase in public and commercial interest in CAM, we are likely to see more funding for research. Much of the research presently funded by the National Institutes of Health (NIH) involves research on substances that can be patented and marketed through a restricted source. Most alternative modalities are in the public domain, therefore capturing research dollars for CAM can be more difficult. However, with the formation of the National Center for Complementary and Alternative Modalities (NCCAM), more funding will likely be generated for well-designed research studies over the next 5 to 10 years (Novey, 2000).

The NIH established the Office of Alternative Medicine in 1992. In 1998 the name was changed to the National Center for Complementary and Alternative Modalities. NCCAM has a fivefold purpose:

1. To facilitate evaluation of various therapies
2. To investigate and evaluate the effectiveness of therapies
3. To provide information on complementary therapies
4. To support research training

NCCAM also funds research to explore the effectiveness of several complementary modalities (Snyder & Lindquist, 2002).

NCCAM has also classified CAM therapies into five domains: (a) alternative systems of care; (b) mind-body therapies; (c) biologic-based therapies; (d) manipulative and body-based methods; and (e) energy therapies.

Alternative systems of care include health care that has been developed apart from the Western approach to health care. Some examples of this would be homeopathy, Native American medicine, acupuncture, and naturopathy. Mind-body therapies are interventions that use several techniques to facilitate the mind's capacity to improve physical symptoms and body functions. Imagery, yoga, prayer, and tai chi are modalities that are classified as mind-body therapies. Biologic-based therapies would be any modality that includes plant-derived preparations, such as herbs, aromatherapy, or any nutritional or food supplement. Manipulative and body-based methods are therapies that are based on manipulation and/or movement of the body, such as chiropractic, massage, or hydrotherapy. Finally, energy therapies focus on energy that comes from within the body or coming out of external sources. Examples of energy therapies would include therapeutic touch, Reiki, or external Qi Gong (Snyder & Lindquist, 2002). Because of the vast number of modalities in each of the domains, this chapter will discuss a few of the more widely used modalities.

Role of the Faith Community Nurse

Because faith community nurses (FCNs) are agents of health promotion within a faith community, they need to be aware of the wide use of complementary therapies that may be used by those patients with whom they will come in contact. FCNs need this knowledge so that they may:

- Provide guidance when obtaining health histories.
- Answer basic questions about complementary therapies and refer clients to reliable information sources.
- Make referrals to competent CAM practitioners.

When performing a routine health history, many patients may not volunteer information about their use of CAM. Some individuals will only share this information if they feel the FCN displays an attitude of acceptance of their use. This information is vital, because many of the herbal preparations may cause interactions with various prescriptive medications. Additionally, using a combination of several alternative modalities may decrease the effectiveness of the other.

Referring patients to a competent therapist can be a difficult task. Unfortunately, licensure, certification, and regulations vary widely from state to state and among various different modalities. For many of the alternative modalities, no governing body currently exists. This can be confusing and frustrating to consumers when trying to find a properly credentialed provider.

A study conducted by Kirksey et al. (2002) described the frequency of CAM therapies used by people with HIV/AIDS to manage their illness and treatment-related symptoms. Of the 422 subjects in the study, more than one third used at least one CAM modality to assist with reducing the side effects associated with the treatment of the disease. Yet health care providers were not the primary sources of information about CAM for these subjects. More than half of the subjects noted that they had learned about these modalities through self-study (e.g., television and print media). Because nurses are involved in holistic practice, being knowledgeable about CAM is important, so that they can help clients alleviate the life-altering symptoms associated with various diseases.

Many of the modalities that have been mentioned have always been a part of nursing practice. This chapter will discuss several very common modalities in CAM. Also included is the background of the therapy, practical applications, credentialing, and what an FCN should look for in a provider when making a referral. A list of Web references is provided at the end of the chapter for various modalities, along with a bibliography and selected research on the modality.

Homeopathy

Background Information

Homeopathy is an alternative medical system that has been around for over 2 centuries, therefore, it is not based on modern technology. Although it has its roots in ancient herbal medicine and alchemy, homeopathy works differently from conventional medicine. Unlike traditional medicine, the homeopathic practitioner is educated to look at the whole person who presents with symptoms. These symptoms are then placed in the context of the patient's whole being. The aim of homeopathy is to promote general health by reinforcing the body's own natural capacity to heal (McCabe, 2000).

According to McCabe (2000), the term *homeopathy* means "similar to the suffering." The homeopathic remedy is a catalyst and is prepared from a variety of sources of plants, animals, and minerals. The remedy is prepared in such a way that the smallest possible amount of the substance is used to stimulate the body's vital force to heal the underlying problem, not just the symptoms.

In traditional allopathic medicine, the patient's symptoms are treated by medication. For example, a runny nose caused by an allergic reaction will be treated by a substance (e.g., antihistamine) that causes the nose to dry up. In homeopathic practice, the runny nose could be treated with Histaminum (histamine), prepared in such a way that only an infinitesimal amount of the histamine remains in the remedy. This stimulates the individual's own natural healing abilities, rather than inhibiting the immune response (Cummings & Ullman, 1997).

The individual responsible for the development of the homeopathic system of medicine was Dr. Samuel Hahnemann at the end of the 18th century. Hahnemann conducted his own clinical experiments searching for treatments using plants and mineral substances. He found that these substances created a tremendous change in humans. However, often these substances were toxic. To create a less toxic treatment, he began to dilute his preparations, ending up with a system that left only a slight trace of the original substance in place. His theorem was that the more diluted the substance became, the less toxic and more potent and more efficient in the treatment of the disease. Hahnemann's *Materia Medica* is a book in which he gathered all of his knowledge that he left behind as his legacy for those practitioners who would follow in his path.

Practical Applications

When visiting a homeopathic practitioner for the first time, the visit can range anywhere from 1 to 2 hours. An extensive case-taking history is completed and a homeopathic remedy is usually given. The homeopathy must match the symptom of the patient as closely as possible to the remedy. The homeopathy must also take into account the psychosocial aspects of the patient and what was happening in the patient's life at the time of the illness (Novey, 2000).

BOX 10-1
Recommended Sources for Homeopathic Products

Boericke & Tafel
Homeopathyworks.com/bandt.htm
Telephone: (800) 876-9505

Boiron
www.boiron.com
Telephone: (800) 258-8823
Consumer Information: (800) 264-7661

Dolisos
www.lyghtforce.com/Dolisos/
Telephone: (800) 365-4767

Hahnemann Pharmacy
www.hahnemannlabs.com
Telephone: (888) 427-6422

Luyties
www.1-800homeopathy.com
Telephone: (800) HOMEOPATHY

Homeopathy has an extensive list of conditions that it can treat. The *Repertory of the Homeopathic Material Medica* (Kent, 1981) is an excellent resource. For a more complete list, see the additional references at the end of the chapter. A few of the acute and chronic conditions are listed below:

Acute conditions: Colds, flu, conjunctivitis, anaphylactic reactions, musculoskeletal injuries, bites and stings, coughs, food poisoning, herpes simplex and zoster, earaches

Chronic conditions: Diverticulitis/diverticulosis, migraine headaches, ulcerative colitis, uterine fibroids, warts, chronic back pain, osteoporosis, sciatica, temporomandibular joint (TMJ), carbon monoxide poisoning

Homeopathic remedies are not herbal medicines. Homeopathic preparations or remedies are regulated and approved by the Food and Drug Administration (FDA). The Homeopathic Pharmacopoeia of the United States (HPUS) has a list of all remedies that can be sold in the United States. The remedies can be found in many health food stores, and the preparations bear the *HPUS* label on the container. Box 10-1 is a list of sources for homeopathic products.

Credentialing

The only certification board that certifies competency in homeopathy in the United States is the Council for Homeopathic Certification (CHC). The designation for this type of practitioner is CHC. Only three states currently license homeopathy: Arizona, Connecticut, and Nevada. Laypersons also practice homeopathy in an unlicensed capacity in all other states. Most other states consider homeopathy a process of diagnosis and treatment and is included in a physician license. This varies from state to state as well (Novey, 2000).

What to Look for in a Provider

Because no one organization is responsible for the practice of homeopathy, the consumer needs to know what to look for in a homeopathic provider. The length of practice and education of the practitioner is a consideration. Novey (2000) recommends that the homeopathic practitioner have at least 5 years of practice. Education programs should have a minimum of 500 hours of classroom training, along with a clinical component. That the practitioner may have a medical license does not guarantee that he or she has adequate background and knowledge of homeopathic principles. The final question that a consumer might ask would be whether the practitioner regularly attends seminars or workshops to keep pace with new developments in the field.

Acupuncture

Background Information

Acupuncture belongs to the category of manipulative and body-based methods. Acupuncture is also part of a larger system of health care called *oriental medicine.* Originating in China, approximately 4,000 years ago, this modality uses needles, which penetrate beneath the skin to reach the nerve endings, with the purpose of relieving pain. This modality is based on principles of the meridians that run through the body to the hands and feet. This modality is not one that can be self-administered, unlike acupressure, which is a massage-like therapy based on pressure points on feet, hands, and ears. Acupressure is primarily a self-care treatment. In Western culture it may be known as reflexology and in Japanese culture as "shiatsu" (Novey, 2000).

Until the 1970s, there was little practice of acupuncture in the United States. The FDA reclassified the needles used by an acupuncturist from an experimental device to a standard medical device to be used by a qualified practitioner in 1994 (Novey, 2000).

The philosophy behind acupuncture is that pain results from blocked *Qi,* or life force. Basic to this is the understanding of the meridians or channels that lie along the planes of fascia between the muscles. On the surface of the body are 14 meridians and 361 acupuncture points. The insertion of the needles opens up the flow of energy through the meridians (Stux & Pomerantz, 1987).

According to Stux and Pomeranz (1987), 228 research studies have been conducted on acupuncture and its role in pain relief. These studies concluded that the acupuncture needles activate small fibers in the muscle that send impulses to the spinal cord. This causes several neurotransmitters to be released (enkephalin, serotonin, beta-endorphins) into the blood and cerebrospinal fluid, which then causes analgesia, or pain relief.

Needles are not the only method of stimulation in acupuncture. In the United States moxabustion is frequently used. Moxa is the leaf of the Artemisia vulgaris plant in a powdered form. The moxa is burned near or on an acupuncture point. Moxa is used to warm the body when the pathology involves cold (Novey, 2000).

Electric stimuli can be used. The TENS unit would be an example of the use of electrical stimuli for pain relief. Attaching electrodes to the handles of the acupuncture needles can deliver a stimulating impulse (Novey, 2000).

Finally, laser is another method of acupuncture stimulation. Still considered experimental in the United States, laser is used widely in Canada and Europe. Laser is used for wound healing and scars (Novey, 2000).

Practical Applications

Acupuncture is highly effective for treating both acute and chronic pain. Box 10-2 provides a partial list of those conditions for which acute and chronic pain can be relieved by acupuncture. The American Academy of Medical Acupuncture (AAMA), founded in 1987, is the national professional society of North American physicians who have incorporated acupuncture into their medical practice. Box 10-3 provides a partial list of conditions that can be effectively treated with acupuncture. A visit to the AAMA Web site (www.medicalacupuncture.org/) will give a more complete list of the conditions treated by medical acupuncturists. Acupuncture can also play a role in preventing illness (Novey, 2000).

Literature spanning over 20 years from 1970 through 1997 supports the use of acupuncture for various categories, such as psychiatric disorders, cardiovascular system, dermatology, headache, to mention a few (Klein & Trachtenberg, 1997).

BOX 10-2
Acute/Chronic Pain Relief from Various Conditions

Sprains and strains	Postsurgical pain
Whiplash injuries	Migraines
Fibromyalgia	Low back pain
Sciatica	Myofascial pain
Arthritis	Reflex sympathetic
Carpal tunnel syndrome	dystrophy
Phantom limb pain	Neck pain

From Novey, D. (2000). *Clinician's complete reference to complementary/alternative medicine.* St. Louis, MO: Mosby.

Credentialing

Acupuncture is licensed in 36 states and the District of Columbia. The National Certification Commission for Acupuncture and Oriental Medicine (NCCAOM) is a nonprofit organization that was established by the profession to create standards of competence and safety, not only in acupuncture, but also in oriental medicine. NCCAOM has a database of over 8,500 active acupuncturists. To be certified one must pass a comprehensive written examination and practical exam. To sit for the examination one must complete an acupuncture program with a minimum of 3 years after a 2-year undergraduate program and 1,350 hours of acupuncture education, which must include 500 clinical hours. An apprenticeship is required as well. Credentials that successful candidates use to practice acupuncture may include Dipl.Ac., Dipl.CH, or Dipl.ABT. Like homeopathy, acupuncture is not restricted to licensed physicians. Some states do require a minimum of 200 hours of formal training and certification. For medical doctors, the AAMA offers a certification examination (Novey, 2000).

What to Look for in a Provider

Acupuncture is a skill that requires both education and years of experience. The acupuncturist should be familiar with various drugs that the client may be taking, in addition to any herbal preparations. When looking for a practitioner of acupuncture, having a good reputation in the community is essential, along with credentialing that was discussed previously (Novey, 2000).

BOX 10-3
Selected Conditions Treated by Acupuncture

Hypertension	Multiple sclerosis
Asthma	Depression, anxiety
GERD	Sore throats
Peptic ulcer disease	Constipation/Diarrhea
Spastic colon	Bladder/Kidney infections
PMS	Sensory disturbances
Endometriosis	Allergies

GERD, gastroesophageal reflux disease.
From Novey, D. (2000). *Clinician's complete reference to complementary/alternative medicine.* St. Louis, MO: Mosby.

Chiropractic

Background Information

Chiropractic is a manipulative body-based therapy whose primary focus is on the spine and its function. Chiropractic care dates back to the 1890s. The roots of chiropractic practice stem from a system of the body's self-healing capacity, similar to that of homeopathy. Like homeopathy, opposition grew between chiropractic and allopathic medicine. Chiropractic was viewed as a more natural approach to healing and opposed the use of medication and surgery. In recent years, scientific study has focused on the use of chiropractic as an effective means to treat back and neck complaints. We are now witnessing collaboration between chiropractors and the medical community (Novey, 2000).

Chiropractors make up the third largest health profession after medicine and dentistry. The majority of chiropractors are in a single full-time practice. Over the past 15 to 20 years, the number of individuals visiting chiropractors has doubled. The demographics of the population that uses chiropractors tend to be between ages 18 and 55 years, men, and people with at least a high school education (Novey, 2000).

Practical Applications

Chiropractic modalities are most known for their treatment of musculoskeletal complaints. The therapeutic treatment that chiropractors provide is often spinal manipulation or termed *adjustment.* However, chiropractic practice also includes counseling for lifestyle changes, rehabilitation, nutrition counseling, and several other interventions (Novey, 2000).

Over 80% of conventional insurance plans in the United States, including preferred provider organization (PPO) and point of service (POS) plans, now include at least some of the cost for chiropractic adjustment (Cherkin & Moore, 1997).

Credentialing

The majority of chiropractors have a private practice or a practice in clinics. In the United States there is a minimum requirement of 2 years of undergraduate study that focuses on science, specifically biology. Most chiropractic schools have a 4-year curriculum. The practice of chiropractic is regulated in all 50 states and in many countries. State licensing boards regulate education and experience. The boards also serve to protect the public safety and welfare. Likewise, licensure for chiropractors is also state specific. The National Board of Chiropractor Examiners conducts a national board exam, which creates some national standards for chiropractic care. Many states require passage of this examination prior to licensure (Novey, 2000).

What to Look for in a Provider

If the chiropractor has been recommended by another health care professional, then it is likely that the chiropractor provides competent care. Chiropractors who are credentialed with several managed care plans may demonstrate that the practitioner had made a commitment to provide a certain standard of care (Novey, 2000).

Reiki

Background Information

Reiki is truly an ancient healing art, which involves energy and touch. Dr. Mikao Usui is credited as the founder of the practice. Usui, a Christian theologian and teacher, was on a quest to find out how Christ was able to heal by touch. The practice of Reiki can be traced back to Japan in the mid-1800s and came to the West by way of Hawaii (Lubeck, Petter, & Rand, 2001). As the practice of Reiki became Westernized in the 1980s and 90s, there have been variations or branches of Reiki that are slightly different from the Usui Reiki that was introduced many years before.

The term *Reiki* means universal life force energy. One's ability to perform Reiki comes from being attuned. This process begins with the technique being passed from teacher to student and dates back to the one who first channeled the technique (Lubeck et al., 2001). Reiki cannot be learned from a textbook alone. A trained professional must make the energy connection. A Reiki therapist is certified by the Master therapist.

Practical Applications

Although validated clinical research on Reiki is limited, a study was conducted in 1997 by Karin Olsen, RN, PhD, from Canada. Her research focused on the use of Reiki as an alternative to opioid use for the management of pain. The study involved 20 clients experiencing pain for various reasons, including cancer. Reiki treatments were given by a second-degree Reiki-certified therapist. Pain levels were measured before and after the treatment. The results showed a highly significant ($p<0.001$) reduction in pain following the Reiki treatment (Olsen, 1997).

Credentialing

No official credentialing exists for the practice of Reiki. The technique must be passed on from practitioner to practitioner. Three training levels are practiced for the Reiki practitioner. The first-degree level is where the student learns hand positions for self-healing and treating others in lying and sitting positions. The second-degree practitioner focuses more on working with others. The use of symbols to strengthen the Reiki energy is the main focus. The third level of Reiki is that of Reiki Master or teacher (Novey, 2000).

When visiting a Reiki therapist, the treatment begins with the patient in the supine position. The patient should not be under the influence of any drugs or alcohols, including caffeine or tobacco (Novey, 2000). The practitioner begins at the head and moves down the body to the feet. No massaging or rubbing occurs, and the movement is passive and can be done several inches above the body. The patient can be fully clothed, because the energy can flow through the clothing. Reiki treatments are preferably performed in a quiet room, keeping light to a minimum. The room should be at a comfortable temperature, and meditation music can be used. All jewelry should be removed, and belts and tight clothing should be loosened (Lubeck et al., 2001). The body can be scanned for disturbances in the energy field. If a hot or cold spot is found, the therapist may ask the patient for feedback about the imbalance. An entire Reiki treatment can last anywhere from 1 to 1.5 hours.

What to Look for in a Provider

The practice of Reiki is not regulated. The most effective way to locate a Reiki practitioner is through referral. As with other treatment modalities discussed, it is prudent to ask therapists how long they have been practicing and what qualifications they possess.

Therapeutic Touch

Background Information

The nursing literature has described physical touch as having five dimensions of caring: physical comfort, mind-body comfort, social interaction, physical comfort, and spiritual sharing (Chang, 2001). Therapeutic touch (TT) is defined as the use of the hand, either on or near the body, with the intention to help or to heal. Therapeutic touch does not need to take place within a religious or spiritual framework, making it different from the laying-on of hands. The practitioner can accomplish two things with the use of therapeutic touch. First, the practitioner can sense various body energies, such as cold or hot, passive or active, blocked or free.

Energies can then be returned to the patient by the TT practitioner, such as warm, soothing, relieving pain (Snyder & Lindquist, 2002).

Research by Candace Pert, PhD (1997), in the field of neurotransmitters, has increased our understanding of how the flow of neuropeptides can affect and interrupt cellular communication. The energy that is exchanged during TT can reestablish the cellular communication and return the individual to a healthy state.

The technique of TT was developed in the 1970s by a professor of nursing, Dolores Krieger. Her research focused on clients who had received TT and had an increase in hemoglobin level compared to a group of clients who had received routine nursing care (Krieger, 1997). Further research has been conducted at the University of Alabama on burn clients who have received TT. Those burn clients who had received TT not only reported significant pain reduction, but also had differences in their lymphocyte count (Turner, 1998).

There are three basic assumptions to TT:

1. Human beings are open systems and energy fields.
2. Illness causes an imbalance in energy flow.
3. Trained practitioners can sense and intervene in the client's energy field to stimulate that individual's own natural healing potential. (Snyder & Lindquist, 2002)

Practical Applications

Therapeutic touch can be used for various chronic disorders, such as chronic fatigue syndrome, fibromyalgia, abuse, or chronic pain. Cancer patients often find therapeutic touch helpful after they have exhausted other forms of treatment.

Credentialing

TT is a rapidly growing modality; however, the practice is not fully standardized. The American Holistic Nurses Association offers certification in healing touch, which is slightly different from TT. The Nurse Healers and Professional Associates Cooperative was formed to promote TT and offer training (Novey, 2000).

What to Look for in a Provider

Most TT practitioners will have a minimum of a professional license as a nurse, physical therapist, or massage therapist. Most have completed a certificate program or informal TT training. According to Mackey (1995), more effective results may be obtained from a practitioner who is doing more than 60 treatments per month. So this might be a question that one would ask before engaging the services of a TT practitioner.

Guided Imagery

Background Information

Guided imagery is a mind-body therapy, which has been in existence for centuries by American Indian tribes, Christianity, Judaism, and Eastern doctrines. It has increased in popularity since the 1970s. According to Bazzo and Moeller (1999), guided imagery is defined as "the process of purposeful use of mental images by working with another person or by listening to an audiotape, to achieve a desired therapeutic goal" (p. 319). Guided imagery uses the powers of the mind to help the body maintain health, heal, or relax. It includes a wide variety of techniques, which involve simple visualization and suggestion. The suggestion can involve using story-telling or metaphors. Using techniques led by a professional, the patient can develop control over aspects of autonomic functioning and return the body to improved balance and health (Bazzo & Moeller, 1999). Because guided imagery is practiced with another person or audiotape, imagery can be practiced as an independent activity (Snyder & Lindquist, 2002).

Guided imagery allows a client to focus his or her attention on images that are associated with the anxiety produced when he or she has achieved a relaxed state of mind.

Practical Applications

Guided imagery is practiced widely to alleviate anxiety and depression, to relieve physical and psychological discomfort, to overcome health-endangering habits (e.g., smoking), and to prepare clients for surgical procedures (Novey, 2000). Guided imagery can be practiced alone by the individual or with a coach or audiotape/videotape. Other applications of guided imagery can include sleep disorders, anxiety disorders, grief therapy, fitness training, and medication compliance.

Because of the natural ability of young children to use their imagination, they are often better at imagery. The literature supports much success in using guided imagery in children to alleviate pain and anxiety. The developmental and cognitive age of the child needs to be considered, and guided imagery techniques may need to be modified (Snyder & Lindquist, 2002).

Credentialing

In 1989 the Academy for Guided Imagery was established to provide training for clinicians. Additionally, the academy wanted to increase awareness among health care professionals and the public about the benefits of imagery and the propagation of research findings. Since 1989, the academy has produced books, audiotapes and videotapes, workshops, and self-study courses for health care professionals and the general public.

The academy offers a 110-hour certificate program specifically for nurses to learn the techniques of guided imagery. The program is divided into four phases. Each phase is an evening and 3 days. Additional practice, including 10 documented imagery sessions, is required to be certified. The training is opened only to registered nurses who hold a valid license (Academy for Guided Imagery, 2004).

What to Look for in a Provider

Several guided imagery techniques for relaxation and stress management can be purchased commercially. For more serious health issues, a health professional who has been trained and certified by the Academy for Guided Imagery should be sought (Novey, 2000).

Herbal Medicine

Background

According to Blumenthal (1999), herbal medicine is defined as products used for medicinal purposes that contain active ingredients that are entirely plant and/or vegetable material. Herbal treatment is developed largely through experimentation, family, and cultural tradition. The first books on herbal medicines were written more than 5,000 years ago by the Chinese (Novey, 2000). Herbal medicines are also referred to as botanicals or phytotherapies.

Historically, most of the herbal use in the United States was based on Native American Indians (Althoff, 1997). The U.S. Pharmacopoeia and National Formulary contains almost 170 herbal medicines that were used by the American Indians. Other herbal preparations in the Pharmacopoeia were used by people of the West Indies, Central and South America, and Mexico (Gillespie, 1997).

The World Health Organization (WHO) estimates that approximately 80% of the world's population still rely on herbal medicines for some aspect of their health. This can be attributed to several reasons. Many individuals cannot afford modern pharmaceuticals. For others, the issue is access to the drugs or physicians who prescribe them (Borins, 1998).

Prevention Magazine conducted a study in 1997 and found that 41% of Americans who used herbals had learned about them from family or friends; 37% from magazines; 35% from books; 13% from health food stores; and 5% from television. Only 9% received information from their health care provider (Johnston, 1997). Only when health care providers become aware of the wide range of alternative therapies being used and are knowledgeable about them, will they be able to advise patients whether the alternative therapy is helping or hindering their care.

Herbal medicines, although not foods or drugs, are still regulated by the FDA. They are classified as dietary supplements. Since the passage of the Dietary Supplement Health and Education Act of 1994, herbal medicines can be sold for stimulating, maintaining, supporting, regulating, and promoting health. They cannot be marketed for treating disease, restoring normal function, or correcting abnormal function. Herbal medicines cannot claim to treat, diagnose, prevent, cure, or mitigate (U.S. Government Printing Office, 1999). For example, a manufacturer can advertise that an herbal preparation supports cardiovascular health but cannot claim that it lowers cholesterol.

Lack of scientific studies exists on the efficacy of herbal supplements. The United States does not have a method to approve therapeutic claims about herbal preparations at the present time. Because herbal medicines cannot be patented in the United States, pharmaceutical companies cannot recover research costs. Most of the research on herbal preparations has been done in Germany. Herbal medicines are prescribed by physicians in Germany for disorders of the central nervous system, respiratory tract, urinary tract, cardiovascular, and gastrointestinal systems (Novey, 2000).

Practical Applications

Nurses must be aware that the patient is using herbal medications, especially in certain situations. Those situations include: (a) a patient with a chronic illness, (b) a patient undergoing a surgical procedure, and (c) a patient using prescription medications. For patients undergoing a surgical procedure, who may be taking gingko biloba, they may be at risk for bleeding tendencies. St. John's Wort, taken by many for mild to moderate depression, can decrease the effectiveness of many prescription medications. Also, nurses need to remind patients who may be taking anticoagulants (e.g., Coumadin) that echinacea may potentiate the action of Coumadin (Scalzo & Cronin, 2001).

Credentialing

No single regulatory body exists for credentialing herbalists. Chiropractors, naturopathic physicians and practitioners of Traditional Chinese Medicine all use herbs to treat various illnesses.

The Global Institute for Alternative Medicine offers a Nurse Master Herbalist Program. This program is a 360-contact hour distance learning program for nurses that is approved by the American Holistic Nurses Association (Global Institute for Alternative Medicine, 2004).

What to Look for in a Provider

The American Herbalist Guild (AHG) has information on how to locate an experienced herbalist in your area. The Web site can be found at the end of the chapter.

Aromatherapy

Background Information

Aromatherapy has its roots in herbal medicine. Although not considered a part of herbal medicine, the essential oils used in aromatherapy come from a plant source. Aromatherapy involves the use of either extracts or essences of oils from flowers, herbs, or trees to promote health and well-being. The effects of aromatherapy can be very effective and work at the cellular, physiologic, and psychological levels (Novey, 2000).

Aromatherapy has been a part of nursing care in Europe, Canada, and the United Kingdom for several years but is a recent addition to nursing care in the United States (Snyder & Lindquist, 2002). A study conducted by Eisenberg et al. (1998) found that of 2,055 adults surveyed, 5.6% indicated that they used aromatherapy.

Two mechanisms of action of aromatherapy include dermal action and olfaction, or smell. Dermal action is when the oils are absorbed through the skin. The dermis and adipose layers of the skin act as the reservoir and then the oils reach the bloodstream. Massage or hot water may actually enhance the absorption of these essential oils. Olfaction, or smell, uses the olfactory bulb and nervous impulses, which travel to the limbic system of the brain. Chemicals in an aroma trigger various responses. The effect of odors on the brain has been established by research (Snyder & Lindquist, 2002).

Practical Applications

Aromatherapy is a very safe complementary therapy that can be used for a multitude of symptoms. Few adverse reactions to aromatherapy have been reported in the literature (Robins, 1999). Aromatherapy can treat symptoms, such as psychological (insomnia, depression), physiologic (pain, infection), or spiritual (care of the dying).

Patients with atopic eczema or sensitive skin should avoid using oils directly on the skin. Essential oils should never be taken by mouth or used on the skin in an undiluted form. Essential oils should be kept away from the eyes. Several essential oils have known carcinogenic activity, such as exotic basil, cade, and yellow and brown camphor. Also, some essential oils should be avoided during the first trimester of pregnancy and, perhaps, avoided completely throughout the duration of the pregnancy (Snyder & Lindquist, 2002).

Credentialing

Presently, no recognized certification or governing body exists for aromatherapists in the United States and no requirement for a person who is administering aromatherapy to be certified or accredited. The National Association of Holistic Aromatherapy (NAHA) is the largest professional organization. The Aromatherapy Registration Council was established in 2000 as a nonprofit organization, which administers a national exam and has a list of those registered aromatherapists.

What to Look for in a Provider

Because of the lack of a regulatory agency for aromatherapists, the consumer should carefully evaluate the practitioner. The Aromatherapy Registration Council has a list of registered aromatherapists.

Summary

This chapter has provided information on a selected number of widely used complementary and alternative modalities. Nursing has traditionally focused on promoting a caring and healing environment, therefore many of these modalities are supported by the nursing paradigm. Because consumers demand a more holistic approach to health that includes complementary modalities, nurses must have the knowledge to provide clients with accurate information about various modalities or refer them to resources. The FCN is in a position to empower individuals to assume more responsibility for their own well-being. Many of the modalities discussed in this chapter require active participation by the client. A similar format is presented for each modality, including background information, practical applications, credentialing, and what to look for in a provider.

Reflect and Discuss

1. Reflect on your own personal feelings about the use of complementary and alternative therapies. Have you used any forms of CAM?
2. Can you be impartial in providing unbiased information to patients who seek to use these modalities?
3. Discuss ways that the FCN might empower individuals to assume responsibility for their own well-being.
4. How will the faith community that you serve view your level of knowledge on complementary and alternative modalities?

Case Study

Maria is a 36-year-old woman who lives with her husband and three children, ages 6, 4, and 2, in a single home in the country. Maria is 5 days postpartum. She is married to a very busy attorney and, prior to the birth of her fourth child, worked 4 days a week. She is now on a maternity leave.

She finds that around early evening she experiences crying episodes. She has always attended daily Mass on her way to work but has not been able to do this since she returned home from the hospital with the new baby. She contacts the FCN and states: "I just can't relax and sleep at night." She reports that she is so tired in the evening that she just cries for hours until she has put all of the children to bed. She states that she is not sure how she will be able to manage this new baby with her three other children when her maternity leave is over in 3 months and she has to return to work. She reports that her husband usually arrives home around 8 PM, when everybody is in bed, and isn't able to help with the bedtime routine.

The FCN asks Maria how she has handled stressful situations before. Maria explains that she has used relaxation tapes when her job made her stressful. "I still have the tapes, but I have been so busy with the new baby that I haven't had a chance to listen to them."

The FCN encourages Maria to listen to her tapes after her husband comes home from work when everyone is in bed and she has some quiet time alone. She also provides Maria with some places where she may purchase some new guided imagery tapes to listen to.

After a week, the FCN calls Maria, who reports that she feels more relaxed and is sleeping much better. The FCN points out that the guided imagery tapes were perhaps useful in relieving some of her anxiety. Together they discuss the usefulness of relaxation/imagery in any number of situations.

References

Academy for Guided Imagery. (2004). *Certification for Nurses*. Available online at: http://www.imageryrn.com/

Althoff, S. (1997). *Consumer guide to alternative medicine*. Lincolnwood, IL: Publications International.

Astin, J. (1998). Why patients use alternative medicine. *Journal of the American Medical Association, 279*, 1548–1553.

Bazzo, D., & Moeller, R. (1999). Imagine this! Infinite uses of guided imagery in women's health. *Journal of Holistic Nursing, 17*(4), 317–330.

Blumenthal, M. (1999). *The complete German commission E monographs. Therapeutic guide to herbal medicines*. Newtown, MA: Integrative Medicine Communications.

Borins, M. (1998). The dangers of using herbs. What your patient needs to know. *Postgraduate Medicine, 104*(1), 91–100.

Chang, S. (2001). The conceptual structure of physical touch in caring. *Journal of Advanced Nursing, 33*(6), 820–827.

Cherkin, D. C., & Moore, R. D. (1997). *Chiropractic in the United States: Training, practice, and research*. Rockville, MD: U.S. Department of Health and Human Services, Agency for Health Care Policy and Research. AHCPR Publication No. 98-N002.

Cummings, S., & Ullman, D. (1997). *Everybody's guide to homeopathic medicines*. New York: Penguin Putnam.

Eisenberg, D., Davis, R., Ettner, S., Appel, S., Wilkey, S., & VonRompay, M. (1998). Trends in alternative medicine in the USA 1970–1997. *Journal of the American Medical Association, 280*, 784–787.

Gillespie, S. (1997). Herbal drugs and phytomedicinal agents. *Pharmacology Times, 63*(12), 53–61.

Global Institute for Alternative Medicine. (2004). Available online at: http://www.gifam.org/courseNMH.htm.

Johnston, B. (1997). One-third of nation's adults use herbal remedies. Market estimated at $3.24 billion. *HerbalGram, 40*, 49.

Kent, J. T. (1981). *Repertory of the homeopathic material medica*. New Delhi: B Jain.

Kirksey, K., Goodroad, B., Kemppainen, J., Holemer, W., Bunch, E., & Corless, I. (2002). Complementary therapy use in persons with HIV/AIDS. *Journal of Holistic Nursing, 20*(3), 264–277.

Klein, L., & Trachtenberg, A. (1997). *Acupuncture bibliography online*. Bethesda, MD: National Library of Medicine. Available online at: http://www.nln.nih.gov/pubs/resources.

Kreitzer, M., & Jensen, D. (2000). Healing practices: Trends, challenges, and opportunities for nurses in acute and critical care. *AACN Clinical Issues, 11*, 7–16.

Krieger, D. (1997). *Therapeutic touch inner workbook*. Santa Fe, NM: Bear.

Lubeck, W., Petter, F., & Rand, W. (2001). *The spirit of Reiki*. Twin Lakes, WI: Lotus Press.

Mackey, R. (1995). Discover the healing power of therapeutic touch. *American Journal of Nursing, 95*(4), 26–32.

McCabe, V. (2000). *Practical homeopathy. A comprehensive guide to homeopathic remedies and their acute uses*. New York: St. Martin's Griffin.

Mitzdorf, U., Beck, K., Horton-Hausknecht, J., Weidenhammer, W., Kindermann, A., & Takaxc, M. (1999). Why do patients seek treatment in hospitals of complementary medicine? *Journal of Alternative and Complementary Medicine, 5*, 463–573.

Novey, D. (2000). *Clinician's complete reference to complementary/alternative medicine*. St. Louis, MO: Mosby.

Olsen, K., & Hanson, J. (1997). Using Reiki to manage pain: A preliminary report. *Cancer Prevention and Control, 1*(2), 113.

Pert, C. (1997). *Molecules of emotion. The science behind mind-body medicine*. New York: Simon & Schuster.

Ray, P. (1997). The emerging culture. Available online at: http://www.demographics.com

Robins, J. (1999). The science and art of aromatherapy. *Journal of Holistic Nursing, 17*(1), 5–17.

Scalzo, R., & Cronin, M. (2001). *Herbal solutions for healthy living*. Brevard, NC: Herbal Research Publications.

Snyder, M., & Lindquist, R. (Eds.). (2002). *Complementary/alternative therapies in nursing* (4th ed.). New York: Springer Publishing.

Stux, G., & Pomeranz, B. (1987). *Acupuncture: Textbook and atlas*. Berlin: Springer-Verlag.

Turner, J. G. (1998). The effect of therapeutic touch on pain and anxiety in burn patients. *Journal of Advanced Nursing, 28*(1), 10–20.

U.S. Government Printing Office. (1999). *Dietary Supplement Health Education Act: Is the FDA trying to change the intent of Congress?* Washington, DC: Author.

Additional Resources

Achterberg, J., & Lawlis, F. (1982). Imagery and health intervention. *Topics in Clinical Nursing, 3* (4), 55–60.

Betts, T. (1996). The fragrant breeze: The role of aromatherapy in treating epilepsy. *Aromatherapy Quarterly, 51,* 25–27.

Birch, S., & Hammerschlag, R. (1996). *Acupuncture efficacy: A compendium of controlled clinical studies.* National Academy of Acupuncture and Oriental Medicine.

Brewitt, B., Vittetoe, T., & Hartwell, B. (1997). The efficacy of Reiki hands-on-healing: Improvements in spleen and nervous system function as quantified by electrodermal screening. *Alternative Therapies, 3*(4), 89.

Buenting, J. (1993). Human energy fields and birth: Implications for research and practice. *Advances in Nursing Science,* (4), 53–59.

Cherkin, D. C., & Moore, R. D. (1997). Chiropractic in the United States: Training, practice, and research. Rockville, MD: U. S. Department of Health and Human Services, Agency for Health Care Policy and Research. AHCPR Publication No. 98-N002.

Clarke, J. H. (1984). *A dictionary of practical material medica* (Vol. 3). New Delhi: B Jain.

Dorn, M., Knick, E., & Lewith, G. (1997). Placebo-controlled, double-blind study of Echinacea pallidae radix in upper respiratory tract infections. *Complementary Therapies Medicine, 5,* 40–42.

Esplen, M., & Garfinkel, P. (1998). Guided imagery treatment to promote self-soothing in bulimia nervosa. A theoretical rationale. *Journal of Psychotherapy Practice & Research, 7*(2), 102–118.

Jacobs, J. (1994). Treatment of acute childhood diarrhea with homeopathic medicine: A randomized clinical trial in Nicaragua. *Pediatrics, 93*(4), 719–725.

Kent, J. T. (1981). *Repertory of the homeopathic material medica.* New Delhi: B Jain.

Komori, T., Fujiwara, R., Tanida, M., Nomura, J., & Yokoyama, M. (1995). Effects of citrus fragrance on immune function and depressive states. *Neuroimmunomodulation, 2,* 174–180.

Lafreniere, K., Mutus, B., Cameron, S., Tannous, M., Giannotti, M., & Abu-Zahra, H. (1999). Effects of therapeutic touch on biochemical and mood indicators in women. *Journal of Alternative and Complementary Medicine, 5*(4), 367–370.

McKinney, C., Antoni, M., Kumar, M., Tims, F., & McCabe, P. (1997). Effects of guided imagery and music (GIM) therapy on mood and cortisol in healthy adults. *Health Psychology, 16*(4), 390–400.

O'Reilly, W. B. (1996). *Organon of the medical art by Dr. Samuel Hahnemann.* Redmond, WA: Birdcage Books.

Peck, S. (1998). The efficacy of therapeutic touch for improving functional ability in elders with degenerative arthritis. *Nursing Science Quarterly, 12*(1), 52–61.

Reilly, D. (1986). Is evidence for homeopathy reproducible? *Lancet, 10*(344), 1601–1606.

Rowe, T. (1998). *Homeopathic repertory, case-taking, and case analysis methodology.* Berkeley, CA: North Atlantic Books.

Terrett, A. (1996). Misuse of the literature by medical authors in discussing spinal manipulative therapy injury. *Journal of Manipulative Physiological Therapy, 18*(4), 203–210.

Triano, J., & Schultz, A. (1997). Loads transmitted during lumbosacral spinal manipulative therapy. *Spine, 22*(17), 1955–1964.

van Tulder, M., Koes, B., & Bouter, L. (1997). Conservative treatment of acute and chronic nonspecific low back pain: A systematic review of randomized controlled trials of the most common interventions. *Spine, 22*(18), 2128–2156.

Zimmerman, M. (1989). Using principles of relaxation, visualization, and guided imagery in the care of persons recovering from addictions. *Addictions Nursing Network, 1*(3), 9–11.

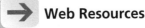 ## Web Resources

http://www.healthy.net/nch   State Associations for Licensed Homeopathic Professionals

http://www.homeopathy~council.org   The Council on Homeopathic Certification (CHC)

http://www.homeopathic.com   Hahnemann College for Heilkunst

http://www.simillibus.com   Resources, Articles, and Links for Homeopathy

http://www.homeopathic.org   National Center for Homeopathy

http://www.nccaom.org   National Commission for the Certification of Acupuncture and Oriental Medicine

http://www.aaom.org   The American Association of Oriental Medicine

http://www.aama~ntl.org/index   The American Academy of Medical Acupuncture

http://www.amerchiro.org   American Chiropractic Association

http://www.chiropractic.org   International Chiropractors Association

http://www.wfc.org   World Federation of Chiropractors

http://www.interactiveimagery.com   The Academy for Guided Imagery

http://www.iaii.org   The International Association of Interactive Imagery

http://www.odp.nih.gov/ods/databases.ibids   Office of Dietary Supplements; International Bibliography Information on Dietary Supplements

http://www.vm.cfsan.fda.gov/~dms/aens   U.S. Food and Drug Administration Center for Food Safety and Applied Nutrition.

http://www.gifam.org/courseNMH.htm   Global Institute for Alternative Medicine

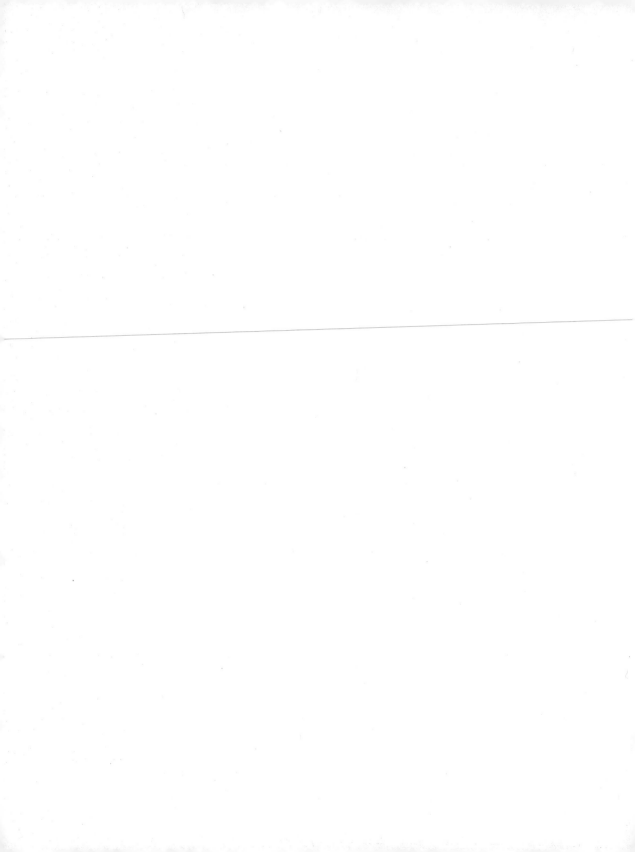

11

Self-care and the Faith Community Nurse

The concept of *altruism* in nursing is a significant part of nursing history (Kozier, Erb, Berman, & Snyder, 2004). Most nurses still enter the profession of nursing because of a desire to help others and to give back to the community. Caring for others is obviously a positive character trait, but many nurses have not learned the importance of taking care of themselves in the process. Nursing students are taught throughout their nursing programs how to care for patients, families, and others, but how many programs teach these same nursing students how to care for themselves? (Slaninka, 2003) This chapter will focus on self-caring behaviors that nurses need to incorporate into their lives to be available both physically and emotionally to the clients whom they will serve as faith community nurses (FCNs).

Nursing has been impacted by early religious values, which called for self-denial and devotion to duty. Nurses prior to the 1800s were not paid for the services that they provided in the home and in the community, and many came from religious orders (Potter & Perry, 2001). This service orientation is still true of today's faith community nurses. Many serve as volunteers in congregations to provide health care counseling, referrals, and education. The role of the faith community nurse by definition has a "service" orientation. Sieg (2004) states that nurses have become accustomed to placing their own needs at the end of a lengthy list of taking care of people and then rarely have time for themselves.

Nurses are clearly very good at caring for other people but rarely think of taking care of themselves. What happened to the latter part of the early Christian value: "Love thy neighbor as thyself"? Unfortunately, people are thought of as selfish when they think to take care of themselves, but unless nurses and other health care professionals learn to take good care of themselves, there will be nothing left to give to anyone else, either professionally or personally. The time has come to acknowledge this fact and to begin to take action (Slaninka, 2003). Nurses need to support one another in their efforts to perform self-caring activities.

Personal Expectations

Real Versus Ideal

Nurses have been socialized into being "all things to all people." In managing dual roles of family and career, responsibilities mount and nurses increasingly become stressed and "burned out," both at home and in the work setting (Keegan, 2001). Some nurses have family obligations, in addition to work, and might spend the week working full-time; bringing work home after hours; cleaning house; cooking meals; taking children to child care, piano lessons, ballet classes, and little league practice; preparing the meals, and helping with homework. Other nurses might be enrolled in educational programs to advance their professional careers. The role of FCN is often above and beyond all of those responsibilities, and nurses begin to wonder whether there are enough hours in the day. Wade (2002) stresses the importance of not forgetting one's self because all of these activities are considered. In an effort to assess self-caring behavior, students at West Chester University perform a self-assessment exercise to identify the things they are presently doing in their lives to take care of themselves, on the first night of class in a course titled, Care of the Inner Self (Table 11-1). This self-assessment is a good starting point to see where one is on the concept of self-care and what needs to be changed to move forward from that spot.

FCNs cannot be all things to all people, so maintaining boundaries becomes very important for self-preservation. Often it is difficult for FCNs to release ownership of their original

---

TABLE 11-1

Care of the Inner Self: Self-assessment

As present or future health care professionals, most of us are very good at taking care of other people, which is often the reason that we have chosen to be nurses. This assessment form will give you an idea of *"how well you take care of yourself."* Briefly answer the following questions as honestly as you can.

1. Do you do any form of exercise? If so, what kind of exercise do you do and how often? (Walking, running, swimming, dancing, biking, etc.)
2. What is the average amount of sleep that you get every night?
   Do you feel rested when you wake up?
3. Do you feel that you generally eat well? High fiber? Low fat?
   Lots of fruits and vegetables?
4. How much water do you drink each day? How much caffeine?
   Is the water that you drink filtered?
5. Do you take any extra vitamin supplements?
   If so, which ones do you take?
6. Do you smoke cigarettes, cigars, or pipes?
   If so, how much?
7. Do you drink alcohol of any kind? Beer, wine, or hard liquor?
   If so, how much?
8. Do you express your feelings openly with someone, or do you keep your feelings to yourself? Do you use a journal to express your feelings?
9. Do you have an appreciation for nature? Do you have plants or flowers in your home or yard?
10. Do you have a pet? If so, what kind?
11. Do you have a spiritual side to your life? Is faith important to you?
12. Do you take the time to get together with friends? How often?
    Are you a member of a club, organization, or support group?
13. What is your relationship status? Single, married, or have a significant other?
    Are you generally satisfied, or are there challenges that add to your stress?
    Do you have relationships in your family of origin that have unresolved issues?
    Does your family serve as a support for you during both joyful and difficult times?
14. Do you take time in your day/week to be alone?
15. Do you ever meditate, do yoga, or tai chi, etc.? If so, how often?
16. Do you do any creative arts? Play an instrument? Write poems, stories, or articles? Draw or paint?
    Do crafts? Dance? Do pottery or ceramics?
17. What kinds of activities do you do for your mind? Crossword puzzles?
    Read a good book? Earn a degree in college? Or other?
18. Do you like to travel? Do you have travel plans in your future?
19. Are there any other things that you believe you do that enhance your life that I have missed on this form? Please comment.

definitions of nursing in other settings. Personal expectations that "they can do everything" for people in the congregation hinders the capacity to even think about the idea of caring for the self. Self-care becomes essential to have any energy left to begin to care for others and perform effectively in the role of the FCN (Knight, 2003).

Another concept that is difficult for the FCN is setting realistic expectations. Idealist expectations that might never be accomplished cause frustration and undermine serenity. When nurses imagine perfect scenarios instead of working toward realistic goals, they risk eventual disappointment. Expectations are productive only when they provide the impetus necessary to set goals and then strive to achieve them. Bringing expectations in line with reality frees the nurses from unnecessary frustration and helps them find satisfaction in their role. An example of unrealistic goals might be when an FCN is assigned to a family in which the primary issue is alcoholism. If the family is in denial on the issue, it might be impossible to guide the family toward AA and Alanon as ultimate resources.

Limiting the Faith Community Setting

Covington (2003) discusses a caring presence as a way of being. FCNs embrace the caring process and are present to provide a therapeutic environment for healing on the physical, emotional, and spiritual level for the members of their faith community. This caring presence offers a context within which spirituality can be expressed and connections can be made with oneself, others, nature, and a higher power. Creating a space for this caring presence is essential in providing quality care and also essential for the preservation of self-care in the nurses themselves.

The role of the FCN is something that needs to be clarified to the entire parish community. Most people are not aware that the role of the FCN is limited to health education, counseling, and referral. Faith community nursing is not what most people think of when they picture a nurse—where the nurse might enter a home, help with a bath, perform a dressing change on a wound, give a client insulin, and/or take a blood sample. FCNs, on the other hand, might receive a call from a parishioner who requires an initial assessment. The nurse would enter the home, perform a nursing assessment through a nursing history and then might provide health information and education, counseling, or possibly make a referral to another health care agency or primary care provider. The congregation must understand the difference so that FCNs do not find themselves outside the boundaries of the parish nurse role. Setting these limits within the congregation is very important, or else the nurse may be pulled into doing "everything that the clients need." If a nurse is not careful, he or she might spend the whole day in the home providing child care, transportation, helping with a bath, making a meal for the family, and helping the children with their homework. The FCN needs to say *no* to requests that are outside the boundaries of nursing practice. This concept needs to be clarified early in the process so that people are not confused on what services the nurse might provide.

Also important is to clarify the limits of the role of the FCN to the spiritual leader of the congregation. Many spiritual communities have limited resources in terms of staff. Most churches have one or two spiritual leaders to handle huge congregations. The minister may find in the nurse a ready "answer to a prayer for help" within the congregation. The spiritual leader may ask the nurse to do things that are not in the FCN job description, and the nurse may be reluctant or feel guilty about saying *no* to the request. Sieg (2004) states the importance of protecting the self from getting into too many things. This issue can cause resentment over time, when the nurse finds that he or she has no time for self-care, and thus may cause compassion fatigue (Henry, 2004). An FCN brochure (Table 11-2) is a good way to communicate the role of the nurse to the congregation, with statements that indicate specifically the role of the FCN. Even with the use of a brochure, parishioners and spiritual leaders might need to be reminded of the limitations of the role of the FCN.

TABLE 11-2

Faith Community Nursing Sample Brochure Information

What is faith community nursing?
Faith community nursing or parish nursing originated in the early 1980s in the Midwestern part of the United States. Faith community nurses (FCNs) serve the faith community by promoting health and wellness within the church. FCNs do not perform home health care or invasive procedures. Referrals can be made to visiting nurses or home health aides for that purpose. You do not need to be a nurse to offer comfort, support, or prayer to anyone. Volunteer training is available for anyone interested in helping with this ministry.

Faith community nursing goals are to:
1. Assess health care needs.
2. Educate the faith community.
3. Offer health information.
4. Use the resources within the community.
5. Offer assessment prevention screenings.
6. Promote growth of the body, mind, and spirit.

Faith community nurses provide:
1. Health teaching.
2. Counseling and phone support.
3. Referral.
4. Assessment of physical, emotional, and spiritual needs.
5. Coordination of transportation needs.
6. Support groups.
7. Blood pressure screenings.
8. Volunteer training.
9. Coordination of meals.
10. Support for caregivers.

Stress Management

Change is a constant in today's health care settings, and nurses as well as other health care professionals are required to adapt quickly to the changes that impact the quality of care that they provide. Decreased length of stay, increased acuity levels, and increased use of technology have all added to the workload of nurses in all settings. The nursing shortage has placed an additional burden on nurses already stressed and overwhelmed in their profession. There is no question that nurses will have these same issues in the faith community. They will need to be involved in activities that will prevent these feelings and to cope with stress that occurs. Lanier (2004) encourages her staff at the MultiCare Regional Cancer Center in Tacoma, Washington, to submit a plan of self-care every year, including goals centered around a healing environment, integrative therapy, meaning and purpose, physical balance, mental balance, emotional balance, and spiritual balance.

Psychoneuroimmunologists continue to investigate the impact of physiologic and psychological stress on the body. Strong evidence exists that stress affects the ability of the body to resist infections and decreases immune function (Bright, 2002). Stress itself is not necessarily harmful to people; rather, it is the interpretation of those stressors that causes the harm to the body. If even a small amount of control is experienced over the stressful situation, or if the situation is seen as challenging rather than difficult, then the stress becomes neutral or even positive for the immune system (Bright, 2002). Nurses can use several techniques to enhance their immune systems.

Most nurses would admit that they have "no time to exercise, don't eat healthy foods, get very little sleep, experience a great deal of stress in their lives, and rarely engage in self-caring behaviors." Needless to say, as nurses they know what they need to do, but they haven't translated that intellectual knowledge into action behaviors to incorporate into their lives. Sieg (2004) states that the more stressed and overwhelmed nurses are, the more they need that break that is rarely taken.

Meditation and Focused Breathing

Meditation and breathing exercises have been described in the professional literature. Ornish (1990) discusses meditation as one of the strategies for reversing heart disease. Kabat-Zinn (1994) uses the concept of mindfulness meditation as he works with clients at the Stress Reduction Clinic at the University of Massachusetts Medical Center. Many hospital settings are incorporating integrative strategies when they teach their clients about stress management. Some health care settings have these resources available to staff as well.

Benson (1975) is one of the pioneers in the area of meditation and is the founder of the Mind-Body Medical Institute in Boston, Massachusetts. He and his associates teach and perform research on the *relaxation response*. Benson describes the relaxation response as including several elements. He describes the importance of beginning with finding a quiet environment and a comfortable position. Benson stresses the need for the person to come to the experience with an open mind and passive attitude. He then instructs the participant to focus on a single syllable or sound and to repeat that sound, focusing on the breath. The participant is encouraged to eliminate any distractions that may find their way into the mind. Incorporating a meditation practice in one's life becomes important because it reduces anxiety, reduces blood pressure, pulse rate, and respirations and provides an overall sense of well-being. Simply "taking a few deep breaths" when feeling stressed can be very effective as a stress management technique.

Kabat-Zinn (1994), founding director of the Center for Mindfulness in Medicine, Health, and Society, teaches a combination of focusing techniques and mindfulness meditation derived from Buddhist meditation methods. This stress reduction program operates as a part of the Center for Mindfulness at the University of Massachusetts Medical School. The major premise of this mindfulness meditation is to be "mindful" and "aware" during the meditation process. Kabat-Zinn begins his workshops by having participants "mindfully" eat a raisin. He urges participants to simply pay attention and focus while eating a raisin. Participants close their eyes and eat the raisin very slowly paying attention to the taste, sound, texture, and smell of the raisin while they eat. By focusing on this simple task, participants can begin to see that this process is really not as difficult as they imagine it to be. This sense of mindfulness can also be adapted to the typical daily activities in which people engage. Washing the dishes, playing solitaire, saying the rosary, making dinner, or taking a walk can all be completed in a "mindful way." The most important concept of this strategy is to try to stay in the present moment. Learning to focus attention on the present and being mindful of that present moment enhances serenity in a unique way (Fontaine, 2000). Reitz (2003) provided a workshop at the Health Ministries Association Conference on "Finding the Sacred Through Movement, Meditation, and Relaxation." She welcomes others to share her mindfulness meditation tips (Table 11-3).

A Sense of Gratitude

There is no question that maintaining a sense of gratitude is easy in faith community nursing when one is confronted in the homes of parishioners with the situations that parishioners cope

TABLE 11-3

Mindfulness Meditation Tips

ENERGY LEVEL FOR MEDITATION

Practice meditation when you have lots of energy. Concentration requires an alert mind; if you are tired, meditation will be a struggle. If you are a "morning" person, meditate in the morning. If you are an "evening" person, try to meditate in the evening.

MEDITATIVE PLACE

Try to find a peaceful place in your home to meditate. Whether it is a corner of a room, or a whole room, decorate it with colors and accents that reflect sacredness for you. If you create an altar, place items upon it that reflect your spirituality and symbolize the presence of God.

MEDITATIVE POSTURE

Sitting is the ideal pose for meditation because energy travels better throughout a straight spine. You may sit on a cushion and lean against a wall, or sit in a chair. Place your legs and hands in comfortable positions. Comfort is more important than struggling with acquired postures. Ideally, hands are placed palms up in lap or on knees to signify receptivity.

TIME LIMITS ON MEDITATION

If you are able to begin your practice by sitting for 20 minutes, two times a day, terrific! If this is difficult, try sitting for 5 minutes, one or two times daily, or less, when first starting out. It is more important to train your mind and body in the beginning to sit daily than it is to make it an endorsee test. If you start small and practice daily, your meditation time will gradually increase on its own.

CONCENTRATION TECHNIQUE

It is helpful to focus your gaze, eyes closed, at the bridge of your nose. This will take practice for it to feel comfortable. Placing the tip of the tongue on the roof of the mouth, behind the teeth, also encourages a sense of being centered.

MEDITATION BREATHING

Begin meditation with a breathing exercise, such as meditation or rhythm breathing. Empty the lungs, breathe in to a count of 8, hold to a count of 4, out to a count of 8, and hold lungs empty for a count of 4. (You may make your own counts; however, the breaths should equal half of the respiratory breaths.) Practice this exercise until you feel your mind begin to settle.

DEALING WITH INTRUSIVE BODY SIGNALS, THOUGHTS, AND EMOTIONS

The purpose of meditation techniques is to give our minds a little action to watch while our brains move into an alpha state. We do not, and cannot, blank the mind. When we sit with our meditation techniques, our consciousness will constantly be invaded by thoughts, emotions, and bodily discomforts. Our job is not to resist these interferences; resistance gives them more energy. Place your errant thoughts and feelings on your mental view screen and imagine them as clouds floating away from you. Scratch the itch or readjust your body if it calls to you. Then return to where you left off in your meditation technique.

TABLE 11-3
Mindfulness Meditation Tips (*continued*)
MINDFULNESS MEDITATION
Fine-tune your hearing; become aware of any sounds outside the room and identify them. Listen for the sounds inside the room. Allow sounds to be a part of your meditation. Become aware of your body and its position. This awareness checklist will aid in your note of being distracted by what is going on around you. Then bring your attention inward and watch the movement of your chest as it expands and contracts to the rhythm of your breaths. Later, move your attention to the bridge of the nose (where your nose joins your forehead), and imagine that you can watch your breath move in and out of your nose. You may want to add a word or short phrase to repeat with your exhalations. Think of this word as a prayer. It is always nice to end with some deep breaths and expressions of gratitude—no matter what you experienced.

with on a daily basis. Nurses enter homes where one might see a terminal cancer diagnosis in a young mother, a father with alcoholism that has impacted the entire family, a child with muscular dystrophy or cerebral palsy, or an elderly woman who has Alzheimer's disease and doesn't recognize any of her family members. FCNs become a lifeline to these families, and the nurses quickly become aware of the blessings in their own lives through their work with others.

Gratitude turns negative energy into positive energy. Gratitude unlocks the fullness of life. Burkhardt and Nagai-Jacobson (2002) describe gratitude as the natural response to one's awareness that life is a gift. It turns what one has into enough and more. It turns problems into gifts, failures into successes, the unexpected into perfect timing, and mistakes into important events. Gratitude makes sense of the past, brings peace for today, and creates a vision of tomorrow. A tool that is particularly effective for accessing gratitude is to make gratitude lists of five things that one is grateful for every day. Keegan (2001) states that a gratitude journal is best done at the end of the day, prior to going to bed. She asks her clients to simply write down the things that occurred that day that caused happiness, even things that might have normally gone unnoticed. At the beginning of this process, one is likely to place on the list things like family members, friends, and so forth, but as the days go on, simpler things will show up on the list of things of gratitude like the sunrise in the morning on a day you have to go to work early or a child's fascination with a flower petal, a puppy cuddling in close to you, or the snow falling in the early evening and the possibility of a snow day. Think: Restore to me the capacity for wonder in the smallest of things that can provide me with a sense of gratitude.

Time Management

People who manage their time effectively usually experience less stress (Kozier, Erb, Berman, & Snyder, 2004). Managing time effectively in this busy world is a real challenge because most people are juggling work, family, and sometimes school responsibilities all at once. There does not seem to be enough hours in the day to keep up with the tasks required. The FCN who feels overwhelmed may need help prioritizing the tasks that need to be completed. The key to time management is to begin to learn to prioritize what is important and must be done today and then to organize your life in such a way to make that happen. Modifications may need to be made to decrease the multiple role demands. A key strategy that will seem paradoxical to the concept of time management is to take a deep breath and relax a bit (Kabat-Zinn, 1994). This deep breathing, if only for a couple of minutes, can help to restore the physical energy that one needs to cope with the many tasks required to be completed in a day.

Making lists of what to do can even become burdensome, but lists are certainly a visual representation of what needs to be done, and ways to begin to manage and prioritize may become clear. One may find that there are things on the list that are not really important at all. Other things on the list can wait for a while and do not need to be done immediately, which then lessens the sense of stress.

Nurses need to learn to delegate to others. In the family situations, delegate the tasks that other family members are able to do competently. Delegate also to the congregational volunteers who are usually eager and willing to help out and to the other FCNs who may have the expertise required to cope with a particular problem that presents itself. Consider the gift of allowing someone to do something rather than the FCN. Consider what a gift that would truly be for the FCN, easing the overwhelmed feeling that is so much a part of life.

One of the strategies that has been found to be very effective is when an assignment is given, to start on it right away. Some of these tasks can be completed quickly if addressed immediately and then the task is no longer on that long list of things that need to be done. The task is done and complete, and a sense of accomplishment is felt for those items instead of a task that is looming in the mind yet to be done.

Finding Personal Peace and Nurturing Spirituality

Important for the FCN is to incorporate some time for personal space and solitude into his or her busy life. Everyone needs some alone time in their week—some people more than others. Solitude regenerates one's physical and spiritual energy that will be needed to serve the parish needs. Also important for the FCN is to be attentive to taking that time for self to allow for the "cup to be filled again." Mauk and Schmidt (2004) talk about the importance of taking a few moments every day to be alone and to reflect on the day's activities. Turning off the radio, television, or CD player, and not answering the phone can provide time for thinking about what is truly important in one's life. This silence can be very powerful as a tool for self-caring.

Nurturing spirituality can be achieved in several ways. One might consider attending daily Mass or worship service when the number of people attending is very small. The services tend to be more intimate and short, which meets the needs of people who want to begin their day with a spiritual presence but also need to get to work. Taking a walk in the morning before the day begins and at the same time saying a rosary or communicating with a higher power during this time can be very peaceful. During this connection, the FCN might ask for guidance and help through the day. Robert Wood Johnson University Hospital at Hamilton (RWJUH) has developed a "Grounds for Healing" by having gardens and art work at the entrances available to staff, patients, and visitors so that people can have a quiet place to sit (Miller, 2003). Taking a walk alone clears the mind of "extra clutter" and allows one to become centered on the mission and purpose for the day.

Music can be used to enhance a nurse's well-being (Mauk & Schmidt, 2004). Music enhances serenity in a way that nothing else can. The selection of music is a very personal thing and what might be soothing and calming to one person would not be to another. The FCN might begin to develop a collection of music that would be helpful in relaxing the nurse at the end of a busy day. The nurse can fill the tub with lavender bubble bath, put in the CD, and just relax the day away.

Storytelling

Communication is a key coping strategy in caring for the self. Although not all FCNs are women, many of them are. The number of male nurses is below 10% of the total population of nurses. New research findings validate something that women have known for years—women tend to connect with other women during stressful times (Taylor, Klein, Lewis, Gruenewald, Gurung, & Updegraff, 2000). These researchers found that women have a different behavioral response to stress than the typical "fight or flight" that was originally assumed. They found that the hormone oxytocin is released as part of the response to stress and encourages women to gather with other women. The sharing that occurs between and among women is clearly a helpful way of venting the issue and also a way of sharing strategies that have worked successfully for others. Members of more formal support groups are introduced to various effective coping strategies during their time with the group. The FCN meetings clearly serve this purpose as nurses gather together to share their "stories." As nurses share their stories, they share the experiences of being a part of making a difference in the lives of their patients (Libster, 2001). This oral tradition has been evident in nursing since the time of sharing stories at change of shift reports in the hospital settings.

Nurses also share the challenges they face as FCNs trying to meet the needs of the congregation and yet not neglecting their own needs in the process. Storytelling is a wonderful way to share with one another and enhance serenity at the same time. Koloroutis and Felgen (2004) talk about the metaphor of the redwood trees and how supporting each other is essential to self-care, much like these majestic trees do for each other in a forest setting. The authors describe the need for nurses to rely on each other and describe the image of the redwood trees as nurses' limbs intertwined with one another reaching toward the sun.

Journal Writing

Communication in writing is another coping strategy for self-care. The therapeutic benefits of writing are well documented in the professional literature. Writing has been used for many years as a teaching tool to reinforce taught material, to summarize key points during a lecture, and to express ideas (Poirrier, 1997). Recently, health care professionals have discovered the value of writing as a clinical intervention. This method can also be used to promote self-caring.

Journals allow the writers to express feelings that they may be having in relation to working with people of the faith community. Daily journal writing is encouraged as an effective coping strategy. Cameron (1992), in her book *The Artist's Way,* encourages everyone to begin their day by writing "three morning pages" in a journal entry. The writer begins to process issues in a different way than one does in oral communication. Journal exercises allow nurses to explore various issues in their lives that might be impacting their ability to care for themselves. Getting emotions down on paper, whether in a journal or a letter, can help a person come to terms with the feelings that they are experiencing and begin to resolve them (Senn, 2001).

Journal writing is voluntary and not graded or judged. Writing in a journal is an opportunity to spell out ideas, beliefs, attitudes, and feelings in whatever style suits a person. Journal writing is spontaneous and honest. It also encourages self-awareness and self-discovery. Looking back on past journals allows people to trace the growth that has occurred and the changes that might have happened in thoughts, attitudes, and behaviors.

There is no wrong way to keep a journal. Journaling is meant to be simply the act of moving the hand across the page and writing down whatever comes to your mind. Nothing is too silly, stupid, or weird to include (Neubauer & Adams, 2000). Trying not to censor one's writing is important; simply thinking of it as a free writing exercise. Some guidelines might be helpful to those who have never considered journal writing as a tool for self-awareness (Table 11-4).

Eliopoulos (2004) states that journaling is a good daily practice for self-nurturing. Senn (2001) shares several strategies for personal journal writing. Neubauer and Adams (2000) make journaling an easy task in their book as well. Mauk and Schmidt (2004) describe journaling as a nonverbal method of capturing personal thoughts on the page and then taking the time to reflect on those thoughts at some point later in time. They say that journaling allows

TABLE 11-4

Guidelines for Journal Writing

1. Write in your journal every day. Choose a time that works for you and make this time a ritual for you.
2. Buy yourself a really nice journal and pen.
3. Choose a comfortable space to write in your journal.
4. Respect the process of awareness that occurs when you write. You may find that in writing something down you are able to think differently than when you talk about something verbally.
5. Write for at least 10 minutes each day.
6. Your journal is meant to be "just for you" to see. You can choose to share what you want with others.

the writer to process ideas and express both negative and positive emotions without interference from anyone else. There is no question that this is a tool that can foster self-caring behaviors.

Nature

Finding a spot in nature that works is another effective strategy in the pursuit of self-care. Kabat-Zinn (1994) uses nature as a site for exercising the mindfulness of his sessions. A walk in the woods can be made into a mindfulness meditation. Instead of quickly walking through the woods, be sure to notice the sights, smells, and sounds in the environment, and the experience will take on a whole new meaning. The nurse might focus on each footstep and become aware of the ability to walk at all. Gratitude comes into play as the FCN considers people in the congregation who are homebound, in wheelchairs, or immobilized in their beds because of stroke. The act of walking can be experienced in such a positive way.

The birds singing in the morning as they greet the day are a joy to listen to; wouldn't it be wonderful if people greeted the day in the same way? A known saying is that the way that a person greets the day indicates his or her attitude toward life. The positive person greets the day by saying, "Good morning, God," whereas the negative person says, "Good God, it's morning."

The beach, for many, is a wonderful place to commune with nature. Nowhere else on earth peaks the five senses in such an extraordinary way. As one walks toward the beach, the smell of the salt air fills the nostrils as one anticipates "hitting the beach" as fast as one can. The feet touch the sand and the shoes come off so that the toes are free to wiggle into the warmth of the sand. Notice the various feels of the sand at different portions of the beach. The sand is finer and hotter on the outer edges. As the water is approached, the sand is firm and, finally, the toes can simply squish into the sand where the water meets the beach. The seagulls are there to greet the day, some with a sense of welcoming the people back to the beach and others wondering how one dare invade their territory. The sight of the waves is something else to behold. The waves thunder toward the shore, and the sound and the sight are incredible. Who can question the existence of God when one spends a day at the beach in this mindful way? The beach is truly an incredible place to commune with nature.

Self-reflection

Wendell Berry said, "The world cannot be discovered by a journey of miles; only by a spiritual journey by which we arrive at the ground at our feet and learn to be at home." Self-reflection is key to an inner peace. In coping with the various issues in the community of the parish, there may be many difficult situations. In the one faith community nursing group in south New Jersey, one member admitted that she felt that her niche was truly to provide transportation to the parish community when needed rather than to do home visits or assessments. Another FCN who had a focus on education agreed to help with any educational programs that the group might decide to give. Another nurse who had a personal experience with the loss of her own husband shared that she would likely be more helpful to grieving members in that she would "definitely understand what they were feeling" because of her own loss. Self-reflection allows the FCNs to have a better sense of where they might best serve the community.

Prayer

The literature on the importance of prayer is increasing. Taylor (2002) shares the effectiveness of prayer as a coping strategy. FCNs often begin and end their meetings with a prayer, asking a higher power to guide them as they attempt to meet the needs of the faith community members. Louis and Alpert's (2000) research compared nurses who were prepared in providing spiritual care with nurses who were not prepared in spiritual care. On the section of the survey that identified "personal sources of spiritual strength" the researchers found that parish nurses ranked prayer (96.6%), talking to someone (86.6%), and reading spiritual resources (72.9%) as the three most used sources for finding strength in coping with their own life struggles. Prayer helps to alleviate anxiety, and it lifts up the spirit. Prayer can also be used as an expression of gratitude (Eliopoulos, 2004). Prayers of thanksgiving encourage a connection with a higher power and contribute to feelings of abundance and blessings in one's life. Prayer and meditation facilitate time for centering and focusing on one's spiritual wellness. A number of communities have planned and developed *labyrinths.* The labyrinth is a kind of spiritual walk intended to clear the mind and give insight to the person on a spiritual journey (Burkhardt & Nagai-Jacobson, 2002). The labyrinth is a path that has one way into the center, and the same path is followed on the return. Linda Clay, congregational nurse in the Church of the Loving Shepherd, was responsible for developing a labyrinth in that church. Parishioners follow the course of the labyrinth into the center in spiritual contemplation to find answers to any questions or concerns that they may have (Fontaine, 2000).

One of the most helpful tools to enhance spirituality is the "God Box." When people find themselves worrying about something over which they have no control, they write on a piece of paper and put it in the God Box. The feeling of turning it over to a higher power is wonderful, and they find that they are able to "let go and let God." Most people who use the God Box quickly find that it is "filled to the brim." Communicating with the higher power in this way acknowledges one's powerless over most situations and allows someone else to take over.

Solitude is essential to self-reflection and prayer, and yet contemporary Western culture makes the act of solitude difficult to attain. Solitude promotes insight as has been recognized by great religious leaders who have retreated from the world and then later shared what has been revealed to them. The desire for solitude is a means of escape from ordinary life and the pursuit of renewal of the mind, body, and the spirit (Storr, 1988). Removal of one's self from the environment promotes self-understanding and contact with one's inner thoughts. Regardless of the nature of the journey, it is important to take the time to be still. The quiet that occurs in this solitude allows a person to listen to the inner voice that is directing him or her along the way of life (Keegan, 1994).

Summary

Nurses in today's health care system are coping with stress more than they ever have before. The nursing shortage and the changes in the health care arena have had a major impact on increasing this stress level for most nurses. Parish nurses are helping to fill the health care needs of people in faith communities, and yet this job is no less stressful than any other nursing position.

Nurses have done a wonderful job of taking care of everyone else in their lives, including patients, family, and friends. Most nurses do not take the time during the day to pay attention to taking care of themselves. This chapter describes this phenomenon and provides various self-care activities that nurses may find helpful in their lives. The chapter provides physical, emotional, and spiritual ideas to incorporate into busy lives. Meditation, breathing exercises, time management, prayer, and solitude are all described as strategies that the FCN might access in the pursuit of self-caring.

Reflect and Discuss

1. Fran was clearly overwhelmed with stress in her retirement. Identify the points in the case study where that phenomenon becomes evident.
2. Identify times in your own life when you have clearly taken better care of others than you have of yourself. What circumstances allowed that to happen?
3. What might Fran have done to prevent this feeling of being stressed and overwhelmed in her retirement?
4. Describe three self-care activities that Fran might incorporate into her life as she copes with this added responsibility.
5. Decide on just one self-care activity that you will include in your life this week. Put it on the calendar and be sure to follow through.

Case Study

Fran is a retired registered nurse living in Ocean City, New Jersey. She worked 40 years as a registered nurse and is finally looking forward to relaxing at the beach in her retirement years. She loved her retirement and was taking long walks on the beach every day, riding her bike, taking a yoga class, connecting with friends, and loving every minute of this well-deserved time "just for her." After about 2 months of relaxation, Fran found that she was getting bored and began to look for part-time employment in nursing. She had heard a bit about faith community nursing and took several classes at the local university to become certified as an FCN. She approached the pastor of her new church about starting a faith community nursing program and found that he was delighted to know that there would be someone to "help him out a bit." Within 6 months Fran had organized a group of six registered nurses to be part of the faith community nursing group, developed a brochure, surveyed the congregation of 2,000 families related to health care needs, organized and provided training for 50 volunteers to help out with the program, had spoken to the youth group and other congregational groups, provided visits to families in the parish, organized blood pressure screenings, provided health education programs on coping with loss issues, and provided other programs.

Whew! Fran was quickly overwhelmed with how much she had to do. She discovered that she was working more hours than she had when she was a full-time nurse, and she wasn't even being paid! She had no time for herself. She had stopped taking her yoga class, wasn't walking on the beach every day, and had no time to have lunch with friends. She was "way too busy" to take care of herself.

References

Benson, H. (1975). *The relaxation response*. New York: William Morrow Publications.

Bright, M. A. (2002). *Holistic health and healing*. Philadelphia: FA Davis.

Burkhardt, M. A., & Nagai-Jacobson, M. G. (2002). *Spirituality: Living our connectedness*. New York: Delmar Publishers, Thomson Learning.

Cameron, J. (1992). *The artist's way: A spiritual path to higher creativity*. New York: GP Putnam's Sons.

Covington, H. (2003). Caring presence: Delineation of a concept for holistic nursing. *Journal of Holistic Nursing, 21*(3), 301–317.

Eliopoulos, C. (2004). *Invitation to holistic health: A guide to living a balanced life*. Sudbury, MA: Jones and Bartlett.

Fontaine, K. L. (2000). *Healing practices: Alternative therapies for nursing*. Upper Saddle River, NJ: Prentice Hall.

Henry, J. (2004). Self-care begets holistic care. *Reflections on Nursing Leadership, 27*(1).

Kabat-Zinn, J. (1994). *Wherever you go, there you are: Mindfulness meditation in everyday life*. New York: Hyperion Press.

Keegan, L. (2001). *Healing with complementary & alternative therapies*. Albany, New York: Delmar Publishers, Thomson Learning.

Keegan, L. (1994). *The nurse as healer*. New York: Delmar Publishers, Thomson Learning.

Knight, C. D. (2003). How do nurses become self-nurturers? Retrieved September 23, 2003, from http://community.nursingspectrum.com/ MagazineArticles.

Koloroutis, M., & Felgen, J. (2004). Holding each other up, a dialogue. *Reflections on Nursing Leadership, (1)*, 44–46.

Kozier, B., Erb, G., Berman, A., & Snyder, S. (2004). *Fundamentals of nursing: Concepts, process and practice* (7th ed.). Upper Saddle River, NJ: Prentice Hall.

Lanier, K. (2004). *The soul of the caring nurse: Stories and resources for revitalizing professional passion*. Silver Spring, MD: American Nurses Association Publication; Nursesbooks.org.

Libster, M. (2001). *Demonstrating care: The art of integrative nursing*. New York: Delmar Publishers, Thomson Learning.

Louis, M., & Alpert, P. (2000). Spirituality for nurses and their practice. *Nursing Leadership Forum, 5*(2), 43–49.

Mauk, K. L., & Schmidt, N. K. (2004). *Spiritual care in nursing practice*. Philadelphia: Lippincott Williams & Wilkins.

Miller, M. S. (2003). Self-care for nurses—Practice what you preach! Retrieved September 23, 2003, from http://community.nursingspectrum.com/ MagazineArticles.

Ornish, D. (1990). *Dean Ornish's program for reversing heart disease*. New York: Random House.

Neubauer, J. R., & Adams, K. (2000). *The complete idiot's guide to journaling*. Alpha Books.

Poirrier, G. P. (1997). *Writing to learn*. New York: National League for Nursing Press.

Potter, P. A., & Perry, A. G. (2001). *Fundamentals of Nursing*. St. Louis, MO: Mosby.

Reitz (June 2003). Finding the sacred through movement, meditation, and relaxation. Workshop presented at the annual Health Ministries Association Conference, Valley Forge, PA.

Senn, L. (2001). *The many faces of journaling: Topics and techniques for personal journal writing*. St. Louis, MO: Pen Central Press.

Sieg, D. (2004). Lost your smile? *Reflections on Nursing Leadership, (1)*, 36–38.

Slaninka, S. C. (2003). Care of the inner self. *Advance for Nurses*, 30–32.

Storr, A. (1988). *Solitude: A return to the self*. New York: Ballantine Books.

Taylor, E. J. (2002). *Spiritual care: Nursing theory, research, and practice*. Upper Saddle River, NJ: Prentice Hall.

Taylor, S. E., Klein, L. C., Lewis, B. P., Gruenewald, T. L., Gurung, R. A., & Updegraff, J. A. (2000). Behavioral responses to stress in females: Tend-and-befriend, not fight-or-flight. *Psychological Review, 107*(3), 411–429.

Wade, C. F. (2002). When giving care, don't forget yourself. Retrieved September 23, 2003, from http://community.nursingspectrum.com.

Additional Resources

Berg, J. A. (1998). Integrative therapies in primary care practices. *Journal of the American Academy of Nurse Practitioners, 10*, 541.

Hong, Y., Li, J. X., & Robinson, P. D. (2000). Balance control, flexibility, and cardio-respiratory fitness among older Tai Chi practitioners. *British Journal of Sports Medicine, 34*(1), 29–34.

Kabat-Zinn, J., Wheeler, E., Light, T., Skillings, A., Scharf, M., & Cropley, T. G., et al. (1998). Influence of a mindfulness meditation-based stress reduction intervention on rates of skin clearing in patients with moderate to severe psoriasis undergoing phototherapy (UVB) and photochemotherapy (PUVA). *Psychosomatic Medicine, 60*(5), 625–632.

Luskin, F., Newell, K., Griffith, M., Holmes, M., Telles, S., & Marvasti, F., et al. (1998). A review of mind-body therapies in the treatment of cardiovascular disease. *Alternative Therapies, 4*(3), 46–61.

McCullough, M. E., Hoyt, W. T., Larson, D. B., Koenig, H. G., & Thoresen, C. (2000). Religious involvement and mortality: A meta-analytic review. *Health Psychology, 19*(3), 211–222.

Newman, M. A. (1999). The rhythm of relating in a paradigm of wholeness. *Image: Journal of Nursing Scholarship, 31,* 227.

Robbins, L. B., Pender, N. J., Conn, V. S., Frenn, M. D., Neuberger, G. B., & Nies, M. A., et al. (2001). Physical activity research in nursing. *Journal of Nursing Scholarship, 33,* 315–321.

Sergerstrom, S. C., Taylor, S. E., Kemeny, M. E., & Fahey, J. L. (1998). Optimism is associated with mood, coping, and immune changes in response to stress. *Journal of Personality and Social Psychology, 74*(6), 1646–1655.

Snyder, M., & Chlan, L. (1999). Music therapy. In J. J. Fitzpatrick (Ed.), *Annual review of nursing research.* New York: Springer.

Young, D. R., Appel, I. J., Jee, S., & Miller, E. R. (1999). The effects of aerobic exercise and Tai Chi on blood pressure in older people. *Journal of the American Geriatric Society, 47*(3), 277–284.

→ Web Resources

http://www.interactiveimagery.com   Academy for Guided Imagery

http://www.aath.org   American Association for Therapeutic Humor

http://www.nhna.org   American Holistic Nursing Association

http://www.paguide.com   Canadian Society of Exercise Physiology

http://www.brightspot.org   Center for the Improvement of Human Functioning

http://www.healthy.net/cmbm   Center for Mind-Body Medicine

http://www.mindfulnesstapes.com   Center for Mindfulness/UMASS

http://www.mbst.com   Center for Mindfulness in Medicine, Healthcare, and Society

http://www.JoyfulNoiseletter.com   Fellowship of Merry Christians, Inc.

http://www.healingtouch.net   Healing Touch International

http://www.heart-net.com   HeartNet International

http://www.refexology-usa.net   International Institute of Reflexology

http://www.mindbody.harvard.edu   Mind-Body Institute

http://www.naha.org   National Association For Holistic Aromatherapy

http://www.goecities.com?Athens/1501/sheckfil.html   Under Shekhina's Wings

http://www.tm.org   Transcendental Meditation Program

IV

Health Promotion and Disease Prevention

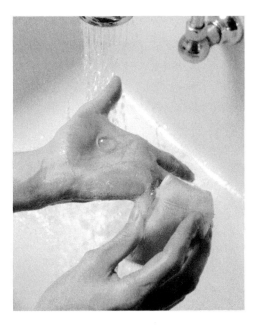

12

Planning Health Promotion/ Disease Prevention Programs

Essential Elements for Faith Community Nursing/ Health Ministry Program Development

The process of developing programs for a faith community nurse (FCN) ministry may seem like a daunting task, especially when one considers that many FCNs function as volunteers on a part-time basis. The most important issue to remember in the development of any faith community ministry is that FCNs need to recruit the help of a health ministry team to aid them in the processes of planning, implementing, and evaluating the programs that address the assessed needs of the congregation. Ideally, a faith community health ministry team is created prior to establishing a faith community nursing program in the congregation. The members of this team could be recruited by recommendations of the clergy, the church council, or by responding positively to a questionnaire distributed to all members of the faith community. The members of this team would work with the FCN to provide the desired and needed services and programs for the members of the faith community.

Many models of faith community health ministry teams exist, and each has unique characteristics that work in each individual situation. Whether or not all members of the health ministry team would require a medical background will need to be determined at the start of the program, and the criteria for being a member of the team will need to be clearly addressed in the planning stages of the process. The size and demographics of each individual faith community will have a significant influence on the types of individuals that become members of the health ministry team. At least one professional nurse should take charge of the health ministry team. Each individual faith community will need to determine its needs and decide if more than one professional nurse is needed to meet the goals and objectives set forth by the health ministry team.

As discussed in Chapter 5, assessment of the faith community is essential before any faith community nursing/health ministry programs are developed. Thorough assessment of the faith community will guide FCNs in addressing the areas of interest and the needs of the members of the congregation, thus setting the stage for a successful program. Assessment of the larger community in which the congregation resides is also essential in the development of faith community nursing. This process helps FCNs learn about the resources available within the community as well as how the members of the faith community represent the culture and needs of the community at large. Once an assessment of the members of the faith community and the community at large is completed, FCNs will need to review the data collected and determine the most commonly addressed needs and desires of the faith community. A good way to initiate a program is to plan an educational activity or event that addresses one of the needs. By doing so, the FCN will be demonstrating awareness of the desires and needs of the members of the faith community. Programs should be directed at meeting the members' needs and not the needs or preferences of the FCN, the health ministry team, or other individuals.

Types of Faith Community Nurse/Health Ministry Programs

Blood pressure screening/monitoring programs are often the first programs initiated by the faith community nursing team. This activity is a good way for FCNs to interact with the members of the congregation and, at the same time, provide a service that is valuable to them. Often this activity is a way for FCNs to provide health teaching to the members whom they serve as well as an opportunity to further assess what additional types of programs the members would like to have regarding their heart health. See Box 12-1 for guidance in developing a blood pressure program in a faith community.

If, as a result of the assessment process, the FCN identifies a need to provide health information addressing various health topics, one way of accomplishing this task would be to develop monthly or seasonal bulletin board displays that focus on some of the desired health topics. Information about various health topics can be obtained from sources, such as pamphlets and posters distributed by local hospitals, health departments, or health-related organizations within the community. Information posted on various Web sites on the Internet is a very convenient source for FCNs to obtain material covering most any health issue. FCNs can use bulletin board displays to creatively relay health information to all age groups in the faith community in a fun, visible, and nonthreatening way.

Many faith communities publish monthly newsletters and distribute them to all members. Faith community nurses could use this publication for the dissemination of health-related information addressing various health topics. When using this type of media, FCNs would need to be sensitive to the educational level of the members of the faith community, because it would be very ineffective to publish literature at a level that is either too simple or too complex for the members to read and comprehend. Most FCNs will be able to determine what educational level is appropriate for the members from information gathered from the initial assessment of the faith community. Another similar media application would be to insert short health-related information segments into the weekly Sunday service bulletin. Again, the use of information from local health facilities and organizations, as well as the Internet, would be an appropriate way for FCNs to provide information to many members without a large cost attached.

Many FCN/health ministry programs are very successful in offering a few services, such as a monthly blood pressure screening, and providing health education to the members of the congregation via bulletin boards and articles in monthly newsletters and Sunday bulletins. To expand the activities of FCN/health ministry programs, FCNs may want to provide health information to the members of the congregation by addressing health issues that are identified in the *Health Observances and Recognition Days* calendar, published by the American Hospital Association (Society for Healthcare Strategy and Market Development of the American Hospital Association, 2002). Each month has health-related observances and recognition days that focus on issues, such as chronic illnesses, safety, health screenings, and the recognition of health care providers. Provided are names of organizations that support every observance listed in the calendar as well as contact information for the majority of the organizations. The use of this calendar would be helpful in initiating ideas for topics for program development as well as providing sources of information regarding many health-related issues (Box 12-2).

This program schedule is just a sample of the various topics and programs that could be developed using the *Health Observances and Recognition Days* calendar. Program development for a period of several years could be developed just from the topics and resources listed in this publication. The programs developed from this source would provide health education for many members of all ages, in various types of faith communities.

To expand on the information presented to the members of the faith community using the *Health Observances and Recognition Days* calendar, the FCN/health ministry team could

---

BOX 12-1
How to Start a Blood Pressure Screening/Monitoring Program in a Faith Community Nursing/Health Ministry Program

1. Review the assessment of the faith community and determine whether there is an interest in a blood pressure screening/monitoring program.
2. Determine whether members of the health ministry team would be able to assist the FCN in taking and recording blood pressures. If no members are able to assist with this task, the parish nurse may consider recruiting help from an outside source (nurse colleagues or FCNs from another congregation close by) or training someone on the health ministry team to take and record blood pressures.
3. Distribute a questionnaire to determine when the members would like to have the blood pressure screening/monitoring program take place. The questionnaire could offer several options to choose from: Once a month; every other month; before Sunday services; after Sunday services.
4. Once the frequency and time for the screening/monitoring are established, contact the church council and the clergy to arrange the best physical site for the screening/monitoring to be held. The site should be convenient for the members, yet offer a quiet environment with a private space for counseling, if necessary.
5. Obtain the needed equipment (blood pressure cuffs, stethoscopes, a notebook, or other source for keeping records of participants and blood pressure readings). The acquisition of this equipment will most probably need the approval of the church council or the church treasurer.
6. Visit the local chapter of the American Heart Association to obtain brochures relating to hypertension. Some chapters of this organization may also have pocket-sized cards to distribute to the individuals to record their blood pressure readings. If wallet cards are not available, the FCN should consider creating and reproducing one similar to the card illustrated here:

ZION LUTHERAN

BLOOD PRESSURE SCREENING/MONITORING PROGRAM

DATE	BLOOD PRESSURE	DATE	BLOOD PRESSURE
_____	_____	_____	_____
_____	_____	_____	_____
_____	_____	_____	_____

7. Post signs in noticeable areas of the building where members meet for services to announce the time and location of the blood pressure screening/monitoring.
8. On the day of the blood pressure screening/monitoring, have volunteers from the health ministry team available to help with registration, distribution of brochures, etc.
9. Encourage participants to return for the next screening/monitoring. The FCN should make herself or himself available to answer any questions and/or schedule a private meeting with participants, if the need arises.
10. After the screening/monitoring is completed, the FCN should schedule a time with the participating members of the health ministry team to discuss the outcome of the event and to plan for changes in the program, if necessary.

---

coordinate with some local chapters of national organizations to provide activities related to the health issues addressed in the program calendar. One example of this would be to contact the American Automobile Association or state or local police departments to organize a bicycle rodeo for the children of the congregation and surrounding community. This activity is often coordinated within the month of May to accompany information regarding bicycle safety. Children participate in obstacle courses set up by these organizations to emphasize safe bi-

BOX 12-2
Health Observances and Recognition Days

The following monthly program schedule of health education programs for adults and youth is an example of how the events from the *Health Observances and Recognition Days* calendar could be used in a faith community nurse/health ministry program.

January

Adults: Healthy eating and weight management

Youth: Proper handwashing

The adult program will focus on making healthy food choices and how this can lead to weight loss and/or weight management. Information for this program can be obtained from the American Dietetic Association, local and state health departments, and some local hospital wellness departments.

The youth program will be presented to the preschool children with an interactive program using poems and actual handwashing practice. The program for the older school-aged children will be presented in a discussion-type session and perhaps a video presentation. Information for this program could be obtained from the American Academy of Pediatrics, some state and local health departments, as well as some local hospital wellness departments.

February

Adults: Heart health

Youth: Child passenger safety

The adult program will focus on a "healthy heart." Common heart disease processes will be described as well as the common treatments for these conditions. Information can be obtained from the American Heart Association, local and state health departments, and some local hospital wellness departments. The case study presents an example of how a discussion-type session can motivate an individual to seek professional medical treatment for a health issue she was ignoring and could have resulted in a negative outcome.

The youth program will focus on the reasons why seat belts are so important in preventing serious injury. Information for these programs can be obtained from the National Highway Traffic Safety Administration and some state and local police departments.

March

Adults: Vision and eye health

Youth: Poison prevention

The adult program will focus on common eye diseases and their treatments. Information for this program can be obtained from the National Eye Institute or local ophthalmologists.

The youth program will address common household items that can be described as potential poisons. Preschool-aged children will participate in an interactive program in which they will describe and point to potential household poisons that are placed in a big box along with other usual household items. Mr. YUK will be explained to them as well as the phrase, "Always ask an adult first." Information for this program can be obtained from the National Poison Prevention Week Council as well as some local and state health departments and local hospital emergency rooms or wellness departments.

April

Adults: Cancer awareness and screenings

Youth: Youth sports injury prevention

The adult program will focus on the common types of cancer as well as the common cancer screenings. Information for this program can be obtained from the American Cancer Society, state and local health departments, and some hospital wellness departments.

The youth program will address (in very simple terms) the common sports injuries that children and adolescents can experience while playing sports. Prevention of injury will be emphasized. Information for this program can be obtained from the National Youth Sports Safety Foundation, Inc., and some local hospital wellness and trauma departments.

BOX 12-2
Health Observances and Recognition Days *(continued)*

May

Adults: Arthritis awareness

Youth: Bicycle safety

The adult program will focus on the types of arthritis and the usual treatments to control arthritis. Information for this program can be obtained from the Arthritis Foundation, some state and local health departments, and some local hospital wellness departments.

The youth program will focus on the importance of safety rules and helmet use in preventing serious injury in bicycle accidents. Information for this program can be obtained from the National Highway Traffic Safety Administration, National Safe Kids Campaign, Automobile Association of America, state and local health departments, some state and local police departments, as well as some local hospital trauma departments.

June

Adults: Hernia awareness

Youth: Fireworks safety

The adult program will focus on the common types of hernias and the treatments usually associated with them. Information for this program can be obtained from local hospital wellness departments as well as local physicians and surgeons.

The youth program will focus on the safety guidelines that should be followed to enjoy fireworks without injury. Information for this program can be obtained from the American Academy of Ophthalmology, the Consumer Products Safety Commission, National Safe Kids Campaign, and local hospital trauma departments.

July

Adults: Dental health

Youth: Safety around the pool and yard

The adult program will focus on dental and oral health issues. Information for this program can be obtained from the Academy of General Dentistry, the American Dental Association, state and local health departments, as well as local dentists and oral surgeons.

The youth program will address the many dangers of pool and backyard play areas. Information for this program can be obtained from National Safe Kids Campaign, some local hospital trauma departments, as well as local pediatricians and family physicians.

August

Adults: Cataract awareness

Youth: Immunization

The adult program will discuss what cataracts are, when they should be treated, and the procedures that are used to restore vision. Information for this program can be obtained from the American Academy of Ophthalmology, some local hospital wellness departments, as well as some local ophthalmologists.

The youth program will focus on the importance of immunizations in preventing many communicable diseases. Information for this program can be obtained from the National Partnership for Immunization, state and local health departments, as well as local pediatricians and family practice physicians.

September

Adults: Cholesterol education

Youth: Head lice

The adult program will focus on what cholesterol is and the prevention and treatment of high cholesterol. Information for this program can be obtained from the National Heart, Lung, and Blood Institute, the American Heart Association, some state and local health departments, as well as some local hospital wellness departments.

(continued)

BOX 12-2
Health Observances and Recognition Days *(continued)*

The youth program will discuss the common occurrence of head lice and the usual prevention and treatment guidelines. Information for this program can be obtained from the National Pediculosis Association, some state and local health departments, some local hospital wellness departments, as well as local pediatricians and family practice physicians.

October

Adults: Breast cancer awareness

Youth: Dental hygiene

The adult program will focus on the importance of early detection of breast cancer and the usual screening guidelines. Information for this program can be obtained from the American Cancer Society, some state and local health departments, as well as some local hospital wellness departments.

The youth program will focus on the importance of good dental hygiene and oral health. Information for this program can be obtained from the American Dental Hygienists Association, the American Dental Association, some state and local health departments, as well as some local dentists.

November

Adults: Diabetes awareness

Youth: Indoor exercise

The adult program will focus on the guidelines to prevent or control the complications of diabetes. Information for this program can be obtained from the American Diabetes Association, the American Association of Diabetes Educators, some state and local health departments, as well as some local hospital wellness departments.

The youth program will address the importance of physical exercise and how indoor exercise programs can be accomplished without a lot of cost and special equipment. Information for this program can be obtained from local chapters of the YMCA and YWCA, the Boys and Girls Clubs of America, some local hospital wellness departments, as well as some local pediatricians and family physicians.

December

Adults: Drunk & drugged driving prevention

Youth: Safe toys and gifts

The adult program will focus on safe behaviors related to the consumption of alcohol and drugs. Information for this program can be obtained from the National Highway Traffic Safety Administration, some state and local police departments, as well as some local hospital trauma programs.

The youth program will focus on dangerous toys, especially those dangerous to children's eyesight. Information for this program can be obtained from Prevent Blindness America, the National Safe Kids Campaign, and some local hospital trauma centers.

---

cycle riding habits as well as to enforce the importance of following traffic safety rules while riding on local streets and rural roads. The use of bicycle helmets is also emphasized, and often some of these organizations have bicycle helmets or coupons for reduced prices on bicycle helmets as rewards for attendance to the rodeo or as prizes for activities they successfully complete while participating in the bicycle rodeo.

Another example of an activity to accompany a program addressed in the monthly calendar would be to have a member of the local chapter of the American Cancer Society visit interested women of the faith community in October in observance of Breast Cancer Awareness Month. Programs that instruct women on how to become more aware of breast health are often very informative and helpful in alleviating the anxiety that many women have about this very personal issue regarding their health. In addition, the representatives of the American

Cancer Society would also be able to discuss the programs available within the local area regarding breast and other cancers. One such program is "Tell A Friend," a program in which volunteer women call one another on the telephone to remind other women to have their annual mammogram performed. The monthly reminders have shown positive results in the early detection of breast cancer in women who participate in the program.

For the months when programs address seat belt safety and other automobile safety issues, FCNs could contact local chapters of the American Automobile Association or some state and local police departments to arrange for representatives to present various programs to a group of interested members of the congregation. One example of a program offered by these organizations is one that addresses the proper installation and use of infant and toddler car safety seats. In this program, representatives actually inspect the child safety seats used by individuals participating in the program for malfunctioning parts and/or improper installation in the vehicles where they are used. Many individuals who participate in this program learn that they are not installing their child safety seats properly and that they are using the wrong size of child seat for their child. This type of activity helps to reinforce the proper use of these safety devices and helps to ensure that children are safer if involved in an automobile accident, the leading cause of childhood deaths in the United States.

When the FCN/health ministry team learns that individuals within the faith community are interested in ongoing health education regarding various health issues, such as weight management, management of chronic diseases, or to participate in activities such as an exercise program or cooking healthy meals, the development of support groups or specific activity groups may be beneficial to those interested members. When these types of programs are planned, it is important that the health ministry team members become involved with some of the activities so that FCNs do not feel that they must be available to every group for every planned activity. It should be understood that FCNs would always be available to provide support and guidance to the members of these various groups; however, attendance at every function is not reasonable or possible in most program settings. FCNs very often stay involved with the groups in some capacity, especially in the formation stages when group members need to develop goals and objectives and look to the FCN for guidance with these tasks. Another task often handled by FCNs is the contacting and networking with organizations within the community as well as with some state and national organizations for the purpose of obtaining health information and resources addressing the health needs of the group. In some parish settings, support groups become self-directed and FCNs basically serve as a consultant to the group members. Durrant and Rieckmann (2003) believe that the strength of support groups, as an intervention, lies in two areas: being able to gain objective insight into personal behavior and realizing that one is not alone in trying to cope with life's problems. Insight comes with the power of the group's feedback, and group membership provides a sense of community.

Health fairs are another activity that may be of interest to the members of the faith community. Health fairs can be big events with lots of activities, or small, with a single focus. Schumann (2003) describes a congregation that had so many expectant parents that she created a baby fair focusing on parent education. Health fairs can be targeted to other specific audiences, such as teens or the elderly. The size of the faith community may determine whether a health fair will be open only to the congregants or whether it will be open to the general community. Small congregations may wish to consider co-hosting a health fair with another church, synagogue, or mosque.

A health fair is an event to:

- Increase health awareness by providing health screenings, activities, materials, demonstrations, and information.
- Increase awareness of local, state, and national health services and resources.

- Motivate participants to make positive health behavior changes.
- Provide immunizations for children and adults.
- Teach self-care practices.
- Identify topics and participants for future health programs.

Patterson (2003) states that health fairs make a health ministry accessible and visible. She reports that a health fair is one of the first events that clergy and health cabinets want to see take place with a new faith community nursing program. Boyes (2001) suggests that health fairs encourage well-being in a festive atmosphere. Exhibits, booths, demonstrations, activities, speakers, exercise classes, nutritious food samples, puppet shows, and health screening can help congregants make healthy lifestyle choices. Boyes describes a health fair that she developed using a theme of wholeness. This theme is congruent with the mission of faith community nursing, and it broadens the scope of the event to include psychosocial and spiritual wellness, in addition to physical wellness.

Wurzbach (2002) describes a model health fair as having four distinct aspects:

1. *Health education:* the first and most important aspect of health education. Health education should be delivered in interactive ways.
2. *Screening:* The longest lines at health fairs are for blood pressure and other screening tests, because people want to know about themselves. The easiest screening tests to arrange are height and weight, blood pressure, anemia, and vision acuity. Screenings that require more resources are screenings for cancer, glaucoma, hearing, cholesterol, and genetic disorders. Whenever laboratory tests are involved, consult public health law for requirements that must be met.
3. *Counseling and referral:* Counseling sessions allow a trained professional to outline actions that need to be taken to improve wellness.
   Counselors can encourage healthy lifestyle changes and appropriate community resources.
4. *Follow-up:* This can be done by mailings or by telephone, provided that the attendee has given prior permission for this contact.

Durban (2003) cautions that a health fair is definitely not something a new FCN should attempt to undertake in the first year. Health fairs require a large amount of planning and organization and are not an activity FCNs should consider, unless many members of the congregation would be willing to help with the many responsibilities necessary to have a successful event. The health ministry team would need to be very actively involved with the planning and organization of the health fair. The FCN should be responsible for assessing the types of venues that will participate in the health fair and be responsible for contacting the organizations that will provide services or information for the assessed needs. Wilson (2000) advises that at least three RNs be available at blood pressure screening tables to avoid lines. She also suggests that church members serve as greeters and guides. Because health fairs require an enormous amount of planning and organization, it is essential that adequate time and volunteers will be available from the point of initial planning to the final cleanup stages on the day the activity takes place. See Box 12-3 for how-to steps to plan a health fair and Box 12-4 for a checklist for success for a health fair.

Rice, Rider, and Pollard (2004) have developed a *Health Fair Planning Guide* that is available free of charge online (see Web Resources). Their suggestions for interactive and creative health education activities are a valuable resource. Each activity is described, and the age groups of suggested target audiences are listed.

Some FCN/health ministry programs offer structured health education programs to the members of the congregation. Often, the Sunday church school hour is used for this purpose at specified times throughout the year. This activity would definitely need the approval and

BOX 12-3
How to Plan a Health Fair

6 to 12 months before the health fair:
- Establish goals and objectives for the health fair.
- Establish a date and time—spring or fall are usually recommended.
- Select a theme.
- Select a chairperson and planning committee members.
- Select and reserve a site that is accessible for people with disabilities.
- Identify possible services, information, exhibits, and activities.
- Create subcommittees, if indicated—clinical, administrative, facilities, food procurement (incentives, promotional items, giveaways, door prizes, and supplies), clerical, and publicity.
- Select health screenings and services to be offered.
- Review liability insurance.
- Determine the level of attendance that can be safely accommodated.

3 to 6 months before the health fair:
- Establish timelines.
- Secure commitments for health care providers and exhibitors.
- Secure volunteers, including greeters, registration table staff, and someone to take pictures during the fair.
- Reserve any required rental equipment.
- Create a referral plan—for use if screening detects a problem that needs immediate attention and/or referral.

3 months before the health fair:
- Order educational materials from organizations.
- Plan and secure prizes, decorations, giveaways, and tablecloths.
- Reserve trash receptacles.
- Make posters and flyers.
- Duplicate printed materials—registration and evaluation forms.
- Provide written confirmation to all participants, including day and time for setup, a map to the location, and general guidelines (including the expectation that all booths will be manned at all times). Ask participants to bring extension cords (if needed), and if they have specific space requirements.
- Publicize "save the date."

1 month before the health fair:
- Meet with committee or subcommittee chairs to review progress of implementation plans.
- Publicize the event to your target audience(s). If the general public is invited, provide a press release to the local newspapers and use public service announcements on local radio and television stations.
- Map out a floor plan of the exhibit stations and a traffic flow.
- Make booth signs.
- Make a program, acknowledging exhibitors, volunteers, donors, etc.

(continued)

BOX 12-3
How to Plan a Health Fair (continued)

• Secure supplies:
  Pens and pencils
  Markers
  Paper clips, rubber bands, tacks, pins, stapler, tape
  Hammer, nails, screwdriver
  Paper
  Batteries
  First-aid kit
  Trash bags
  Paper towels
  Tissues
  Camera
  List of participants with telephone numbers

cooperation of the church council, and clergy, as well as the education department of the faith community. Planned health-related activities or education sessions could be planned for the youth, with age appropriateness being a key component. Examples of this would be proper handwashing and poison prevention programs for the preschool-aged children. School-aged children may enjoy a program about playground, sports, and bicycle safety. Teenagers may be interested in the prevention of sports injuries, safe driving practices, exercise plans, and information about choosing healthy foods. Programs for adults could be developed in response to a questionnaire that asks the participants what types of programs would be of interest to them. The FCN could obtain information from community resources, if necessary, or provide the necessary information and guidance by a discussion type of format. These types of formal health education programs would require a considerable amount of planning and organization; however, the positive outcomes that may result would be well worth the effort.

Using *Healthy People 2010* as a Planning Guide for Program Development

The planning and development of many of the programs discussed thus far could be accomplished using the *Healthy People 2010 Initiatives* (Healthy People, 2004). These initiatives, developed by the U.S. Department of Health and Human Services, are a nationwide health promotion and disease prevention agenda that aims to improve the health of all people and eliminate health disparities in the United States in the first 10 years of the 21st century. Many focus areas addressed in these initiatives target the chronic diseases that are prevalent in American society today. Examples include heart disease, hypertension, diabetes, cancer, asthma, obesity, and so forth. Faith community nurses will probably realize that many of the assessed needs of the faith community involve the conditions addressed in these initiatives, and the programs they develop will be helping to meet the objectives of these initiatives to reduce or eliminate these focus areas by 2010.

BOX 12-4
Checklist for a Successful Health Fair

1. *Site.* Consider access roads, restroom facilities, parking, lighting, and access for persons with disabilities.
2. *Layout.* Plan a single entry point and have participants register as they enter. Allow extra space around screening areas for lines to form and space for activities to occur. Have adequate numbers of screeners to prevent long lines. Consider privacy issues and noise. Set up the space the evening before the fair, if possible.
3. *Materials.* Make a list of needed equipment: electrical equipment, tables, chairs, microphones, and last-minute supplies, including a first-aid kit.
4. *Registration.* Have greeter usher people to the registration table. Prepare registration forms to include any needed consents (i.e., follow-up) and program evaluation forms. Programs can be distributed at the registration table, and evaluation forms can be collected at the exit (an incentive is a nice touch).
5. *Photos.* Have someone take pictures throughout the event. These will record the health fair and provide publicity for the next one.
6. *Timing.* Check the community calendar before scheduling your health fair. Try not to conflict with other community activities that could affect attendance. The event should not last longer than 4 hours. When you schedule the fair, consider the target audience. An internal fair, open only to the members of the faith community, may work best after a worship service.
7. *Exhibitors.* Confirm all participants by telephone the week before the fair. Remind them to arrive for setup at least 30 minutes before the fair opens and reconfirm any special space or equipment needs.
8. *Giveaways.* Plastic bags make it easier for participants to collect printed information. Other giveaways should support the theme of the event.
9. *Directions.* Post signs to direct people to parking, restrooms, registration areas, etc.
10. *Cleanup.* There should be a committee just for this function. There should be clear guidelines as to the time frame for cleanup and how the space is to be left after the fair.
11. *Thanks.* Everyone involved should be formally thanked in writing. Exhibitors should be sent an evaluation form.
12. *Evaluation.* Registration will provide attendance data. Provider will report number of people who screened positively and required medical attention and/or referral. Analyze responses of attendees and exhibitors.

The following example of a program to include Diabetes Self-Management Education (DSME) in an FCN/health ministry program could be used as a guide to develop a similar program in a faith community, thus addressing a health issue very prevalent in American society today. Faith community nurse programs that provide DSME would provide a support system as well as valuable information opportunities for parish members with diabetes. FCNs would need to involve all interested members of the church community to support a DSME program. Success would rely heavily upon the resources available within the church community and the ability of the FCN to integrate community resources into the program. Many resources within many larger communities would be a source of printed information and professionals willing to provide information sessions. Networking with the local chapter of the American Diabetes Association (ADA), the local health department, and local hospitals would be very valuable in initiating and maintaining a successful DSME program in a faith community setting.

To start a DSME program, the FCN would need to assess the interest and needs of the church community as the first step in the process. A simple questionnaire included in the congregational newsletter or the Sunday bulletin would be an effective way for the FCN to assess the interest of the members of the faith community as well as the types of information and services the members would like to receive regarding diabetes. The FCN's understanding of members' needs is important so that an appropriate program can be developed to address the specific needs identified by the members of the congregation. Additionally, FCNs will need to respect the diverse cultures prevalent in many communities and be sensitive to the cultural issues that affect the health knowledge and health outcomes of the individuals whom they serve. FCNs are in a unique position that allows them the opportunity to address these cultural diversities in their approaches to the education and care that they provide for the individuals in the faith communities where they serve.

If the assessment reveals that the needs of the church community essentially involve information regarding diabetes and its management, the FCN could obtain this information from the ADA or the local health department. Bulletin boards, posters, and inserts for the church publications could reflect the information obtained from these organizations. If these community resources are not immediately available to the FCN, information from these organizations can be accessed from their Web sites on the World Wide Web. Most FCNs have very limited financial resources for the purposes of reproducing printed materials; therefore, it would benefit the FCN to access these materials directly from these community or national resources whenever possible.

After reviewing the assessment, the FCN may realize that the members of the congregation are interested in other activities relating to diabetes that will require more than obtaining information from local resources. Members may be interested in a support group or personal information on how to manage their diabetes. If a support group were targeted, the FCN would again start by assessing the members for the best time and place to gather together for this purpose. This assessment could be accomplished through a questionnaire. Once a time and place are established, the FCN would meet with these interested individuals and again assess what the majority of the members would like to experience in this group setting. The FCN would provide the members with information to support the topics that they would like to discuss as well as provide support to the group.

The FCN should always refer the individuals' medical management of diabetes to their health care provider. An FCN could provide clarification of the disease process, the complications of the disease, as well as clarification of recommended self-care behaviors, such as routine blood glucose monitoring, adherence to medication regimes, foot care, and the importance of professional follow-up and eye exams. Individual instruction should be limited to supporting the individuals' self-care, as directed by their health care provider. The support to these individuals could be accomplished by providing them with printed materials and, if appropriate, referral to other organizations such as the ADA or a local hospital-based diabetes program.

The FCN could provide telephone follow-up with interested members to encourage the use of recommended self-management behaviors, such as regular blood glucose monitoring, adherence to recommended medication and diet regimes, participation in a regular exercise program, foot care, and continued follow-up with a health care professional. The FCN could also encourage the members of a diabetes support group to become involved with encouraging each other in the recommended self-care practices of diabetes management. Although these activities would require considerable time and commitment from the FCN, the benefits of such activities would most probably delay or reduce the complications that result from unmanaged diabetes.

The use of the Internet to provide information and support to the individuals of the faith community is also a media source that FCNs should consider when planning DSME and other types of programs for the members of the faith communities where they serve. Many faith communities have established Web sites for their particular congregations, and FCNs may be able to recruit skilled individuals from within the congregation to help them set up a site that allows for information to be posted as well as the opportunity to provide online support services via a chat room environment. This media source will only continue to expand in the future; therefore, FCNs should take advantage of the many opportunities that the Internet may offer in providing education and support to the individuals in the faith communities where they serve.

A faith community nursing program could also be an appropriate setting for blood glucose screenings for the members of the congregation. The FCN would need to network with the local chapter of the ADA, or a hospital wellness department, to determine whether diabetes screening could be supported by these organizations and that proper follow-up care would be available for those individuals who have abnormal blood glucose levels. This program would require a substantial time commitment on the part of the FCN as well as the members of the faith community. Once the resources and services for the actual screening were located, the FCN and the health ministry team would need to organize all of the other aspects of the activity. The members of the congregation could be recruited for many of the activities, such as setting up the area to be used, providing volunteers to register individuals for screening, and so forth. The FCN would need to provide the opportunity for individuals to ask questions concerning their results and be prepared to make the appropriate referrals, if necessary.

Periodic evaluation of the DSME program would be beneficial for future expansion of the program or as a means of addressing program elements that are not effective. This evaluation could be accomplished by the distribution of a questionnaire to all members of the congregation involved in the DSME program or the use of focus or discussion groups with the individuals involved in the program.

FCNs could consult with one another as well as with other agencies in the community so that they are able to share new ideas and current recommendations for diabetes management to the members of the faith communities where they serve. This networking with other FCNs and community resources would be a great opportunity for FCNs to connect with individuals involved in policy development that focuses on public health issues, such as diabetes and other chronic illnesses. FCNs are in a unique position to practice in an environment where they can observe, on a very personal level, how chronic diseases such as diabetes affect the daily lives of the individuals and communities where they serve. This type of interaction gives FCNs a unique perspective on chronic health concerns that would be essential in the development of new policies concerning these public health issues in America today.

Faith community nurses have innumerable opportunities to implement programs in faith communities that will positively impact critical health issues currently burdening the health of American society. The program just described could be expanded to address other chronic illnesses, such as heart disease, asthma, obesity, and so forth. These types of programs support standards 1–6 of the professional standards of faith community nursing (American Nurses Association & Health Ministries Association [ANA-HMA], 2005).

These standards can be addressed through the development of programs, such as DSME. In this type of program structure, FCNs help individuals to set achievable health outcomes, help individuals plan their care to achieve these outcomes, and assist the individuals to implement plans to facilitate desired outcomes. DSME programs and similar programs that address other chronic health issues implemented by FCNs have the potential to substantially decrease the costs of these chronic diseases to both the individuals they serve and the society as a whole.

Faith community nurses are in a position to provide education and services to individuals, which will result in positive outcomes for individuals with chronic diseases, such as diabetes. If every FCN/health ministry program implemented some element of DSME in their faith community, the positive impact that could result is very encouraging. FCNs should understand that their role in the community health setting is highly valuable, and that even programs conducted on a small scale in small faith communities will make a positive impact on the health of the individual faith community as well as the health of American society.

Summary

Program development is a very critical element in the success of a faith community nursing/health ministry program. Every FCN/health ministry is unique and, for this reason, no two programs will be the same. The individuality of faith communities as well as the individuality of FCNs only emphasize the fact that an FCN/health ministry program in one faith community can serve as only a guide to other faith communities looking to develop their own FCN/health ministry programs. What does remain constant in the development of health education/health promotion programs is the need to develop a faith community ministry team to aid FCNs in the planning, implementation, and evaluation processes required for a successful health ministry. The process of a successful FCN/health ministry program is one that requires FCNs to assess the needs of the faith community, recruit the help of a dedicated health ministry team, plan programs that address the assessed needs of the faith community, provide programs that support the assessed needs of the faith community, and continually evaluate the programs for components that require expansion of services or, in contrast, eliminate components that are no longer effective or necessary.

Successful FCN/health ministry programs are very valuable to both the individuals within the faith community and to the community at large. FCNs have the opportunity to address the health needs of the individuals whom they serve in a unique practice setting. Regardless of size or complexity, FCN/health ministry programs provide the opportunity for individuals to learn about and practice healthy lifestyles that are essential in reducing the critical health issues that affect many Americans today.

Reflect and Discuss

1. Describe why it is essential to use assessment data in planning faith community nurse/health ministry programs.
2. What are some examples of community resources that would be helpful in the development of health education programs in a faith community?
3. Describe some ways that a large urban faith community nurse/health ministry program would differ from one located in a rural setting. How would the two programs be similar?
4. Describe how FCNs can make an impact on the overall health of the American society.

Case Study

Emily Walker is an FCN in a suburban community Christian church with 350 members. After the distribution of a questionnaire to the members of the congregation, Emily assessed the need to provide health education to the members of the adult Sunday church school class regarding heart disease. Emily obtained information brochures from the local chapter of the American Heart Association as well as the local hospital wellness department.

During the first session, Emily presented the signs and symptoms of heart disease to the members of the class. The information presented to the members included the typical as well as the not so typical symptoms that individuals may experience with heart disease.

After the program, a middle-aged woman approached Emily and stated to her that she was so thankful for the information from the day's program. She had recently been troubled with a strange sensation in her upper abdomen, sometimes accompanied by nausea, and the feeling of fatigue. The woman reported that she would be making an appointment with her doctor the next day.

Several weeks passed before Emily had the chance to see this woman again. The woman reported that she had Emily to thank for possibly saving her life. After seeing her physician the week after the program, the woman was scheduled for some diagnostic heart tests and immediately had a cardiac catheterization and the placement of a stent into one of her main coronary vessels. Her physician informed her that she was a fortunate woman to have avoided the potential for a very serious heart attack. The woman told Emily that had she not attended the program and learned, the symptoms she was trying to deny and pass off as something minor could have been fatal. She also informed Emily that it was so nice to get this very vital health information from someone she trusted and in such a relaxed atmosphere. The woman asked to be a member of the health ministry team and has been very supportive of all of the programs that Emily presents to the members of the congregation.

This type of scenario is not uncommon for FCNs to experience. The information that individuals receive as a result of an FCN/health ministry program can lead to healthy choices and lifestyle changes that positively affect the health of the members of the faith community. These types of experiences encourage FCNs to continue to practice in faith communities.

References

American Nurses Association & Health Ministries Association. (2005). *Faith Community Nursing: Scope and standards of practice.* Silver Springs, MD: ANA.

Boyes, P. (2001). Church health fairs: Partying with a purpose. *Journal of Christian Nursing, 18*(3), 17–19.

Durban, E. (2003). Making health ministry accessible and visible: The health fair. In D. L. Patterson (Ed.), *The essential parish nurse: ABCs for congregational health ministry.* Cleveland, OH: The Pilgrim Press.

Durrant, L., & Rieckmann, T. (2003). Facilitating support groups. In R. J. Bensley & J. Brookins-Fisher (Eds.), *Community health education methods* (2nd ed.). Sudbury, MA: Jones and Bartlett Publishers.

Patterson, D. L. (2003). *The essential parish nurse: ABCs for congregational health ministry.* Cleveland, OH: The Pilgrim Press.

Rice, C. A., Rider, L., & Pollard, J. M. (2004). *Health fair planning guide.* Available online at: http://fcs.tamu.edu/health/health_fair_planning_guide/htm.

Schumann, R. (2003). A spirit of commitment and creativity. In S. D. Smith (Ed.), *Parish nursing: A handbook for the new millennium.* New York: Haworth Press.

Society for Healthcare Strategy and Market Development of the American Hospital Association. (2002). *Health observances and recognition days* [Brochure].

U.S. Department of Health and Human Services (US-DHHS). (2000). *Healthy people 2010.* Washington, DC: Author.

Wilson, L. (2000). Implementation and evaluation of church-based health fairs. *Journal of Community Health Nursing, 17*(1), 39.

Wurzbach, M. E. (Ed.). (2002). *Community health education and promotion* (2nd ed.). Gaithersburg, MD: Aspen Publishers.

→ Web Resources

http://www.agd.org/   Academy of General Dentistry
http://www.health.gov/NHIC/NHICScripts/Entry.cfm?HRCode=HR2388   American Academy of Ophthalmology

http://www.aap.org/   American Academy of Pediatrics

http://www.aap.org/family/healthfairkit/htm
    American Academy of Pediatrics Health Fair Kit

http://www.aadenet.org/   American Association of
    Diabetes Educators

http://www.csaa.com/home/   American Automobile
    Association

http://www.cancer.org/docroot/home/index.asp
    American Cancer Society

http://www.ada.org/   American Dental Association

http://www.adha.org/   American Dental Hygienists
    Association

http://www.diabetes.org/home.jsp   American Diabetes
    Association

http://www.eatright.org/Public/   American Dietetic
    Association

http://www.americanheart.org   American Heart
    Association

http://www.arthritis.org/   Arthritis Foundation

http://www.bgca.org/   Boys and Girls Clubs of America

http://www.cdc.gov/   Centers for Disease Control and
    Prevention

http://www.cpsc.gov/   Consumer Products Safety
    Commission

http://www.nei.nih.gov/   National Eye Institute

http://www.nhlbi.nih.gov/   National Heart, Lung, and
    Blood Institute

http://www.nhtsa.dot.gov/   National Highway Traffic
    Safety Administration

http://www.partnersforimmunization.org/   National
    Partnership for Immunization

http://www.headlice.org/   National Pediculosis
    Association

http://www.poisonprevention.org/   National Poison
    Prevention Week Council

http://www.safekids.org/   National Safe Kids
    Campaign

http://www.nyssf.org/   National Youth Sports Safety
    Foundation

http://fcs.tamu.edu/health_fair_planning_guide/
    activity_ideas.htm   Texas A&M University
    Health Fair Planning Guide

http://www.ymca.com/index.jsp   YMCA

http://www.ywca.org/   YWCA

Health Education

13

The health educator role is one of the most extensively developed roles in faith community nursing practice. In the health educator role, the faith community nurse (FCN) empowers the client (individual, family, or faith community) to incorporate health and healing practices from its faith perspective to achieve desired outcomes. FCNs minister within the concept of stewardship of one's body and personal health as a responsibility to God and respect for his creation. The FCN approaches health education with respect for the dignity of all persons. The FCN recognizes the responsibility to care for each person as a child of God. Christian FCNs believe that through Jesus Christ, life is found. Jesus Christ's example and teaching point to the way of life, based on the Gospel (Christian Medical Commission, 1990, 2002).

Van Dover and Bacon (2003) studied parish nurses, using a grounded theory approach to explain the process that parish nurses or FCNs use to provide spiritual care to people under their care. The theory emerged from a core category of "Bringing God Near" (BGN). The essence of the spiritual care process of parish nurses is bring God near to their patients/clients. It begins with the nurse's focus on facilitating integration of body, mind, and spirit as part of the healing process. Stages in the process include: trusting God, forming relationships with the patient/family, opening to God, taking action, and experiencing results. Van Dover and Bacon concluded that the BGN reveals that spiritual caregiving is a unique way that nurses care, and that the person of the nurse is one way for God's healing love and care to be offered to the patient. The theory of Bringing God Near is highly relevant to the health educator role of the FCN.

The new *Faith Community Nursing: Scope and Standards of Practice* (American Nurses Association & Health Ministries Association [ANA-HMA], 2005) addresses the health education role of the FCN, specifically in Standard of Practice 5B: Health Teaching and Health Promotion. This standard states that, "The faith community nurse employs strategies to promote health, wellness, and a safe environment" (ANA-HMA, 2005, p. 15). The measurement criteria for this standard are presented in Box 13-1.

FCNs may choose to personally provide health education programs, or they may choose to arrange for other appropriate professional people to conduct them. The resources available in the faith community and time constraints will certainly affect these decisions. This chapter will provide resources for the FCN who chooses to prepare his or her own health education programs and guidelines for using a speaker.

Theoretical content and formal practicum experiences related to teaching and learning activities vary greatly across nursing educational curricula. The inclusion or exclusion of formal content about teaching and learning in undergraduate and graduate nursing education programs has also varied over time. With this in mind, this chapter will provide the theoretical base for health promotion and behavior change and basic, how-to information about teaching methods, materials, and evaluating learning outcomes. For the seasoned educator, the chapter should provide a theoretical review and some new resources. For the novice educator, the chapter will serve as a coach's playbook.

BOX 13-1
Measurement Criteria for Standard 5B: Health Teaching and Health Promotion

The FCN:

1. Provides health teaching that addresses such topics as spiritual practices for health and healing, healthy lifestyles, risk-reducing behaviors, developmental needs, activities of daily living, and preventive self-care.

2. Uses health promotion and health teaching methods appropriate to the situation, the faith community, and the patient's spiritual beliefs and practices, developmental level, learning needs, readiness, ability to learn language or communication preference or culture.

3. Supports the beliefs and practices of the faith community when selecting information and programs.

4. Evaluates health information resources for use within faith community nursing for accuracy, readability, comprehensibility by patients, and congruence with patients' spiritual beliefs and practices.

5. Seeks ongoing opportunities for feedback and evaluation of the effectiveness of health education and health promotion strategies used.

(ANA-HMA, 2005, p. 15.)

Health Behavior and Change

Since the late 1960s there have been federal initiatives for health promotion and disease prevention. *Healthy People 1990, 2000,* and *2010* provide objectives for the nation's health. The overarching goals of *Healthy People* are quality of life and decreasing health disparities for the American people. In the last 30 years, there have been positive changes in the health of Americans. These changes include: fewer deaths from coronary artery disease and cancer, improved control of hypertension, a decrease in mean population cholesterol levels, fewer alcohol-related automobile accidents, fewer adults using tobacco products, and more women having routine mammograms. Fifty percent of the original *Healthy People 2000* objectives related to eliminating health disparities have been achieved (National Center for Health Statistics, 2001).

On the negative side, more children and adults are overweight, diabetes incidence has sharply increased, more teens are sexually active, seat belt usage is only at 67% (with 85% being the target), 20% of children under age 3 have not had basic immunizations, 16% of adults over age 65 do not have health insurance, and 70% of adults over age 50 have not been screened for colorectal cancer (National Center for Health Statistics, 2001).

Health promotion is behavior motivated by the desire to increase well-being and actualize human potential (Pender, Murdaugh, & Parsons, 2002). *Health education* is defined as, "Any combination of planned learning experiences based on sound theories that provide individuals, groups, and communities the opportunity to acquire information and skills needed to make quality health decisions" (Wurzbach, 2002, p. 6). Faith-based health education combines the concepts of whole health or Shalom with health promotion. Faith-based health education is health education delivered in the context or worldview of the faith tradition. As such, it integrates and incorporates the use of prayer, Scripture, and devotional worship into health education.

Glanz, Rimer, and Lewis (2002) state that health education includes instructional activities and strategies to change behavior as well as organizational efforts, policy directives, economic supports, mass media, and community-level programs. The goal of health education is for the target person or group to make informed and voluntary changes in behavior that affect health in a positive way. Health education encourages positive lifestyle behaviors that prevent acute and chronic disease, decrease disability, and enhance wellness. Glanz et al. (2002) state that two ideas are key to health education. The first idea is that behavior is affected by multiple levels of influence, which include individual, interpersonal, organizational, community, and public policy factors. The second key idea is that reciprocal causation occurs between individuals and environments—behavior *influences* and *is influenced* by the social environment. The concept of reciprocal causation can help explain the positive correlation found between religion and health.

The field of health education has posited many theoretical approaches and models about health-related behaviors. Glanz et al. (2002) suggest that different theoretical approaches are suited to different contexts. They report that the constructs that cut across the theories of health education include:

- The importance of the individual's worldview.
- Multiple levels of influence on behavior.
- Behavioral change as a process.
- Motivation versus intention.
- Intention versus action.
- Changing behavior and maintaining change.

The faith-based approach is a critical worldview element to faith community nursing. The faith-based worldview provides both the rationale and the incentive for the health promotion and disease prevention activities related to the stewardship of one's body.

The Health Belief Model

The Health Belief Model (HBM) has been the most popular model for the past 5 decades. The HBM was developed in the 1950s by a group of social psychologists in the U.S. Public Health Service who were trying to explain why people were not using free services available for tuberculosis screening. Later the model was extended to include people's reactions to symptoms and adherence (or not) to medical regimens. Janz, Champion, and Strecher (2002) classify the HBM as a value-expectancy theory. According to the HBM, the person has a desire to avoid illness or to get well from an illness (value). Also a belief is that a specific health action available to the person would prevent or ameliorate illness (expectation). The expectancy is further delineated in terms of the individual's estimate of personal susceptibility and the severity of the illness (Fig. 13-1). Many believe that most people will take action to prevent, to screen for, or to control ill health conditions, if they regard themselves as susceptible to the condition, if they believe the condition could have serious consequences, if they believe that a course of action available would be of benefit to decrease their susceptibility or to decrease the severity of the conditions, *and* if they believe that the barriers and costs of taking action are outweighed by the benefits (p. 47). Numerous research studies, both retrospective and prospective, show that perceived barriers are the most powerful HBM dimensions in explaining or predicting health protective behaviors. Perceived susceptibility has also been an important predictor of preventive behaviors.

Theories of health behavior are important to FCNs because they provide guidance in planning activities that will influence positive behavior changes. The FCN can use the HBM as well as Pender's Health Promotion Model (that follows) as a basis for health education planning. Several other theories of health behavior have been proposed and also have relevance for faith community nursing practice. Space prevents a detailed discussion of these theories, but the major ones are presented briefly in Table 13-1.

Pender's Health Promotion Model

The initial version of Pender's Health Promotion Model (HPM) first appeared in the nursing literature in the early 1980s. It was proposed as a framework for integrating nursing and be-

INDIVIDUAL PERCEPTIONS MODIFYING FACTORS LIKELIHOOD OF ACTION

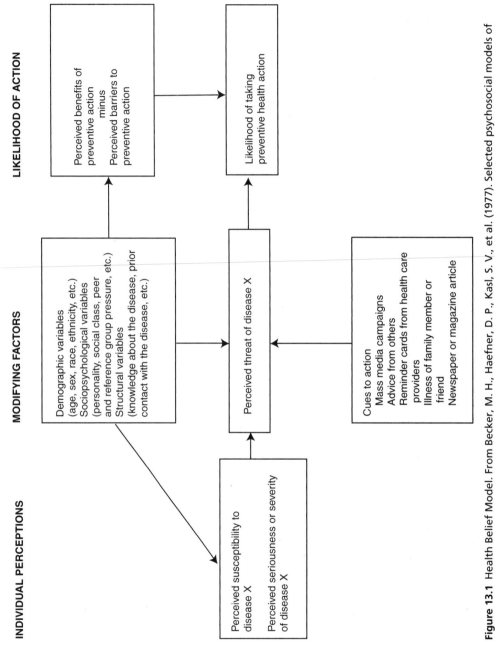

Figure 13.1 Health Belief Model. From Becker, M. H., Haefner, D. P., Kasl, S. V., et al. (1977). Selected psychosocial models of individual health-related behaviors. *Medical Care, 15,* 27–46. Used with permission.

TABLE 13-1

Models of Health Behavior

TITLE	AUTHOR(S)	DESCRIPTION
Theory of Reasoned Action (TRA) & Theory of Planned Behavior (TPB)	Fishbein & Ajzen (1975)	Attitudes and subjective norms influence behavioral intention, which is the immediate determinant of behavior. These relationships are depicted as follows: • *Behavior is a function of intention to perform the behavior.* • *Intention is a function of attitude toward behavior plus subjective norm for behavior.* This theory is based on the assumption that both attitudes and subjective norms are amenable to change and that there are no barriers to performance of the intended behavior. Ajzen (1991), in a critique of the TRA, suggested that behavior may not be completely under the control of the individual, and he added a third variable of *perceived behavioral control* to the original concepts of attitudes and subjective norms and named this extended theory the Theory of Planned Behavior (TPB).
The Transtheoretical Model	Prochaska & DiClemente (1984)	Health-related behavior change progresses through five stages, regardless of whether the client is trying to quit an unhealthy behavior or to adopt a healthful behavior. These stages include: 1. *Precontemplation:* The client is not thinking of making any health-related life changes. 2. *Contemplation:* The client is seriously considering quitting or adopting a behavior in the next 6 months. 3. *Planning or preparation:* The client, who has tried to quit a negative behavior or to adopt a positive behavior in the past year, is seriously thinking about making a contemplated change within the next month. 4. *Action:* This stage covers a period of 6 months during which the client has made the behavior change and it has persisted. 5. *Maintenance:* This stage begins 6 months after action has started and continues indefinitely. Prochaska proposes that different processes of change are appropriate at different stages of behavior change. She describes five experiential process and five behavioral processes. She states that experiential processes, which are internally focused on behavior-linked emotions, values, and cognitions, are much more important than behavioral processes for understanding and predicting progress in the early stages of change, and that behavioral processes are more important to the later stages.
Social Cognitive Theory	Schwarzer (1992) Bandura (1997)	This theory explains behavior in terms of a three-way dynamic, reciprocal way in which personal factors, environmental influences, and behavior interact. A premise of this theory is that people learn through their own experiences and by observing the actions of others.

(continued)

TABLE 13-1

Models of Health Behavior *(continued)*

TITLE	AUTHOR(S)	DESCRIPTION
The Interaction Model of Client Health Behavior (IMCHB)	Cox (1982)	This theory focuses on characteristics of the client and factors external to the client to explain actions related to risk reduction and health promotion. Client background variables included in the model are demographics, social influences, previous health care experience, and environmental resources. These background variables and the intrinsic motivation, cognitive appraisal, and affective response of client, in regard to a particular behavior, interface with elements of client-professionals interaction (affective support, health information, decisional control, and professional-technical competencies) to affect health outcomes. Critical elements of health outcomes are the use of health services, clinical health status indicators, severity of health care problems, adherence to the medical regimen, and satisfaction with care.
The Integrative Model	Fishbein (2000)	The integrative model of health behavior begins with external variables of demographics, attitudes toward targets, personality traits, and other individual differences modified by behavioral beliefs and their evaluative aspects, normative beliefs and motivation, and efficacy beliefs, which then result in attitude, norms, self-efficacy, skills, intention and environmental constraints, and, ultimately, to behavior. One can clearly see the evolution from the TRA to the TPB and, finally, to this integrative model.

havioral science perspectives on factors influencing health behaviors. The initial model has been replaced by the revised model depicted in Figure 13-2. The HPM is defined as a competence or approach-oriented model. Unlike the HBM, it does not address fear and threat as a source of motivation for healthy behavior. Because fear and threat as motivators are of limited usefulness when working with children and adolescents, the HPM model can be used across the life span (Pender, Murdaugh, & Parsons, 2002). The HPM is excellent for planning health promotion programs in faith community settings.

The HPM integrates several constructs from the expectancy-value theory of motivation with social cognitive theory, within a nursing perspective of holistic human functioning. The variables in the HPM model and their interrelationships are presented in Box 13-2.

Interventions for Health Behavior Change

Increasing healthy behaviors and decreasing risky or negative health behaviors of the faith community are a major challenge for the FCN. Pender et al. (2002) have identified behavior change strategies based on health behavioral theories and models. These strategies will be presented briefly.

Raising Consciousness

Consciousness-raising is an important element in health behavior change. Through seeking and gaining information, observing others, and interpreting information in view of one's own

INDIVIDUAL CHARACTERISTICS AND EXPERIENCES

BEHAVIOR-SPECIFIC COGNITIONS AND AFFECT

BEHAVIORAL OUTCOME

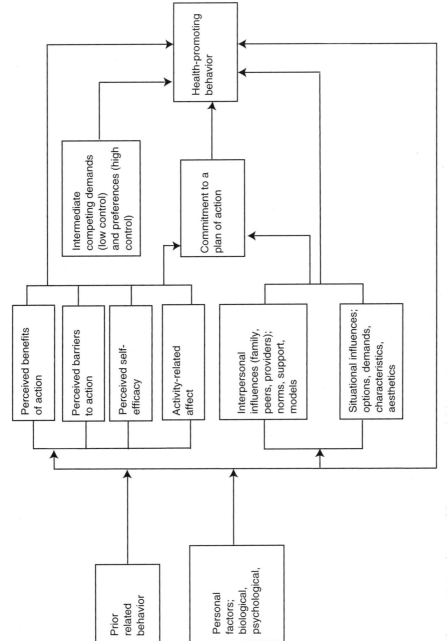

Figure 13.2 Pender's Health Promotion Model (revised). From Pender, N. J., Murdaugh, C. L., & Parsons, M. A. (2002). *Health promotion in nursing practice* (4th ed.). Upper Saddle River, NJ: Prentice-Hall. Used with permission.

BOX 13-2
Variables of the Health Promotion Model

INDIVIDUAL CHARACTERISTICS AND EXPERIENCES

- Prior related behavior: Empirical studies indicate that often the best predictor of behavior is the frequency of the same behavior in the past. Habit strength accrues each time the behavior is repeated.
- Personal factors: biological (age, body mass index, pubertal status, menopausal status, aerobic capacity, strength, agility, and balance); psychological (self-esteem).
- Self-motivation and perceived health status and sociocultural (race, ethnicity, acculturation, education, and socioeconomic status).

BEHAVIOR-SPECIFIC COGNITION AND AFFECT

This set of variables within the HPM is considered to be of major motivational significance and, as such, constitutes the critical core for nursing intervention. Measuring change in these variables is essential to determine whether such changes actually result from the intervention.

- Perceived benefits of action—61% of studies of the HPM reported empirical support for the importance of perceived benefits in influencing health behaviors. Anticipated benefits of action mentally reinforce the consequences of behavior.
- Perceived barriers to action—79% of studies of the HPM provided empirical support for the importance of barriers as a determinant of health promoting behavior. Barriers may be real or imagined. They consist of perceptions concerning the unavailability, inconvenience, expense, difficulty, or time requirements of a particular action. When people are unready to act and barriers are high, action is unlikely to occur.
- Perceived self-efficacy—86% of studies of the HPM provided support for the importance of self-efficacy. When a person feels efficacious and able to perform an action or behavior, he or she is likely to encourage others to engage in target behavior.
- Activity-related affect—consists of three components: emotional arousal to the act itself (act-related), the self acting (self-related), and the environment in which the action takes place (act-context). The resultant feeling state is likely to affect whether the behavior will or will not be repeated. Because this is a new variable, few studies have explored the contribution of this construct.
- Interpersonal influences—57% of studies of the HPM model provided empirical support for the importance of interpersonal influences on health promoting behavior. Primary sources of influence are family members, peers, and health care providers. Interpersonal influences can also include the expectations of significant others, social support, and modeling.
- Situational influences—56% of studies of HPM provided empirical support for situational influences as significant predictors of health promoting behavior.

COMMITMENT TO A PLAN OF ACTION

This element initiates a behavioral event and will carry an individual through the intended action, unless a competing demand intervenes that the individual does not resist. Commitments can be strengthened by using nurse-client mutual goal-setting and by formal contracts for behavioral changes.

IMMEDIATE COMPETING DEMANDS AND PREFERENCES

Immediate competing demands and preferences refer to alternative behaviors that intrude into consciousness as possible courses of action immediately prior to the intended act of health promoting behavior.

BEHAVIORAL OUTCOME—HEALTH PROMOTING BEHAVIOR

Health promoting behavior, which should result in improved health, is the endpoint or outcome in the HPM.

From Pender, N. J., Murdaugh, C. L., & Parsons, M. A. (2002). *Health promotion in nursing practice* (4th ed., pp. 69–74). Upper Saddle River, NJ: Prentice-Hall. Used with permission.

circumstances, an awareness of the potential benefits of adopting a healthy behavior or quitting a negative behavior can be enhanced. FCNs can raise consciousness in various ways—by providing written health-related information, programs, screenings, and individual counseling, to name a few. Risk appraisals and risk-reduction counseling also raise consciousness. Materials need to be culturally specific and age and literacy-level appropriate to be effective.

Reevaluation of Self

Self-reevaluation results from a state of client dissatisfaction with self as a result of recognizing inconsistencies between self-standards (values and beliefs) and behaviors. Adherence to standards that individuals set for themselves (and those standards that faith communities set for their members) increases self-concept through feelings of pride and satisfaction, whereas violating these personal standards results in negative feelings of guilt and self-censure. The FCN can assist clients with self-reevaluation by suggesting the things that would be possible to do or to achieve after making a behavior change. Spiritual care, prayer, use of Scripture, and the relationship of faith and health can easily be integrated into this strategy.

Promoting Self-efficacy

Self-efficacy refers to beliefs in personal capabilities to carry out a given behavior. *Task* self-efficacy refers to beliefs in being able to carry out progressively more demanding tasks. *Regulatory* self-efficacy refers to beliefs in being able to overcome barriers to engage in a desired behavior. Prayer and the use of Scripture are important elements to this strategy. The most powerful motivator for self-efficacy is successful performance of a behavior. Thus, whenever feasible, the FCN should facilitate the client's successful performance of a target behavior and give the client positive feedback. The FCN can also help clients overcome barriers by suggesting specific strategies for successful performance. These strategies are particularly relevant to smoking cessation, weight loss programs, exercise programs, and for stress reduction. The FCN can also assist clients by modeling the target behavior.

Enhancing the Benefits of Change

Planning for rewards or reinforcement of positive behavior change is important, because when positive reinforcement is given, the behaviors are more likely to be repeated. Positive reinforcement provides the most effective motivation for behavioral change. Reinforcement can be tangible, social, self-generated, or spiritual. Immediate and continuous reinforcement is highly desirable, especially in the early phases of behavior change. Intermittent reinforcement applied later stabilizes the behavior and makes it more resistant to extinction.

Controlling the Environment

Modifying the environment to stimulate and to support behavioral change is important for positive behavioral change. Often environmental cues will trigger certain behaviors. Learning what specifically triggers both positive and negative behaviors provides strategies for planning and intervention.

Dealing with Barriers to Change

The FCN's role is to assist the client in minimizing real and perceived barriers to healthful behaviors. This can be done by assessing the situation, clarifying information, correcting misinformation, and providing supportive services.

Maintaining the New Behavior

The maintenance stage of health behavior change presents special challenges for the client and the FCN. Not only does a new behavior need to be sustained in the environment where it was learned, but it needs to be generalized to other situations.

Habit formation facilitates maintenance of behaviors.

The Health Education Process

Assessing the Congregation as an Audience

Assessing the congregation as an audience is the first step in planning a health education event for individuals, families, or communities. Faith community assessment data will be helpful to the FCN in assessing the target audience. The congregational survey provides the FCN with quantitative information about the:

- Incidence and types of chronic diseases that exist in the faith community.
- Demographics of the faith community (ages, educational level).
- Formal committees and standing groups within the faith community.
- Interests of the faith community members about specific health topics.
- Scheduling preferences of the membership.

Barnes, Neiger, and Thackeray (2003) state that *audience analysis* includes needs, wants, motivational and resistance points, general attitudes, behaviors, and preferences related to health problems—what they know, what they fear, and how they will likely react to specific methods related to the health problem. Audience analysis is an attempt to get inside the head and heart of the target audience. FCNs prepare health education programs using audience (congregational) analysis to develop interventions that ring true with congregants and to produce the intended effects. Barnes et al. (2003) define *channel analysis* as the process that helps determine which communication methods will most likely appeal to the target audience. This includes the setting where the audience is most easily reached, the method(s) in which they receive most of their information, and their preferences for communication methods. Channel analysis assists the FCN plan successful health education programs for the faith community.

Kitchie (2003) reports that although nursing assessment of needs, readiness, and styles of learning is the first and most important step of instructional design, it is the step most often neglected. Good assessments ensure that optimal learning will occur with the least amount of anxiety for the learner. Good assessments also increase motivation to learn by focusing on what the learner feels is most important to know or to be able to do.

A learning need is a gap between what someone knows and what someone needs to know because of a lack of knowledge, attitude, or skill.

Assessing learning needs includes the following steps:

1. Identify the learner.
2. Choose the right setting to collect the data.
3. Collect the data from the targeted learners.
4. Prioritize needs for knowledge as mandatory, desirable, or possible.
5. Determine the availability of educational resources and the number of materials needed.

In reality, the FCN makes an assumption that people are interested and ready to learn, by their attendance at the health program or event. Despite preference survey data, it is often impossible to predict who or how many people will actually attend a given program. Even when pre-registration is required, attendance numbers can be fluid. If instructional materials and/or handouts will be used, plan to have extra copies available. The FCN does need to plan programs with consideration of the following key elements: age level, literacy level, and cultural issues.

AGE CONSIDERATIONS

Teaching principles differ for children and for adults. Helpful for the FCN is to review the principles and apply them in program planning.

Preschool-age Children

Morrison (2001) suggests the following principles for teaching health promotion to preschool-age children:

- Children learn best through all their senses.
- Teachers should show love and respect for all children.
- Good teaching is based on theory, philosophy, goals, and objectives.
- Children's learning is enhanced through the use of concrete materials.
- Teaching should be centered on the child.
- Teaching should move from the concrete to the abstract.
- Teaching should be based on the children's interests.
- Keep teaching sessions short, no longer than 15 minutes.
- Use storytelling as a method.
- Give children tangible rewards as reinforcers of learning.

School-age Children and Teens

Bastable and Rinwalske (2003) recommend the following strategies for teaching school-age children and teenagers:

- Use diagrams, models, pictures/videotapes, and printed materials as adjuncts to teaching methods.
- Use materials that show peers.
- Clarify terminology.
- Use analogies.
- Encourage participation.
- Provide reinforcement.
- Share decision making where appropriate.
- Suggest options.
- Be flexible.

Adults

Knowles (1990) coined the term *andragogy* to describe his theory of adult learning.

Education in this framework is learner-centered rather than teacher-centered and is a collegial relationship rather than an expert to novice relationship. The emphasis for adult learning is related to life tasks and social roles. Adults need to see the benefits that they will gain from the learning activity for it to be relevant. Adults are self-directed and come to the learning experience with a wealth of previous experience and knowledge. Adults are quicker than children at grasping relationships, but they tend to be more resistant to change. Knowles, Holton, and Swanson (1998) provide the following principles for teaching adults:

- Learners need to know why they need to learn something before undertaking it.
- Learners seek self-direction.

- Learners have various life experiences that need to be incorporated into learning experiences.
- Learners become ready to learn the things that they need to know to cope effectively with real-life situations.
- Learners have a life-centered or problem-centered orientation to learning.
- Learners are motivated to learn by intrinsic motivators, such as a sense of satisfaction.

Hansen and Fisher (1998) suggest the acronym TEACH as a guideline for patient education:

T = **T**une in to the learner's thoughts and needs and address the learner's priorities for learning first.

E = **E**dit information to focus on "must know" content.

A = **A**ct on teachable moments. Teach at every opportunity.

C = **C**larify often and verify your assumptions by seeking frequent feedback from the learner.

H = **H**onor the learner as a partner by building learning on the learner's prior experiences and sharing the responsibility for the educational process.

Literacy Level

Literacy is an umbrella term that is used to describe socially required and expected reading and writing skills, including the ability to understand printed/written materials commonly encountered in daily living. Doak, Doak, and Root (1996) state that the commonly accepted definition of literacy is the ability to read, understand, and interpret information written at an eighth grade level. They define *low literacy* as the ability of adults to read, write, and comprehend information between the fifth and eighth grade levels of difficulty, and they define *functional illiteracy* as reading, writing, and comprehension below a fifth grade level.

Fisher (1999) categorizes literacy into three general kinds of tasks:

- *Prose tasks*—tasks that measure reading comprehension and the ability to extract themes from newspapers, magazines, poems, and books.
- *Document tasks*—tasks that assess the ability to interpret documents, such as insurance reports, consent forms, and transportation schedules.
- *Quantitative tasks*—tasks that assess the ability to work with numerical information embedded in written materials, such as computing restaurant bills, interpreting paycheck information, or counting calories.

The 1992 National Adult Literacy Survey showed that 23%, or 40 to 44 million adult Americans, are at the lowest literacy level (Level 1) and that 25% to 28%, or 50 million people, demonstrated skills at the next higher level of proficiency (Level 2). This means that 50% of Americans fell into the two lowest levels of literacy. A Level 3 proficiency is the minimal standards needed to function in the workplace. The survey provides specific age-related and racial/ethnic findings. The literacy proficiencies of young adults were lower in the 1992 survey than in the 1985 survey. Older adults were more likely than middle-aged or younger adults to demonstrate limited literacy skills. Black, Native American/Pacific Islander, and Hispanic adults were more likely than white adults to perform in the lowest levels. Of all the racial ethnic groups, Hispanic adults reported the fewest years of schooling (a mean of just over 10 years). Nearly half of all adults in the lowest level were living in poverty (http://www.nces.ed/gov/naal/resources/execsumm.asp). The National Assessment of Adult Literacy 2003 (NAAL) project is underway, and data have been collected from a sample of 18,000 American adults. The results of this recent survey will be released in summer 2005.

The 2003 survey has added a scale that measures a health literacy component (http://www.nifl.gov/nifl/webcasts/200040803/webcast08-03.html).

Health literacy refers to how well an individual can read, interpret, and understand health information. The AMA Ad Hoc Committee on Health Literacy (1999) defined health literacy as, "a constellation of skills, including the ability to perform basic reading and numerical tasks required to function in the health care environment" (p. 553). Clearly, functional illiteracy and low literacy significantly affect both motivation to learn and compliance to medical regimens (Bastable, 2003). Research findings about the abilities of patients to meet the literacy demands of written materials related to their care are presented in Box 13-3.

With this information in mind, the FCN needs to carefully assess printed educational materials and self-prepared material for literacy levels. Doak et al. (1996) recommend that instructional materials be written at the fifth grade level. Bastable (2003) reports that over 40 formulas are available to measure readability levels of printed educational materials. She cautions that although these measures can predict a level of reading difficulty of material based on sentence structure and word length, they do not take into consideration the client-specific variables that affect the reader or the actual content of the materials. Readability formulas are mathematical equations derived from multiple regression analysis that describe the correlation between the author's writing and the reader's ability to comprehend them.

The Spache Grade Level Score (Spache, 1953) focuses on evaluating materials written for children at grade levels 1 to 3. The SMOG Formula (McLaughlin, 1969) is a valid, simple, and fast method of assessing readability of materials from grade 4 to college level. This method is based on 100% comprehension of materials read; so if the SMOG formula rests reading materials at an eighth grade level, it means that all readers able to read at the eighth grade level would comprehend the material.

Most computerized word processing software packages will asses the readability of written material. In Microsoft Word XP, readability statistics are an option in the spell-check tool. Word XP uses the Flesch Formula (Flesch, 1948) to provide the *Reading Ease Score* of the document. This formula rates text on a 100-point scale; the higher the score, the easier the text is to read. Most documents would aim for a score of 60 to 70. Word XP also provides the *Flesch-Kincaid*

BOX 13-3
Research About Literacy and Written Health Education Materials

Estey et al., 1991	Materials written at the fifth grade level were understood better than those written at the ninth grade level.
Jolly et al., 1993; Williams et al., 1996; Duffy & Snyder, 1999; Lerner et al., 2000	Emergency room instructional materials written at the 10th grade level were out of the readable range for most clients.
Winslow, 2001	A significant mismatch exists between the reading ability of older adults and the readability of documents related to their health services offered through local, state, and federal programs.
Davis et al., 1990; Lerner, 2000	A discrepancy exists between average client reading comprehension levels and the readability demand of printed educational materials used in ambulatory care settings.
Davis et al., 1990; Doak et al., 1998	Standard institutional consent forms require college-level reading comprehension.
Meade et al., 1992; Doak et al., 1998; Brownson, 1998	More than half of the American Cancer Society literature reviewed was written at the12th grade level or higher.

BOX 13-4
Writing User-friendly Educational Materials

- Write in a conversational style, using the personal pronoun *you* and the possessive pronoun *your, yours.*
- Write in an active voice using the present tense.
- Put the most important information first and highlight with boldface or italics.
- Use short words with only one or two syllables as much as possible.
- Write one concept per paragraph.
- Convert medical terms into lay terms.
- Write out words instead of using medical abbreviations.
- Use numbers and statistics sparingly.
- Keep sentences short.
- Define terms clearly, and use the terms consistently.
- Use a simple, easy-to-read font.
- Use lots of white space between paragraphs.
- Use culturally appropriate pictures.

Grade Level Score, in which a score of 7.0 means that the text is written at a seventh grade level.

Box 13-4 provides some basic linguistic, motivational, organizational, and content principles to keep in mind when preparing written educational materials.

Cultural Issues

Spector (2004) states that all aspects of human behavior can be interpreted through the lens of culture and that everything in life can be related to and from the context of culture. Culture is the medium of our individuality—the way we express ourselves. Culture is also the medium of social relationships.

As previously discussed in Chapter 6, heritage consistency is a concept that was developed by Estes and Zitzow (1980) to describe the extent of which one's lifestyle reflects his or her respective tribal culture. The theory has been expanded to study the degree to which a person's lifestyle reflects his or her traditional culture. The values indicating heritage consistency exist on a continuum, and a person can possess value characteristics of both a consistent heritage (traditional) and an inconsistent heritage (acculturated). The concept of a cultural continuum allows for individual differences within cultures and negates the idea of cultural stereotypes. Heritage consistency includes a determination of one's cultural, ethnic, and religious background.

The following definitions were developed by the Office of Minority Health (2001):

- *Culture*—"the thoughts, communications, actions, customs, beliefs, values, and institutions of racial, ethnic, religious, or social groups" (p. 131).
- *Ethnicity*—"a group of people that share a common and distinctive racial, national, religious, linguistic, or cultural heritage" (p. 131).
- *Religion*—"a set of beliefs, values, and practices based on the teachings of a spiritual leader" (p. 132).

Spector (2004) reminds us that religious teachings in relation to health help present a meaningful philosophy and set of practices within a system of social controls having specific values, norms, and ethics. These are related to health in that adherence to a religious code is conducive to health and spiritual harmony (p. 12). Different cultural backgrounds create different attitudes and reactions to illness and affect how people express themselves orally and nonverbally. Culture also guides the way an ill person is defined and treated. Illness may be viewed as a punishment for the violation of a religious code or for sinful behavior. Religion also determines the role that faith plays in the person's response to treatments and to the recovery process.

Faith communities can be culturally homogeneous or culturally diverse. An FCN in a culturally diverse faith community will need to understand the cultures of the target population and make cultural assessments prior to providing health education. An advantage in a faith community setting is the common bond of a shared belief system; however, culturally congruent communication will be essential to health education.

> **BOX 13-5**
> **Strategies for Cultural Competence**
>
> - Understand yourself—your values and biases.
> - Create an inclusive environment by using inclusive language at the appropriate literacy level.
> - Understand the culture of the target population.
> - Greet people formally unless invited to do otherwise.
> - Be sensitive to cultural roles related to decision making about health care.
> - Respect folk practices, unless they are harmful.
> - Develop facilitation skills.
> - Avoid body language and gestures that may be misunderstood.
> - Provide people with adequate personal space.
> - Choose educational materials wisely.
> - Diversify teaching techniques and learning styles.

The concept of *cultural competence* was presented in Chapter 6. The first step in providing culturally competent care is to be aware of one's biases, one's lack of knowledge, and to be open to personal consciousness-raising about people of other cultures. Box 13-5 presents strategies for cultural competence and Box 13-6 provides cross-cultural Web resources.

When and Where to Teach

The "when" of conducting a health education program will depend on the data collected from the faith community regarding their preferences for days and times for health programs. Specific health programs can be planned using the health calendar described in Chapter 12. For example, February is "Heart Health" month and October is Breast Cancer Awareness month. In addition to congregational assessment data, the FCN should be aware of major local events and national events that may conflict with the planned event. The FCN should also be aware of vacation periods when many congregants would be out of town.

The "where" for health education programs will be dependent upon the physical facilities of the church, temple, or mosque. Ideally, the size of the room should comfortably accommodate the expected size of the audience. If there will be small group discussions or breakout groups, the room needs to be large enough to accommodate that activity, or additional spaces need to be available. Depending upon the setting, rooms may need to be reserved in advance for specific activities. Who will set up and break down the room(s) will be a function of the faith community staffing or volunteers and needs to be clearly assigned in the planning stages of the program.

Spaces used for educational programs should be well ventilated, temperatures controlled, and have adequate electrical outlets to accommodate audiovisual equipment. Spaces should have adequate lighting, have an adequate sound system, and be accessible for persons with disabilities. If screening activities will be a part of the program, provision of privacy for the actual screening procedures is important. Portable screens can be used to create private spaces, if separate rooms are not available.

When planning programs for young children, Sunday school rooms with small scale furniture are appropriate. If only a large room is available, individual "classrooms" can be created with area rugs.

BOX 13-6
Web Resources for Cross-cultural Information

Asian American/Pacific Islander American Health Forum
http://www.apiahf.org
CDC on the Move Against Health Disparities
http://www.kaisernetwork.org/health_cast/hast_index.cfm?display=details&hc+52
Center for Research on Ethnicity, Culture, and Health
http://www.sph.umich.edu/crech/
Congress of National Black Churches (CNBC)
http://www.cnbc.org
Cross Cultural Health Care Program
http://www.xculture.org/index.cfm
Midwest Latino Health
http://www.uic.edu/jaddams/mlhrc/mlhrc.html
National Alliance for Hispanic Health
http://www.hispanichealth.org
National Asian Pacific Center on Aging
http://www.napca.org
National Council of La Raza
http://www.nclr.org
National Heart, Lung, and Blood Institute Strategic Plan to Address Health Disparities
http://www.nhlbi.nih.gov/resources/docs/plandisp.htm
Native American Cancer Research
http://www.memebers.aol.com/natancan/
Resources for Cross Cultural Health Care
http://www.diversityRx.org
Symposium on Diversity in Health Professions
http://www.iom.edu/IOM/IOMHome/nsf/Pages/nickens+symposium

Program Goals, Behavioral Objectives, and Evaluation

Mager (1997) developed the system for writing behavioral objectives that serve to guide teachers to make appropriate instructional decisions and assist learners in understanding what they are expected to know. The terms *goals* and *objectives* are sometimes used interchangeably; however, they have distinct and different meanings. A *goal* is a broad, global statement describing the outcome of a program or event. An *objective*, on the other hand, is short-term and measures a single, specific *behavior* that the learner (not the teacher) will be able to perform. An objective is the intended result of instruction not the process of instruction itself. Objectives are derived from and are consistent with goals. Each objective should describe *one* expected behavior and state specifically *how* it will be measured. Objectives should use verbs that have few interpretations of meaning, such as: *apply, choose, list, predict, compare, define, demonstrate, recall, recognize, write, select,* or *state*. For example:
     At the end of the health education program, the learner will be able to:

1. Describe the signs and symptoms of an impending heart attack.
2. List emergency measures to be taken when a heart attack is suspected.

3. List the steps to perform CPR.
4. Demonstrate the performance of CPR on a model.

Bloom, Englehart, Furst, Hill, and Krathwohl (1956) developed the *Taxonomy of Educational Objectives* as a tool for systematically classifying behavioral objectives. This taxonomy has become widely accepted as a standard aid for planning and evaluating learning. It is divided into three broad categories or domains: cognitive, affective, and psychomotor. Although the domains are described as separate entities, they do, in fact, occur interdependently. The *cognitive domain* involves the acquisition of information and refers to the learner's thinking processes. Objectives in this domain progress from simple to complex across six levels: knowledge, comprehension, application, analysis, synthesis, and evaluation. Objectives for most faith community health education programs will be written at the knowledge, comprehension, and application levels.

The *affective domain* involves feelings and increasing commitment to feelings expressed as emotions, interests, attitudes, or values. This domain is divided into levels that specify the depth of emotional responses to tasks or the degree to which attitudes are incorporated into one's value system. The levels in the affective domain are receiving, responding, valuing, organization, and characterization.

The *psychomotor domain* involves learning to perform skills that require fine and gross motor abilities. Simpson (1972) divides the psychomotor domain into seven levels: perception, set, guided response, mechanism, complex overt response, adaptation, and origination. Learning to administer an injection to walk with crutches is an example of using psychomotor skills. Verbs commonly used to measure each level of each domain are presented in Box 13-7.

Educators have made strong arguments for and against the use of behavioral objectives. The most powerful argument in favor of using behavioral objectives is to provide a frame for evaluating the outcome(s) of the teaching–learning process. Preparing behavioral objectives also helps the teacher organize content.

Although the science of evaluation and testing and measurement in education is a college-level course in itself, the FCN will most likely rely on pretest/posttest and evaluation instruments to assess the success (or failure) of a health promotion program. A pretest measures the learner's knowledge before the educational program, and a posttest measures the learning that occurred as a result of the educational program. Pretests can be informal or formal. An informal pretest is simply to ask the group what they know about a given subject and have people call out responses. A formal pretest is a written quiz. Formal pretests are more intimidating to participants, but intimidation can be lessened by having the participants do the pretest anonymously. Evaluation instruments are usually created by the teacher (although generic instruments can be purchased) and given at the end of the learning experience. These instruments, or tools, ask the learners to rate their satisfaction with their ability to perform each of the program objectives. These tools may also ask the learners to rate instructional methods, the setting, and any other variables that the teacher wishes feedback about. Maintaining records of attendance and an analysis of evaluation data for each program presented provide the FCN with feedback about the success (or lack of success) of health education programming. It also documents an important part of faith community nursing practice. Summaries of these data should be included in the FCN's annual report to the congregation/health ministry committee.

Instructional Methods

Instructional methods are the "how" teaching or instruction is delivered to the learner. Decisions about instructional methods will be made based on various variables, such as how

BOX 13-7
Commonly Used Verbs According to Domain

COGNITIVE DOMAIN

Knowledge	choose, circle, define, identify, label, list, match, name, outline, recall, recognize, report, select, state
Comprehension	describe, discuss, distinguish, estimate, explain, generalize, give example, locate, recognize
Application	apply, demonstrate, illustrate, implement, interpret, modify, order, revise, solve, use

AFFECTIVE DOMAIN

Receiving	accept, admit, ask, attend, focus, listen, observe
Responding	agree, answer, conform, discuss, express, participate, recall, relate, report, try
Valuing	assert, assist, attempt, choose, complete, disagree, follow, help, initiate, join, propose, volunteer
Organization	adhere, alter, arrange, combine, defend, explain, express, generalize, integrate
Characterization	assert, commit, discriminate, display influence, propose, qualify, solve, verify

PSYCHOMOTOR DOMAIN

Perception	attend, choose, describe, detect, differentiate, distinguish, identify, isolate, perceive, relate, select, separate
Set	attempt, begin, develop, display, position, prepare, proceed, reach, respond, show, start, try
Guided response	align, arrange, assemble, attach, build, change, choose, clean, compile, construct, demonstrate, examine, find, insert, locate, measure, mix, open, operate, practice, remove, repair, replace, transfer
Adaptation	adapt, alter, change, convert, correct, rearrange, reorganize, replace, revise, shift, substitute, switch
Origination	arrange, combine, compose, construct, create, design, exchange, reformulate

Adapted from Linn, R. L., & Miller, M. D. (2005). *Measurement and assessment in teaching* (9th ed.). Upper Saddle River, NJ: Pearson Prentice-Hall.

active or passive the learner is and how much control the teacher wishes to maintain during the learning experience.

Cohen (1991) states that learners retain:

- 5% from lecture;
- 10% from reading;
- 20% from audiovisual materials;
- 30% from demonstration;
- 50% from discussion;
- 75% from practice by doing; and
- 90% by teaching others.

Based on this information, the FCN will want to focus on learning activities that use a mixture of instructional styles with as much active learning as possible. Box 13-8 lists traditional and nontra-

BOX 13-8
Instructional Methods

TRADITIONAL	NONTRADITIONAL
Lecture	Gaming
Discussion	Simulation
One-to-one instruction	Role-playing
Demonstration and return	Role modeling
Demonstration	Self-instruction
	Computer-assisted instruction
	Distance education

ditional teaching methods. The methods most germane to faith community nursing practice will be discussed in-depth.

LECTURE

Lecture is the most economic and efficient instructional method because a large number of people can be reached at the same time in a reasonable period of time. This method is unidirectional, flowing from the teacher to the learner. The learner has a passive role in this approach. All of the learners receive the same information at the same time, regardless of their ability or their learning needs. Fitzgerald (2003) states that lecture is relatively ineffective in influencing affective and psychomotor behaviors.

Lectures are organized with an introduction, a body, and a summary or conclusion. The introduction portion of a lecture engages the learner with the topic and builds rapport between the speaker and the audience. Introductions can begin with a story or anecdote, an important fact, or a statistic about the content. In the introduction, review the learning objectives for the presentation. If using a pretest, the audience will begin by doing that activity.

The body of the lecture contains the content of the presentation and is usually ordered according to a prepared outline. Examples should be used throughout to help the audience link new information with familiar information. Keep the purpose of the presentation and the objectives in mind when developing content. Remember the KISS principle (**K**eep **I**t **S**imple **S**uzy). Although it is tempting to provide large amounts of content, information overload can be overwhelming to learners, and key information related to the purpose of the program may get lost.

The conclusion or summary of a lecture should review and summarize the key points that the audience will take home with them. If a posttest will be used, have the audience complete it at the end of the lecture. Time may be allotted at the end of the lecture for the purpose of questions and answers. Be sure to repeat questions asked, so that the entire audience can hear the question. Box 13-9 provides resources for preparing presentations.

Starver and Shellenbarger (2004) advise that speakers should dress for a professional look and avoid wearing distracting or dangling jewelry. They also advise the use of a confident tone of voice, using increasing and decreasing volume and voice animation to help emphasize important points. Speaking clearly and slowly allows the audience to take notes during the presentation. Body language communicates messages to the audience, so facing the audience is important during the

---

BOX 13-9
Resources for Preparing Presentations

Center for Research on Learning & Teaching
http://www.crit.umich.edu/tsmain.html
PBS Teacher Source
http://www.pbs.org/teachersource/health.thm
Center for Application of Prevention Technologies
http://www.open.org/westcapt/bestprac.htm
Health Finder
http://www.healthfinder.gov
Health Teacher with WebMD
http://www.healthteacher.com/
Guidelines for Health Education and Risk Reduction
http://www.aepo-xdv-ww.epo.cdc.gov/wonder/-prevgui/p0000389/p0000389.htm
Association for Supervision and Curriculum Development
http://www.ascd.org
Resources for School Health Educators
http://www.indiana.edu/~aphs/hlthk-12.html
Health Teacher
http://www.healthteacher.com

presentation rather than facing a screen. And most importantly, they advise the presenter to relax, smile, and make eye contact with the audience.

GROUP DISCUSSION

Group discussion is one of the most commonly used instructional methods. This method is both learner- and subject-centered. Groups can be small or large, depending upon the learning objectives. Fitzgerald (2003) reports that group discussion is an effective method for teaching in both the affective and cognitive domains. The teacher's role is to keep the group on track and to facilitate accomplishment of the learning objectives. Group discussion stimulates the learner to think through the issues and share their views with the other members. This method is an active form of learning that is more economical than teaching individuals.

A support group is a powerful tool in modifying or changing behavior. It consists of a group of two or more individuals that meets to achieve agreed-upon goals. Support groups function to provide information, comfort, and connectedness with others who are experiencing similar circumstances (Durrant & Rieckmann, 2003). They are economical and serve both interpersonal and educational gains. Facilitating a support group requires knowledge of the unique needs of the target population and a good understanding of the group process.

ONE-TO-ONE INTERACTION

In individual instruction, the teacher has the ability to assess the learning needs of the learner and to tailor the instruction specifically to meet individual needs. It allows for mutual goal-setting and negotiating a time frame for learning and/or behavioral change to take place. Individual instruction is effective for all domains of learning. This type of instruction is labor intensive and therefore expensive. The FCN frequently uses one-to-one instruction in the health educator and counselor roles.

DEMONSTRATION AND RETURN DEMONSTRATION

Because the FCN is usually not doing "hands-on" nursing care, there are some educational programs where demonstration and return-demonstration will be effective instructional methods. Cooking and first-aid classes are two common examples in which demonstration and return-demonstration would be appropriate.

GAMING

Gaming is an instructional method that requires that the learner participate in a competitive activity with preset rules. The game can be reality based or a fantasy, as long as it is designed to accomplish the behavioral objectives. The goal of the game is to apply knowledge and to practice skills. Fitzgerald (2003) defines gaming as fun with a purpose.

Because gaming is highly active, the retention of information learned is increased. In this method, the teacher explains and clarifies the rules, distributes game materials, and facilitates the game process. At the completion of the game, the teacher debriefs the players by encouraging discussion of the experience, answering questions, and summarizing key points.

Games can be purchased or designed to meet specific needs. The formats of popular games like Jeopardy! and Trivial Pursuit can be adapted for special content.

When planning to use games, be sure to consider group size, time constraints, and the educational and literacy levels of the participants. Prior to using gaming in a real situation, pilot test the game with a small group. Pilot testing gives you the opportunity to assess user difficulty in following the rules or directions of the game as well as how long it takes the group to complete the game.

Assessing and Using Instructional Materials

Instructional materials are tools and aids, both print and audiovisual, that supplement rather than replace actual instruction. Instructional materials should both facilitate and reinforce learning. The use of different instructional materials or a multimedia approach assist individuals with different learning styles to retain information.

Hainsworth (2003) states that appropriate choices of instructional materials depend on the characteristics of the learner, the characteristics of the media, and the characteristics of the task. She suggests the mnemonic LMAT: **L**earner, **M**edia, and **T**ask.

- *Characteristics of the **Learner:*** Choose the media that best meets the needs of your audience. Consider their perceptual abilities, literacy level, developmental level, and learning styles.
- *Characteristics of the **Media:*** Choose media that is consistent with the subject content and learning objectives. Consider a multimedia approach, if financial resources allow.
- *Characteristics of the **Task:*** Task characteristics are defined by the learning objectives, the learning domain, and the complexity of the behavior required by the task.

COMPONENTS OF INSTRUCTIONAL MEDIA

The delivery system, the content, and the presentation are the three major components of media (Frantz, 1980; Weston & Cranston, 1986). Each component will be addressed separately.

Delivery System

The *delivery system* consists of both the actual form of the materials (print, video, music, etc.) and the hardware required to present the material. In a lecture, the person giving the lecture is the delivery system. The lecture may be supplemented with other delivery systems, such as PowerPoint slides or videotapes. The choice of the delivery system is independent of the content of the lesson. The choice is influenced by the size of the target audience, the pacing of the lesson, and sensory aspects most suitable to the target audience.

Content

The *content* is the lesson, the actual information to be conveyed to the target audience. When selecting media, the FCN should consider the accuracy of the information, the appropriateness of the media for the content, and the readability of the materials.

In faith-based health education programs, prayer, the use of Scripture, and devotional worship are integrated into the program content. The International Parish Nurse Resource Center (IPNRC), the Health Ministries Association, and denominational Web sites are all excellent resources and sources of literature and media about the integration of faith and health. See the Additional Resources section at the end of the chapter.

Presentation

The *presentation* describes the way the content is delivered. Weston and Cranston (1986) state that the form of the message is the most important element to consider when selecting instructional materials. They describe the form of the message as occurring on a continuum from concrete to abstract. Concrete-form stimuli are real—for example, giving an injection to a person or to a teaching model. Illusionary representations are less real—looking at a video or a picture of someone giving an injection. The most abstract, or symbolic, representations are numbers and words. Reading or being told about how to give an injection would be an abstract example.

Types of Instructional Materials

Written Materials

Books, leaflets, pamphlets, brochures, handouts, and instruction sheets are the most commonly used written media for health instruction. The advantages of using written materials include:

- Availability of the information to the learner as a reference.
- Acceptability and familiarity to consumers.
- Wide variety.
- Low cost.
- Portability.
- Ability to individualize for different audiences. (Hainsworth, 2003, p. 394).

The disadvantages to written materials include:

- Abstractness.
- They provide no feedback.
- Proper reading level is essential to learning. (Hainsworth, 2003, p. 394)

Written materials can be commercially prepared or self-composed. Obviously, commercially prepared materials have the advantage of being ready to use. With self-composed materials, the FCN has the ability to individualize instructions for a specific person; however, time constraints will most likely preclude doing this. All written instructional materials need to be assessed for content accuracy, reading level, clarity, audience appropriateness, cultural appropriateness, and, ultimately, for cost. Written materials should be "easy on the eyes." Font sizes should consider both younger and older readers. There should be good contrast between the paper color and the font color so that the font can be clearly seen.

Goldman and Schmalz (2001) caution that written materials should be assessed for "ISMs." Is there anything in the piece (in words or pictures) that might be interpreted as ageism, classism, "homophobism," racism, or sexism? Does the piece perpetuate or support any myths or stereotypes?

Demonstration Materials

Demonstration materials include many types of nonprint media, including models and equipment, displays, posters, diagrams, illustration, charts, bulletin boards, and chalk or marker boards. As with written tools, demonstration materials need to convey appropriate and accurate information that is culturally appropriate, at the appropriate reading level for the target audience. Posters and bulletin boards are commonly used methods for FCNs to provide health information and education to the congregation.

Audiovisual Materials

Audiovisual materials stimulate the visual and auditory senses and increase the learner's ability to retain information. As with any teaching aids, audiovisuals need to be previewed for accuracy of content and audience appropriateness. Another issue is the cost of the hardware and software materials.

Slides, overhead transparencies, audiotapes, and computer outputs and videos/DVDs that can be projected onto a screen are the most commonly used audiovisuals. The hardware available to the FCN will determine what audiovisual media can be incorporated into programs.

> ## BOX 13-10
> ## How to Prepare Slides for Presentations
>
> 1. Limit each slide to one concept.
> 2. Use the 6-by-6 rule: There should be 6 or fewer lines per slide and 6 or fewer words per line.
> 3. Use single words (nouns and verbs) and short phrases.
> 4. Slide headings, font size, and style should be consistent throughout the presentation.
> 5. Title fonts should be large—38 to 40 points.
> 6. Text fonts should be a minimum of 24 points.
> 7. Use a light-colored font with a dark background or vice versa.
> 8. Cool colors, such as blue, green, and purple, are best for backgrounds.
> 9. Warm colors, such as yellow, are better for text.
> 10. Use two to three colors per slide, and keep the colors consistent throughout the presentation.
> 11. Show no more than two slides per minute.
> 12. Use easy-to-read fonts, such as Ariel, Century Gothic, Lucida Sans, or Tahoma.
> 13. Use animation and transition sound effects sparingly—they get to be annoying quickly!
> 14. Adjust size and resolution of photographs for clarity.

Health education audiovisual materials can be purchased, rented, or borrowed from various sources. Organizations, such as the American Heart Association and the American Cancer Society, are resources for borrowing audiovisual software.

If the hardware resources are available, the FCN can prepare health educational programs using Microsoft's PowerPoint, a presentation software package. PowerPoint slides are easy and economical to prepare, and they provide a professional result. If the technology is available, PowerPoint presentations can greatly enhance presentations because they provide the visual stimulation of words and pictures. How-to Box 13-10 provides suggestions for preparing presentation slides.

Electronic Resources

The use of technology in health education reflects the use of technology in everyday American life. Cetron and Davies (2001) predict that by 2010, 95% of the people in the industrialized, and half of those in the developing, world, will be online and wired for high speed access. Web-based information can be obtained quickly and at a reasonable cost in one's home and is available free of charge in public libraries. Ease of information access via the World Wide Web has created both an information explosion and information overload. Faith community nurses often serve as facilitators of learning rather than providers of information, and they assist faith community members to critically evaluate the information they find on the Web.

Humes (1999) defines *information literacy* as "the ability to access, evaluate, organize, and use information from a variety of sources." So, if clients are going to use the vast array of Web-based information, they must be able to first locate the information they want, judge whether it is trustworthy, and decide how they will use it to meet their needs. Information literacy is different from *computer literacy,* the ability to use computer hardware and software (Association of Colleges and Research Libraries, 2000).

Sopczyk (2003) suggests that although consumers do not have the professional background to evaluate health-related information, they can be taught some steps to develop information literacy skills and to identify which Web sites are useful and which are problematic. She suggests the following steps:

1. Reduce a topic or a problem to a searchable command that can be used with a search engine.

2. Categorize Web pages according to their purpose. A client should be taught to consider the person or organization responsible for the Web site. For example, a drug company's purpose is to market its drugs; the American Heart Association's purpose is to provide health promotion information.
3. The purpose of the Web pages provides data about potential bias of information.
4. Judge whether the information found is accurate and reliable. Consider the credentials of the author(s), check the date the page was posted, and compare like sites for similarity of information.
5. Identify resources to answer questions or verify assumptions made about the content of a Web page.

In later text, a case study describes using the Web as a resource for health information.

Many guidelines and instruments evaluate Web sites, and several organizations endorse them. One of the best-known and oldest is the Health on the Net Foundation (HON), which is a Geneva-based nonprofit foundation established in 1996. HON has issued its logo to more than 20,000 Web pages that meet the following eight standards that comprise the HON code (2004):

- *Authority:* Health care advice should be given only by health care professionals.
- *Complementarity:* Information provided is designed to support, not replace, the relationship between patients and their health care providers.
- *Confidentiality:* Data related to users, including identity, are kept confidential.
- *Attribution:* Information is supported by clear references to source data, and links are provided to access them. The date when a Web page was last modified is clearly displayed.
- *Justifiability:* Any claims relating to the benefits/performance of a specific treatment, commercial product, or service are supported by appropriate, balanced evidence.
- *Authorship:* Information is provided in a clear, easily readable manner. Contact addresses for further information are provided, and the Webmaster's address is displayed clearly on the site.
- *Sponsorship:* All organizations that own the site are clearly identified.
- *Advertising:* Advertisements are clearly identified so as not to be confused with any health care information given in the site.

To further assist nurses in judging the validity and reliability of Web-based resources, the Health Information Technology Institute (HITI) has developed seven criteria to evaluate health information. These criteria are more stringent than HON's, and they include:

- *Credibility:* Evaluating for credibility includes identifying the source for the medical information, its currency, relevance, and the editorial review process of the information (such as HON). The name and logo of the organization should be clearly displayed, and credentials of authors should be given. The date of revision should be displayed.
- *Content:* This should be accurate, complete, and have the appropriate disclaimer stating that the information provided does *not* substitute for the consultation of a health care professional.
- *Disclosure:* If any information is solicited from users, a clear statement of the use of the information needs to be prominently displayed.
- *Back linkages:* Check links for relevance and for their relationship to the original site. The currency of links and the ease of using links should also be examined.
- *Design and interactivity:* Design speaks to the layout of the Web site and includes accessibility, logical organization, and internal search capacity. Interactivity means that a user can send comments through a link or e-mail address.
- *Caveats:* It should be clear whether a Web site is presenting information about a disease or whether it is representing a product to be sold. If a site claims to do both, it raises a red flag.

Using a Guest Speaker

Depending on the size and resources of the health ministry and the faith community, volunteer (or paid) guest speakers may be used to provide health education programs. Guest speakers are experts about the topics that they will present, and their time is valuable. When the guest speaker is volunteering his or her time for a presentation, the FCN needs to make the event as user-friendly as possible for the guest speaker. The FCN also has the responsibility to see that people do attend. Nothing is as upsetting to a program organizer and to a guest speaker as the lack of an audience. Box 13-11 presents the steps for planning a successful event.

BOX 13-11
Steps for Planning an Event

Three months prior to the event

1. Determine the objectives for the event. This will be done based on the analysis of assessment data about the health education needs of the faith community.
2. Consider the potential number of participants.
3. Consider potential dates and times for the event to be held, and check the availability of rooms.
4. Contact the guest speaker and confirm a date and time for the event. Ask if the guest speaker has any hardware needs for the presentation. Be clear about who will provide the hardware.
5. Reserve a room of the appropriate size, and arrange for hardware as needed.

One month prior to the event

6. Reconfirm the date and time with the guest speaker. Obtain copies of handouts to be duplicated.
7. Publicize the event by inserts in the worship bulletin, by flyers on bulletin boards, and by paid advertising (if desired).
8. Ask the faith community leader to encourage members to attend the event.
9. Register participants (optional).
10. Create a program evaluation form.
11. Solicit volunteer help, if needed.

One week before the event

12. Reconfirm date and time with the guest speaker.
13. Review room setup plans.
14. Make any signs needed.
15. Duplicate handouts, if needed.

Day of the event

16. Place any needed signs.
17. Test hardware as necessary.
18. Meet and greet guest speakers and participants.
19. Administer and collect evaluation forms.

Post-event

20. Review program evaluation forms.
21. Write a thank-you note to the guest speaker and any persons who volunteered to assist with the event.

Summary

This chapter provides content about health behavior and change. It discusses how the FCN uses the health educator role to connect faith, health, and healing for the members of the faith community. FCNs minister within the concept of stewardship of the body and personal health as a responsibility to God. Care and responsibility for and to each other as children of God is a central tenet of a faith community. FCNs can use the Health Belief Model (HBM) and Pender's Model for Health Promotion in planning health education activities.

Interventions for health behavior change were discussed. FCNs can use the intervention strategies of raising consciousness, reevaluating self, promoting self-efficacy, enhancing the benefits of change, controlling the environment, dealing with barriers to change, and maintaining the new behavior. The FCN can integrate the concepts of wholeness, Shalom, and whole health into each of the intervention strategies. Spiritual care, use of Scripture, and prayer can be used in each strategy as well.

The health education process was discussed in detail. Faith community assessment, which includes age considerations, literacy level, and cultural issues, were presented and their relevance to faith-based health education was discussed. Instructional methods were discussed, including the methods of lecture, small group discussion, one-to-one teaching, demonstration, and gaming. Advantages and disadvantages of the methods were discussed.

The assessment of educational materials section of this chapter provides information about the use and evaluation of written, demonstration, audiovisual, and electronic resources. The case study provides application of the evaluation of Web-based resources.

This chapter also reviews important educational principles, such as assessment of readiness to learn, cultural competence, teaching conceptually from simple to complex, mixing passive and active, and visual and oral educational methods to enhance learning retention. It advises FCNs to choose methods and materials that support the purpose and the learning objectives of the instructional event.

Reflect and Discuss

1. A Sunday school teacher is concerned about the hygiene behaviors of her first grade class and asks the FCN to provide a lesson on the importance of handwashing. Describe four principles to consider in planning this lesson. How would you evaluate the effectiveness of the learning?

2. The faith community nurse in an African American church is aware that African American men rarely use screening services for prostate cancer. How would the nurse plan a successful program to provide screening this population?

3. The faith community survey has indicated that over 10% of the members are providing care for an elderly parent in their homes. What educational events might the FCN consider for this population?

4. The assistant pastor has approached the faith community nurse with concerns about suspected recreational drug use by some of the teenagers in the congregation. The FCN community nurse has very little experience with working with drug-related issues. What steps can this nurse take to meet this identified need in the congregation?

Case Study

Mr. Cole has been medically treated for hypertension for 2 years. During a post-service coffee hour conversation with the FCN, Mrs. Maine, he relates that he has discontinued his medication and replaced it with "something better." When Mrs. Maine explores what Mr. Cole is doing to manage his hypertension, he reports that he found a Web site promoting the use of hawthorn, an herbal product to control high blood pressure. He reports that he is feeling "just great" but admits that he has not had his blood pressure assessed since making this change.

Mrs. Maine suggests that he come to her office for a blood pressure check, and she finds his pressure to be elevated. She asks if Mr. Cole can show her the Web site that he used to make his medication decision.

Mr. Cole sits down at the computer and accesses the Web site for the ABC Botanical Company. Mrs. Maine points out that the purpose of this company's Web site is to make sales of their products and that it may be presenting a biased picture to the consumer. She encourages Mr. Cole to see his physician and discuss the treatment for his hypertension. She also suggests that Mr. Cole be more critical in evaluating Web-based information. She provides him with a handout that provides the following suggestions:

How to Evaluate a Web Site

1. *Top domain:* Consider the top domain because it gives a clue to the purpose of the Web site: *.org* identifies a nonprofit organization.

   .gov identifies a government site.

   .com identifies a commercial site.

2. *Accuracy:* Check for obvious errors in spelling and punctuation. Be alert to narrative that states that research has *proven* something—research lends support, shows a lack of support, or has no effect on a premise—it does not *prove* anything.

3. *Authority:* What is the reputation of the organization represented on the Web site? If the Web site has an author, what are the author's credentials? Are statements referenced to other authoritative works?

4. *Objectivity:* Although information is rarely neutral, consider possible biases.

5. *Currency* or *timeliness*: It is often difficult to tell the true date of Web-based information. Well-designed pieces carry the date when they were last updated. Test the links—if they are working, the site is usually current.

6. *Coverage:* Is the Web site for lay or professional readers? Does it tell you which? Is the coverage appropriate to the target audience?

7. *User-friendliness:* How difficult or easy is the site to navigate? Is a plug-in required?

From Thede, L. Q. (2003). *Informatics and nursing* (2nd ed., pp. 100–102). Philadelphia: Lippincott Williams & Wilkins. Used with permission.

 References

Ajzen, I. (1991). The theory of planned behavior. *Organizational Behavior and Human Decision Processes, 50*, 171–211.

American Nurses Association & Health Ministries Association. (2005). *Faith community nursing: Scope and standards of practice.* Silver Springs, MD: ANA.

Association of Colleges & Research Libraries. (2000). *Information literacy competency standards for higher education.* Available online at: http://www.ala.org/acrl/ilintro.html.

Bandura, A. (1997). *Self-efficacy: The exercise of control*. New York: WH Freeman.

Barnes, M. D., Neiger, B. L., & Thackeray, R. (2003). Health communication. In R. J. Bensley & J. Brookins-Fisher (Eds.), *Community health education methods: A practical guide* (2nd ed., pp. 51–82). Sudbury, MA: Jones and Bartlett Publishers.

Bastable, S. B. (2003). Literacy in the adult patient. In S. B. Bastable, *Nurse as educator* (2nd ed., pp. 189–232). Sudbury, MA: Jones and Bartlett Publishers.

Bastable, S. B. & Rinwalske, M. A. (2003). Developmental stages of the learner. In S. B. Bastable, *Nurse as educator* (2nd ed., pp. 119–169). Sudbury, MA: Jones and Bartlett Publishers.

Bloom, B. J., Englehart, M. S., Furst, E. J., Hill, W. H., & Krathwohl, D. R. (1956). *Taxonomy of educational objectives: The classification of educational goals, handbook 1: Cognitive domain*. New York: David McKay.

Brownson, K. (1998). Educational handouts: Are we wasting our time? *Journal for Nurses in Staff Development, 14*(4), 176–182.

Cetron, M. J. & Davies, O. (2001). Trends now changing the world. *The Futurist, 35*(2), 27–40.

Christian Medical Commission. (1990/2001). *Healing and wholeness: The churches' role in health*. Geneva, Switzerland: World Council of Churches; Roswell, GA: Health Ministries Association.

Cohen, M. (1991). A comprehensive approach to effective staff development: Essential elements. Presented at Education Development Center, Cambridge, MA.

Cox, C. (1982). An interaction model of client health behavior: Theoretical prescription for nursing. *Advances in Nursing Science, 5*, 41–56.

Davis, T. C., Crouch, M. A., Wills, G., Miller, S., & Abdehou, D. M. (1990). The gap between patient reading comprehension and the readability of patient education materials. *Journal of Family Practice, 31*(5), 533–538.

Doak, C. C., Doak, L. G., Friedell, G. H., & Meade, C. D. (1998). Improving comprehension for cancer patients with low literacy skills: Strategies for clinicians. *CA-A Cancer Journal for Clinicians, 48*(3), 151–162.

Doak, C. C., Doak, L. G., & Root, J. H. (1996). *Teaching patients with low literacy skills* (2nd ed.). Philadelphia: Lippincott.

Duffy, M. M., & Snyder, K. (1999). Can ED patients read your patient education materials? *Journal of Emergency Nursing, 25*(4), 294–297.

Durrant, L., & Rieckmann, T. (2003). Facilitating support groups. In R. J. Bensley & J. Brookins-Fisher (Eds.), *Community health education methods* (2nd ed., pp. 111–136). Sudbury, MA: Jones and Bartlett Publishers.

Estes, G., & Zitzow, D. (1980, November). Heritage consistency as a consideration in counseling Native Americans. Paper read at the National Indian Education Association Convention, Dallas, TX.

Estey, A., Musseasu, A., & Keehn, L. (1991). Comprehension levels of patients reading health information. *Patient Education and Counseling, 18*,165–169.

Fishbein, M. (2000). The role of theory in HIV prevention. *IDS Care, 12*(3), 273–278.

Fishbein, M., & Ajzen, I. (1975). *Belief, attitude, intention and behavior: An introduction to theory and research*. Reading, MA: Addison-Wesley.

Fisher, E. (1999). Low literacy levels in adults: Implications for patient education. *Journal of Continuing Education in Nursing, 30*(2), 56–61.

Fitzgerald, K. (2003). Instructional methods. In S. B. Bastable (Ed.), *Nurse as educator* (pp. 355–388). Sudbury, MA: Jones and Bartlett Publishers.

Flesch, R. (1948). A new readability yardstick. *Journal of Applied Psychology, 32*(3), 221–223.

Frantz, R. A. (1980). *Selecting media for patient education. TCN Education for self care*. Rockville, MS: Aspen Publishers.

Glanz, K., Rimer, B. K., & Lewis, F. M. (Eds.). (2002). *Health behavior and health education* (3rd ed.). San Francisco: Jossey-Bass.

Goldman, K. D., & Schmalz, K. J. (2001). Tool 1: Deja view: Criteria for previewing educational materials. *Health Promotion Practice, 2*(2), 109–111.

Hainsworth, D. S. (2003). Instructional materials. In S. B. Bastable (Ed.), *Nurse as educator* (pp. 389–426). Sudbury, MA: Jones and Bartlett Publishers.

Hansen, M., & Fisher, J. C. (1998). Patient-centered teaching from theory to practice. *American Journal of Nursing, 98*(1), 56–60.

Health Information Technology Institute (1999). *Criteria for assessing the quality of health information on the Internet*. Available online at: http://www.hitiweb.mitretek.org/docs/policy.html.

Health On the Net Foundation. (2003). *HON code of conduct for medical and health related Web sites*. Available online at: http//www.hon.ch/HONcode/Conduct.html.

Humes, B. (1999). *Understanding information literacy*. Office of Educational Research National Institute on Postsecondary Education, Libraries, and Lifelong Learning. Available online at: http://www.ed.gov/pubs/UnderLit/.

Janz, N. K., Champion, V. L., & Strecher, V. J. (2002). Health belief model. In K. Ganz, B. K. Rimer, & F. M. Lewis (Eds.), *Health behavior and health education* (3rd ed., pp. 44–157). San Francisco: Jossey-Bass.

Jolly, T., Scott, J. L., Fried, C. F., & Sanford, S. M. (1993). Functional illiteracy among emergency department patients: A preliminary study. *Annals of Emergency Medicine, 22*(3), 573–578.

Kitchie, S. (2003). Determinants of learning. In S. B. Bastable (Ed.), *Nurse as educator*. Sudbury, MA: Jones and Bartlett Publishers.

Knowles, M. S. (1990). *The adult learner: A neglected species* (4th ed.). Houston, TX: Gulf Publishing.

Knowles, M. S., Holton, E. F., & Swanson, R. A. (1998). *The adult learner: The definitive classic in adult education and human resource development* (5th ed.). Houston, TX: Gulf Publishing.

Lerner, E. B., Jehle, D. V., Janicke, D. M., & Moscati, R. M. (2000). Medical communication: Do outpatients understand? *American Journal of Emergency Medicine, 18*(7), 764–766.

Mager, R. F. (1997). *Preparing instructional objectives* (3rd ed.). Altanta, GA: Center for Effective Performance.

McLaughlin, G. H. (1969). SMOG-grading: A new readability formula. *Journal of Reading, 12,* 639–646.

Meade, C. D., Diekmann, J., & Thornhill, D. G. (1992). Readability of American Cancer Society patient education literature. *Oncology Nursing Forum, 19*(1), 51–55.

Morrison, G. W. (2001). *Early childhood education today* (8th ed.). Upper Saddle River, NJ: Merrill Prentice-Hall.

National Center for Health Statistics. (2001). *Healthy People 2000: Final review.* Hyattsville, MD: Public Health Service.

Office of the Minority Health. (2001). *National standards for culturally and linguistically appropriate services in health care.* Washington, DC: USDHHS.

Pender, N. J., Murdaugh, C. L., & Parsons, M. A. (2002). *Health promotion in nursing practice* (4th ed.). Upper Saddle River, NJ: Prentice-Hall.

Prochaska, J., & DiClemente, C. C. (1984). *The transtheoretical approach: Crossing traditional boundaries of change.* Homewood, IL: Dow Jones-Irwin.

Schwarzer, R. (Ed.). (1992). *Self-efficacy: Thought control of action.* Washington, DC: Hemisphere Publishing.

Simpson, E. J. (1972). The classification of educational objectives in the psychomotor domain. In M. T. Rainer (Eds.), *Contributions of behavioral science to instructional technology: The psychomotor domain* (3rd ed.). Englewood Cliffs, NJ: Gryphon Press, Prentice-Hall.

Sopczyk, D. (2003). Technology in education. In S. B. Bastable (Ed.), *Nurse as educator* (pp. 427–463). Sudbury, MA: Jones and Bartlett Publishers.

Spache, G. (1953). A new readability formula for primary grade reading materials. *Elementary School Journal, 53*(7), 410–413.

Spector, R. E. (2004). *Cultural diversity in health and illness* (6th ed.). Upper Saddle River, NJ: Pearson Prentice-Hall.

Starver, K. D., & Shellenbarger, T. (2004). Professional presentations made simple. *Clinical Nurse Specialist, 18*(1), 16–20.

van Dover, L. J., & Bacon, J. M. (2003). A theory of spiritual caregiving in parish nursing practice. Fourteenth Sigma Theta Tau International Research Congress, July 12, 2003, St. Thomas, V.I. Available online at: http://stti.confex.com/stti/inrc14/techprogram/session_1871.htm.

Weston, C., & Cranston, P. A. (1986). Selecting instructional strategies. *Journal of Higher Education, 57*(3), 259–288.

Williams, D. M., Counselman, F. L., & Caggiano, C. D. (1996). Emergency department discharge instructions and patient literacy: A problem of disparity. *American Journal of Emergency Medicine, 14*(1), 19–22.

Winslow, E. H. (2001). Patient education materials: Can patients read them, or are they ending up in the trash? *American Journal of Nursing, 101*(10), 33–38.

Wurzbach, M. E. (Ed.). (2002). *Community health education and promotion: A guide to program design and evaluation* (2nd ed.). Gaithersburg, MD: Aspen Publishers.

Additional Resources

Baker, B. (2001). *Teaching P.R.A.Y.E.R.* Nashville, TN: Abingdon Press.

Barnes, L.L., & Sered, S. S. (2004). *Religion and healing in America.* New York: Oxford University Press.

Bliss-Holtz, J. (2003). On the net: How to surf the World Wide Web for health information and avoid the wipeouts. *Advance for Nurses, 5*(21), 43–44.

Carson, V. B., & Koenig, H. G. (2004). *Spiritual caregiving: Healthcare as ministry.* Philadelphia: Templeton Foundation Press.

Chaves, M. (2004). *Congregations in America.* Cambridge, MA: Harvard University Press.

Culture, health, and literacy: A guide to health education materials for adults with limited English literacy skills. Available free from World Education: (617) 482–9485.

Cusveller, B., Sutton, A., & O'Mathuna, D. (2003). *Commitment and responsibility in nursing: A faith-based approach.* Sioux Center, IA: Dordt College Press.

English, L. M., & Gillen, M. A. (2000). *Addressing the spiritual dimension of adult learning: What educators can do.* San Francisco: Jossey-Bass.

Evans, A. R. (1999). *Healing church.* Available online at: http://www.eden.edu/bookstore.

Everist, N. C. (2002). *Church as a learning community.* Nashville, TN: Abingdon Press.

Finck, M. D. (2005). *Stretch and pray: A daily discipline for physical and spiritual wellness.* Minneapolis: Augsburg Fortress.

Gangel, K. O., & Wilhoit, J. C. (Eds.). (1998). *Christian educator's handbook on adult education.* Grand Rapids, MI: Baker Books.

Graber, M. A., Roller, C. M., & Kaeble, B. (1999). Readability levels of patient education material on the World Wide Web. *Journal of Family Practice, 48,* 58–61.

Gregory, J. M. (1995). *Seven laws of teaching.* Grand Rapids, MI: Baker Books.

Griffin, J. L. (Ed.). (2000). *Blessed by the spirit.* Available online at: http://www.eden.edu/bookstore.

Griffin, J. L., & Matheus, R. (1998). *Child in the congregation* (2nd ed.). Available online at: http://www.eden.edu/bookstore.

Griggs, D. L. (2003). *Teaching today's teachers to teach.* Nashville, TN: Abingdon Press.

Hall, D. W., & Koenig, H. G. (2003). *Healing bodies and souls: A practical guide for the congregation.* Minneapolis, MN: Augsburg Fortress.

Halverson, D. (2003). *Teaching and celebrating Christian seasons.* St. Louis, MO: Chalice Press.

Klug, L. (Ed.) (1998). *All will be well: A gathering of healing prayers.* Minneapolis, MN: Augsburg Fortress.

Kotecki, J. E., & Chamness, B. E. (1999). A valid tool for evaluating health-related WWW sites. *Journal of Health Education, 30,* 56–59.

Krych, M. (2004). *The ministry of children's education: Foundations, contexts, and practices.* Minneapolis, MN: Augsburg Fortress.

Livsey, R. C. (1999). *Courage to teach: A guide for reflection and renewal.* San Francisco: Jossey-Bass.

Mattessich, M., Murray-Close, M., & Monsey, B. (2001). *Collaboration: What makes it work* (2nd ed.). St. Paul, MN: AH Wilder Foundation.

McNamara, J. W. (1997). *Health cabinet.* Available online at: http://www.eden.edu/bookstore.

Miller, L. W. (2004). *Faith and health: A framework for Christian nurses.* Victoria, BC: Trafford Publishing.

Myers, M. E. (2002). *Parish nursing speaks.* Available online at: http://www.eden.edu/bookstore.

O'Brien, M. E. (2001). *The nurse's calling: A Christian spirituality of caring for the sick.* Mahwah, NJ: Paulist Press.

O'Brien, M. E. (2003). *Prayer in nursing.* Sudbury, MA: Jones and Bartlett Publishing.

Oermann, M. H., & Wilson, F. L. (2000). Quality of care information for consumers on the Internet. *Journal of Nursing Care Quality, 14,* 45–54.

Pealer, L. N., & Dorman, S. M. (1997). Evaluating health-related Web sites. *Journal of School Health, 67,* 232–235.

Rankin, S. H., & Stallings, K. D. (2001). *Patient education: Principles and practices* (4th ed.). Philadelphia: Lippincott.

Ray, K. (2002). *The nimble collaboration: Fine tuning your collaboration for lasting success.* St Paul, MN: AH Wilder Foundation.

Roberts, P., Priest, H., & Bromage, C. (2001). Selecting and utilizing data sources to evaluate health care education. *Nurse Researcher, 8*(3), 15–29.

Roehlkepartian, J. (2004). *101 great games for infants, toddlers, and preschoolers.* Nashville, TN: Abingdon Press.

Rotundo, J., & Rotondo, M. (2002). *Presentation skills for managers.* New York: McGraw-Hill.

Rowe, L. (2004). *On call: Encouragement for nurses.* Grand Rapids, MI: Baker Books.

Saarmann, L., Daugherty, J., & Riegael, B. (2000). Patient teaching to promote behavioral change. *Nursing Outlook, 48*(6), 281–287.

Spindt, J. (2004). *To serve as Jesus served: A guide to social ministry for congregations.* Minneapolis, MN: Augsburg Fortress.

Striepe, J. (2000). *C.A.R.E.: Congregations affirming relationships everywhere.* Available online at: http://www.eden.edu/bookstore.

Teach, L. (1998). Health related Web site evaluation form. Available online at: http://www.sph.emory.edu/WELKLNESS/instrument.html.

Vogel, L. J. (1991). *Teaching and learning in communities of faith.* San Francisco: Jossey-Bass.

Watkins, W. D. (2004). *The transforming habits of a growing Christian.* Bloomington, MN: Bethany House.

Winer, M., & Ray, K. (1994). *Collaboration handbook: Creating, sustaining and enjoying the journey.* St. Paul, MN: AH Wilder Foundation.

Yate, M., & Sander, P. (2003). *Knock 'em dead business presentations.* Avon, MA: Adams Media Corporation.

→ Web Resources

http://www.aed.org/publications/news/fall95/disease_prev.html   Academy for Educational Development—*ABCs of human behavior for disease prevention*

http://www.ahrq.gov/data/infoqual.htm   Agency for Health Care Policy & Research: Assessing Quality of Internet Health Information

http://www.ahrq.gov/clinc/prevenix.htm   Agency for Healthcare Research and Quality: Guide to Clinical Preventive Services

http://www.alcoholics-anonymoous   Alcoholics Anonymous

http://www.aap/org   American Academy of Pediatrics

http://www.aarp.org   American Association of Retired Persons

http://www.caner.org   American Cancer Society

http://www.adaf.org   American Dietetic Association

http://www.aha.org   American Heart Association

http://www.ama-assn.org/adolhlth/recommend/monogrf1.htm   AMA Guide for Adolescent Preventive Services

http://www.lungusa.org   American Lung Association

http://www.brightfutures.org   Bureau of Maternal/Child Health: Bright Futures

http://www.cdc.gov   Centers for Disease Control

http://www.xculture.org/index.cfm   Cross Cultural Health Care Program   March of Dimes

http://www.fda.gov   Food and Drug Administration

http://www.healthfinder.gov   Gateway to Consumer Health info

http://www.thecommunityguide.org   Guide to Community Preventive Services

http://www.thecommunityguide.org   Evidence-based findings for health education

http://www.healthypeople.gov   Healthy People 2010

http://www.healthtouch.com   Info on prescription and OTC drugs

http://www.presentersuniversity.com   In Focus Corporation. Visual design guide

http://www.navigator.tufts.edu   Links to diet & nutrition sites http://www.mchb.hrsa.gov   Maternal Child Health Bureau

http://www.cancernet.nci.nih.gov   National Cancer Institute

http://www.cdc.gov/nccdphp/index.htm   National Center for Chronic Disease Prevention and Health Promotion

http://www.ncemch.org   National Center for Education in MCH

http://www.cdc.gov/nchswww   National Center for Health Statistics

http://www.niddk.nih/gov/health/diabetes/ndic.htm   National Diabetes Clearinghouse

http://www.health.gov/nhic   National Health Information Center

http://www.nhlbi.nih.gov   National Heart, Lung, and Blood Institute—Education Programs Info Center

http://www.nih.gov/ninr   National Institute of Nursing Research

http://www.epa.gov/nlic.htm   National Lead Information Center

http://www.nmchc.org   National MCH Clearinghouse

http://www.omhrc.gov   Office of Minority Health

http://www.nih.gov/ormh   Office of Research on Minority Health

http://www.cdc.gov/tobacco   Office on Smoking and Health

http://www.plainlanguage.gov   Plain Language

http://www.diversityrx.org   Resources for Cross Cultural Health Care

http://www.raceandhealth.hhs.gov/glance.htm   Race and Health Home Page

http://www.health.gov/scipich/   Science Panel on Interactive Communication

14

Proposal Writing

This chapter will provide the faith community nurse (FCN) with the necessary skills to identify potential funding sources, to prepare a written proposal to request funding, and to manage a funded program. The process of proposal writing is grounded in the conviction that a partnership should develop between the nonprofits, such as faith communities, and the donor. The Foundation Center says that this is truly an ideal partnership because the nonprofits have the ideas and capacity to solve problems but no dollars with which to implement them. Corporate, foundation, and public donors have the financial resources but not the other resources needed to create programs. Bringing the two sectors together results effectively in a dynamic collaboration (http://fdncenter.org/learn/short-course/prop1.html).

What Is Proposal Writing?

Writing a proposal is simply the act of making a written request for money. In the faith community setting, proposal writing might fund the purchase of health screening equipment or the provision of health programming, or it might support a portion of the FCN's salary. A proposal is the written document prepared to apply for funding. The public or private source to which the proposal is submitted is called a *funder*. Grant writing is a competitive process in which the proposal that makes the best case for funding is awarded the funding. In colloquial language, this is called, "getting a grant." Successful grant writers use the art of persuasive writing—coupled with a great idea (which is clearly supported by data), pitched to the right funding source, at the right time. Prayer and good luck are both part of the mix for success. The case study presented at the end of the chapter describes the first steps that an FCN might take in considering writing a proposal to a potential funder.

What is the right funding source? All funding sources provide eligibility criteria. These criteria detail *who* may request funding and for what *purposes* the monies may be used. These criteria are *not* negotiable. Successful proposals closely match the intent of the funder's use for the monies available. The better the match between the faith community's mission and purpose and the funder's preferences for funding, the more likely the project will be awarded funds. For example, the Templeton Foundation provides funding support to scholars who study the relationship between religion and science, so a successful proposal to this foundation would be in that area of research.

Sources of Funding

Sources of funding can be public or private. Public sources include federal, state, and local governments. Private sources can be individuals, foundations, corporations, professional, and philanthropic organizations. Public sources of funding solicit proposals from the general public and special interest groups by providing formal requests for proposals (RFPs) or requests for application (RFAs). The RFPs are printed in the *Federal Register* and posted on the Web sites of the various governmental agencies. RFPs provide the eligibility criteria and the deadlines for proposal submission. The RFP will also indicate the Web site from which an application and directions for the application can be downloaded.

In general, grant proposals to public funding sources are longer and require a considerably greater degree of detail and evaluation methodology than proposals to private sources. Public funding awards generally provide more monies for longer periods of time than private sources. Public grant proposals always limit the number of pages that a proposal can contain. Exceeding the specified length may result in a categorical denial or the removal of the pages that exceed the limit. Proposals to public funders are usually peer reviewed and scored according to a scoring formula. The proposal receiving the highest numerical score is funded first, with subsequent proposals funded until the monies appropriated are used. A proposal may be approved but not necessarily funded. This occurs, if the money resource runs out before an approved proposal is reached. Box 14-1 provides public Web resources that will be of interest to the FCN.

Public funding sources provide workshops and contact persons to educate people about the process of grant writing. Even if you are not funded the first time that you submit a proposal, you can revise and resubmit your proposal in the next funding cycle.

Private funding sources may or may not provide RFPs. Guidelines and instructions can usually be found at the organization's Web site. Some private funding sources require a letter of inquiry (usually with a short summary of the proposed program). The letter of inquiry must receive approval before a fully developed proposal will be considered. Foundations generally accept proposals two to four times per year, and some foundations accept proposals by invitation only. Proposals to private sector funders are generally shorter and less detailed than those going to public funders. Reading the annual report of private funding sources provides valuable information about the "typical" amounts of monies awarded, to whom they have been awarded, and for what purpose. The annual report also describes the mission of the foundation or organization. The mission of the applicant and the mission of the funding organization should be congruent. Local corporations and foundations (including hospital foundations) often prefer to support local constituencies. Local sources of funding are a good starting place for investigating funding sources for faith communities. Box 14-2 lists additional Web sites for funding sources of interest to the FCN. Box 14-3 lists major publications related to grant writing and finding funding sources.

Regional associations of grantmakers (RAGs) often publish a standard or common application form that grantseekers can use for all participating foundations. The forms incorporate headings that structure the way a proposal is written and the information that must be

---

BOX 14-1
Public Funding Sources for Faith Community Nursing

Catalog of Federal Domestic Assistance   http://12.46.245.173.pls/portal30/CATALOG.GRANT_PROPOSAL_DYN.show

CDC National Prevention Information Network   http://www.cdcnpin.org

Center for Faith-Based & Community Initiatives   http://www.hhs.gov/fbci/funding.html

Center for Faith-Based & Community Initiatives Grants Guide   http://www.hhs.gov/fbci/guide

Federal Procurement Data Center   http://www.fpdc.gov

Federal Register   http://www.access.gpo.gov/su docs/aces140.html

Grant Catalog   http://www.whitehouse.gov/government/fbci/grantcatalog2004.pdf

Guidance to Faith-Based & Community Organizations Partnering with the Federal Government   http://www.whitehouse.gov/government/fbci/guidance/index.htm

National Institutes for Health   http://www.nih.gov

State and Local Government Links   http://www.statelocalgov.net/index.cfm

---

BOX 14-2
Funding Resources for Faith Community Nurses

Grants, Etc.   http://www.ssw.umich.edu/resources/index2.html?collection=grants
Nonprofit Grantwriters   http://www.nonprofitgrantwriters.com
The Foundation Center   http://www.foundationcenter.org
The Grantsmanship Center   http://www.tgci.com

---

included. RAGs are not staffed to provide foundation information to the public and should not be used as a first line of research to find foundations in your area. A listing of regional associations is available at http://fdncenter.org/funders/cga/index.html.

Elements of a Proposal

The format of a proposal should follow the instructions provided by the funder to the letter. Not following instructions and misinterpreting instructions are two of the "fatal flaws" that face proposal writers. Using word processing is almost a necessity in this process, and all writing should be backed up on both a hard drive and on removable diskettes or CDs. Kenner and Walden (2001) recommend working for longer rather than shorter blocks of time and environmental management (quiet work spaces, accessible materials) to maximize one's writing productivity. Although different funders may specify different sequencing of sections, a proposal generally has the following elements:

- Cover sheet
- Summary of the proposal
- Budget and budget justification
- Problem statement
- Project description
  - Goals and objectives
  - Methods
  - Staffing/Administration

BOX 14-3
Major Publications Related to Grant Writing and Finding Funding Sources

Chronicle of Philanthropy: http://www.philanthropy.com.
Federal Grants and Contracts Weekly (Arlington, VA)
Foundation Directory; Foundation Directory Supplements; Foundation Grants Index; National Data Bank of Foundations; National Guide to Funding for Children, Youth, and Families; Corporate Foundation Profiles. New York: Foundation Center.
Foundation News and Commentary: http://www.Cof.org.fnc/fncindex/html.
Fund Raiser's Guide to Human Service Funding (2nd ed.). Washington, DC: Taft Group.
Grantsmanship Center Magazine: http://www.tgci.com/publications/pub.htm.
Marquis Who's Who. (2004). *Annual Register of Grant Support.* Indianapolis, IN: Author.

- Evaluation
- Sustainability
- Capacity
- Funding preferences (if applicable)
- Checklist
- Appendix

Cover Sheet

The cover sheet for any public grant proposal is presented in Figure 14-1. Each application packet contains explicit instructions for the completion of this form. Some grant programs instruct the writer to leave some of the boxes blank, so read the directions with care. All forms should be completed in a 12-point font size, using an easy-to-read font, such as Times New Roman. Where signatures are required they should be signed in black ink.

Summary of the Proposal

The summary of the proposal is limited to one page in public proposals and often to less than one page in proposals to the private sector. It must be carefully crafted to engage the interest, enthusiasm, and curiosity of the reader. Successful summaries motivate the reader to continue on and read the whole proposal. The summary statement is the first, and sometimes the only, part of a proposal that is actually read. Here is where you sell your idea to the reader.

The summary statement should include:

- *Problem:* a brief statement of the problem or need that the faith community assessment has identified (1 to 2 paragraphs);
- *Solution:* a short description of the proposed program. It should include what will take place and how many people will benefit from the program, how and where it will operate, for how long, and who will staff it (1 to 2 paragraphs);
- *Funding requested:* an explanation of the amount of grant money required for the program and what your plans are for in-kind and future funding; and
- *The faith community and its expertise:* a brief statement of the name, history, purpose, and activities of the faith community, emphasizing the ability of the health ministry to implement the proposed program.

The summary statement should be written as the *last* step of the proposal writing process. Once all of the parts of the proposal have been developed and written, the summary should be written. If the proposal has been written by a group of people, who each write a part, it should be read in its entirety by the person who will write the summary. Also helpful is to have the summary read by a few people who are not familiar with the project to see what, if any, questions arise.

Budget and Budget Justification

A budget is a financial planning tool. It tells the funder how much money the project will cost and how the money will be spent. Read the directions of the RFP with care because some programs do *not* allow requests for certain kinds of expenditures. *Direct costs* are those costs directly related to the operation of the project. *Indirect costs* are the expenses, or overhead, such as the costs of utilities and facilities maintenance. Some federal grant programs will allow an indirect cost of 8% of the total amount requested. Most private sources of funding do not support indirect costs.

Form Approved Through 05/2004

Department of Health and Human Services Public Health Services **Grant Application** *Do not exceed character length restrictions indicated.*	**LEAVE BLANK—FOR PHS USE ONLY.**	
	Type	Number
	Review Group	Formerly
	Council/Board (Month, Year)	Date Received

1. TITLE OF PROJECT *(Do not exceed 56 characters, including spaces and punctuation.)*

2. RESPONSE TO SPECIFIC REQUEST FOR APPLICATIONS OR PROGRAM ANNOUNCEMENT OR SOLICITATION ☐ NO ☐ YES
   (If "Yes," state number and title)
   Number: Title:

3. **PRINCIPAL INVESTIGATOR/PROGRAM DIRECTOR**	New Investigator ☐ No ☐ Yes	
3a. NAME *(Last, first, middle)*	3b. DEGREE(S)	
3c. POSITION TITLE	3d. MAILING ADDRESS *(Street, city, state, zip code)*	
3e. DEPARTMENT, SERVICE, LABORATORY, OR EQUIVALENT		
3f. MAJOR SUBDIVISION		
3g. TELEPHONE AND FAX *(Area code, number and extension)* TEL: FAX:	E-MAIL ADDRESS:	

4. HUMAN SUBJECTS RESEARCH ☐ No ☐ Yes	4a. Research Exempt ☐ No ☐ Yes If "Yes," Exemption No.		5. VERTEBRATE ANIMALS ☐ No ☐ Yes	
	4b. Human Subjects Assurance No.	4c. NIH-defined Phase III Clinical Trial ☐ No ☐ Yes	5a. If "Yes," IACUC approval Date	5b. Animal welfare assurance no.

6. DATES OF PROPOSED PERIOD OF SUPPORT *(month, day, year— MM/DD/YY)*		7. COSTS REQUESTED FOR INITIAL BUDGET PERIOD		8. COSTS REQUESTED FOR PROPOSED PERIOD OF SUPPORT	
From	Through	7a. Direct Costs ($)	7b. Total Costs ($)	8a. Direct Costs ($)	8b. Total Costs ($)

9. APPLICANT ORGANIZATION Name Address	10. TYPE OF ORGANIZATION
	Public: ⟶ ☐ Federal ☐ State ☐ Local
	Private: ⟶ ☐ Private Nonprofit
	For-profit: ⟶ ☐ General ☐ Small Business
	☐ Woman-owned ☐ Socially and Economically Disadvantaged
	11. ENTITY IDENTIFICATION NUMBER
Institutional Profile File Number (if known)	DUNS NO. Congressional District

12. ADMINISTRATIVE OFFICIAL TO BE NOTIFIED IF AWARD IS MADE Name Title Address Tel: FAX: E-Mail:	13. OFFICIAL SIGNING FOR APPLICANT ORGANIZATION Name Title Address Tel: FAX: E-Mail:

14. PRINCIPAL INVESTIGATOR/PROGRAM DIRECTOR ASSURANCE: I certify that the statements herein are true, complete and accurate to the best of my knowledge. I am aware that any false, fictitous, or fraudulent statements or claims may subject me to criminal, civil, or administrative penalties. I agree to accept responsibility for the scientific conduct of the project and to provide the required progress reports if a grant is awarded as a result of this application.	SIGNATURE OF PI/PD NAMED IN 3a. *(In ink. "Per" signature not acceptable.)*	DATE
15. APPLICANT ORGANIZATION CERTIFICATION AND ACCEPTANCE: I certify that the statements herein are true, complete and accurate to the best of my knowledge, and accept the obligation to comply with Public Health Services terms and conditions if a grant is awarded as a result of this application. I am aware that any false, fictitious, or fraudulent statements or claims may subject me to criminal, civil, or administrative penalties.	SIGNATURE OF OFFICIAL NAMED IN 13. *(In ink. "Per" signature not acceptable.)*	DATE

PHS 398 (Rev. 05/01)   Face Page

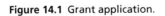

Figure 14.1 Grant application.

When preparing the budget, make additional copies of forms to use as worksheets. Write clear notes on how you computed line items, and keep these worksheets for future reference. These worksheets are actually the only documentation of how the final numbers were developed. They will be a valuable resource tool for monitoring the project once it is underway, and for reporting at the end of the grant period (http://fdncenter.org/-learn/shortcourse/prop2.html).

The federal budget form (Figure 14-2) divides the budget into the following categories:

- Personnel
- Consultants
- Equipment
- Supplies
- Travel
- Other

The form in Figure 14-2 details the allocation of funds for Year 1 of a multiyear project. Less detailed financial projections for subsequent years are placed on the form in Figure 14-3. Private funding sources usually use these or a modification of these budget categories. Narrative budget justification follows the budget forms and gives detailed information about how and why the monies will be spent.

PERSONNEL

The personnel category lists the project personnel by title, tells what percentage of a full-time position will be used by the project (if the FCN nurse will give the project 25% of her time, which would equal 10 hours per week), and lists the salary and benefits—adjusted according to the percentage time used for the project. For example, if the full-time salary is $40,000 per year, $10,000 would be allotted for salary, plus 25% of the salary ($2,500) for the cost of employee benefits would be budgeted for the FCN. In most proposals, the personnel line of the budget is the most expensive.

The budget justification should provide the reader with the rationale for the use of professional and nonprofessional personnel. For example, it should discuss why it is important that the FCN be a registered nurse who has preparation in faith community nursing. Salaries should be justified as being representative of the rates paid in the geographical region where the project is located.

CONSULTANT COSTS

If a consultant is necessary for the success of the project, include the total cost on the budget line, and explain the need for a consultant in the budget justification. Costs will include a per diem rate as well as related travel expenses (if indicated).

EQUIPMENT

The equipment line of the budget is the *total* amount of money needed for the equipment required for the project to meet its objectives. For example, if a project goal is to provide primary care services to children, equipment would include such things as scales, thermometers, an audiometer, eye charts, developmental testing kits, otoscope/ophthalmoscopes, a glucometer, blood pressure equipment, and exam tables. Related office equipment would be included, such as a computer and table.

The budget justification should list equipment to be purchased. Equipment priced over $500 should be discussed individually in the narrative. For example, the purchase of an audiometer and why it is needed would be addressed individually. The cost of a specific brand and model number should be provided. This level of detail demonstrates to the funder that you know

Principal Investigator/Program Director (Last, First, Middle):

DETAILED BUDGET FOR INITIAL BUDGET PERIOD DIRECT COSTS ONLY					FROM		THROUGH	
PERSONNEL *(Applicant organization only)*		TYPE APPT. *(months)*	% EFFORT ON PROJ.	INST. BASE SALARY	DOLLAR AMOUNT REQUESTED *(omit cents)*			
NAME	ROLE ON PROJECT				SALARY REQUESTED	FRINGE BENEFITS	TOTAL	
	Principal Investigator							
SUBTOTALS				→				
CONSULTANT COSTS								
EQUIPMENT *(Itemize)*								
SUPPLIES *(Itemize by category)*								
TRAVEL								
PATIENT CARE COSTS	INPATIENT							
	OUTPATIENT							
ALTERATIONS AND RENOVATIONS *(Itemize by category)*								
OTHER EXPENSES *(Itemize by category)*								
SUBTOTAL DIRECT COSTS FOR INITIAL BUDGET PERIOD					$			
CONSORTIUM/CONTRACTUAL COSTS			DIRECT COSTS					
			FACILITIES AND ADMINISTRATIVE COSTS					
TOTAL DIRECT COSTS FOR INITIAL BUDGET PERIOD *(Item 7a, Face Page)*				→	$			
SBIR/STTR Only: FEE REQUESTED								

PHS 398 (Rev. 05/01)   Page _____

Figure 14.2 Federal budget form.

exactly what you want and why. Lower priced equipment items can be grouped under one category. For example, "physical assessment equipment: $350 for (6) eye charts and (6) B/P cuffs."

SUPPLIES

The line of the budget designated for supplies represents the total amount of money requested for the supplies necessary to the success of the project. Supplies are consumable materials. Using the previous pediatric primary care example, supplies would include tongue depressors, glucometer testing strips, syringes and needles, alcohol wipes, and exam table paper.

Principal Investigator/Program Director (Last, First, Middle):

BUDGET FOR ENTIRE PROPOSED PROJECT PERIOD
DIRECT COSTS ONLY

BUDGET CATEGORY TOTALS		INITIAL BUDGET PERIOD *(from Form Page 4)*	ADDITIONAL YEARS OF SUPPORT REQUESTED			
			2nd	3rd	4th	5th
PERSONNEL: *Salary and fringe benefits. Applicant organization only.*						
CONSULTANT COSTS						
EQUIPMENT						
SUPPLIES						
TRAVEL						
PATIENT CARE COSTS	INPATIENT					
	OUTPATIENT					
ALTERATIONS AND RENOVATIONS						
OTHER EXPENSES						
SUBTOTAL DIRECT COSTS						
CONSORTIUM/ CONTRACTUAL COSTS	DIRECT					
	F & A					
TOTAL DIRECT COSTS						

TOTAL DIRECT COSTS FOR ENTIRE PROPOSED PROJECT PERIOD *(Item 8a, Face Page)* ————	$

SBIR/STTR Only Fee Requested				

SBIR/STTR Only: Total Fee Requested for Entire Proposed Project Period (Add Total Fee amount to "Total direct costs for entire proposed project period" above and Total F&A/indirect costs from Checklist Form Page, and enter these as "Costs Requested for Proposed Period of Support" on Face Page, Item 8b.)	$

JUSTIFICATION: Follow the budget justification instructions exactly. Use continuation pages as needed.

Figure 14.3 Budget for entire proposed project period.

In the budget justification, the estimates of needed supplies should correlate with the expected number of clients to be served in the project. This would be an educated guess, and both writer and the reader are aware that this is so. Logical groups of supplies can be consolidated and priced. For example, the heading "office forms" with a related price would be a logical grouping.

TRAVEL

Funding for travel required for the success of the project may be requested. Travel costs include room and food expenses, conference fees, and transportation. Costs should be budgeted for full-fare transportation and full room cost. In the budget justification, state *why* the attendance at this conference is important to the success of the project. Also state that discounted prices will be requested for transportation and room costs.

OTHER

The "Other" line on the budget includes expenses necessary to the success of the project that do not fit into any of the categories listed. Such expenses might include advertising and printing costs. Again, provide the total cost on the budget form and an explanation of the need. Provide detailed costs for these requests as well as the rationale for their need in the budget justification.

Problem Statement

The problem statement section of the proposal should paint a picture of the proposed program for the reader. It should be written in clear, understandable terminology. The applicant for funding rarely gets to meet face to face with the funder, so what is written in the proposal needs to be clear, accurate, and complete.

The problem statement identifies the conditions, problems, or issues that lead you to propose a program or plan of action. It provides a strong rationale for *why* funding should be provided. This information should be factual and supported with *appropriate* statistics. The problem or needs statement does not propose a solution, but rather it lays the foundation for the action that the rest of the proposal will present as a solution. A strong foundation is essential to a successful proposal, and it constitutes a critical element. If the potential funder is unimpressed with the problem/need statement, there is no reason to read further. The problem/need that the proposal addresses should be clearly linked to a funding priority or goal(s) of the funder. According to Coley and Scheinberg (2000), an effective problem statement does four things:

1. It uses supportive evidence to clearly describe the nature and extent of the problem or need facing the target group that you wish to serve.
2. It illuminates the factors contributing to the problem or the circumstances creating the need.
3. It identifies current gaps in services or programs.
4. Where applicable, it provides a rationale for the transferability of the "promising approaches" or "best practices" that are proposed. (p. 32)

Karsh and Fox (2003) caution that too many proposal writers assume that the existence of the problem and the wisdom of the solution are obvious to the reader. This assumption is false. Competing proposal writers carefully document their problem or need by formally using one or more of the following methods:

- A variety of economic and demographic statistics about the target population to be served and the community where it resides. Census data and state health department biostatistics are appropriate to use—but use *only* those that are specifically relative to your problem or need. Discuss the ways the numbers are relevant, making the connection clear to the reader. Data should be current and accurate with the sources of data cited accurately and completely.
- Relevant, up-to-date research, trends, and literature.

- Results of needs assessments.
- Focus groups results.
- Waiting lists for similar programs.

A case can also be made for the effect(s) of nonintervention on the target population and the community as a whole. The actual costs, both to quality of life and monetary, of prevention/intervention versus nonintervention can be compared.

A solid rationale demonstrates to the reader that the proposal writer has a thorough understanding of the problem and of the target population's needs. It demonstrates that the proposal writer is knowledgeable about the types of interventions that can be successful in addressing the identified problem or need. The rationale should persuade the reader that the proposal writer's approach is a solid choice to address the problem/need identified. It also indicates to the reader that there is knowledge about potential barriers to success.

Coley and Scheinberg (2000) suggest that the problem statement section can be divided into four subsections. The first of these describes the nature and extent of the need/problem. This section should provide a clear picture of the incidence of the problem—the number of people affected, their age, gender, educational level, and ethnicity. The incidence in the faith community should then be compared to the incidence of the need or problem with the geopolitical community, state, or national incidence.

The second subsection would address the factors contributing to the need or problem. They may include:

1. A lack of skill, knowledge, or awareness
2. Debilitating attitudes or harmful values
3. Physical or mental challenges and limitation
4. Dysfunctional or problem behavior
5. Limited resources or access to services
6. Institutional or systemic barrier, including fragmented services
7. Policies, practices, or laws that have negative consequences (Coley & Scheinberg, 2000).

The causes of the needs and problems can also be discussed in terms of socioeconomics or culture, as appropriate. For example, the culture of poverty will have a number of contributing factors related to population needs. In this subsection, avoid circular reasoning. The absence of a program is *not* the cause of a problem or need. The need or problem must be addressed in relation to contributing factors.

The third subsection addresses the impact of the need or problem on the client, the client's family, the faith community, and the community at large. Specifically state what benefits can be expected from the implementation of the proposed program. Discuss both quantitative (objective measures, such as affected numbers of persons, measurable increases or decreases in incidence or effect) and qualitative (subjective measures of quality of life) impacts to the target population.

The last subsection would present the theoretical perspectives that have been useful in designing interventions, the successful approaches used in other places, and the likely barriers to resolving the problem. Briefly compare strategies and consider the unique needs of the faith community population.

Project Description

The project description is the detailed description of the proposed project. It includes goals and objectives, method or implementation plan, and staffing and administration. Each of these areas will be discussed individually.

GOALS AND OBJECTIVES

Goals are statements about the intended mission or purpose of a program. They are typically broad in scope and are *not* measurable. Most proposals identify only one or two goals, and instances occur when the funder actually provides the program goals within the context of funding priorities.

Objectives, on the other hand, are very specific, achievable, measurable outcomes that are essential for achieving expected program goals within a specified time frame. Each goal may have several related objectives. Nurses are very familiar with writing measurable, expected outcomes, using action verbs (reduce, increase, decrease, promote, demonstrate) to indicate the expected direction of the change in knowledge, attitude, behavior, skills, or conditions.

Program objectives can be *process* or *outcome* objectives. Process objectives relate to the *activities* needed to implement the program not to the outcomes expected for the program recipients. Process objectives are concerned with *how* the program is implemented. Examples of process objectives are described:

- Two domestic violence prevention groups will be formed by the faith community within the first 4 months of the program.
- A minimum of 25 people will participate in monthly blood pressure screening.

Outcome objectives are used to describe the *expected benefits* to program recipients. An outcome objective specifies a target group and identifies what is expected to happen to them as a result of the intervention or approach. The outcome objective also indicates the time frame in which the outcome will occur. Changes may occur in behavior, skill level, attitudes, values or beliefs, knowledge, or in improved conditions.

Examples of outcome objectives would be:

- After 1 year of programming, the domestic violence rates will decrease by 20%.
- Seventy-five percent of identified hypertensive congregants saw a physician within 1 month of the screening.

Coley and Scheinberg (2000) report that well-stated outcome objectives provide:

- A time frame.
- The target group.
- The number of program recipients.
- The expected measurable results or benefits.
- The geographical location or service location.

METHODS OR IMPLEMENTATION PLAN

The goals and objectives explain to the reader exactly what the expected outcomes of the program will be. The methods section details the specific activities that will take place to achieve the objectives. It enables the reader to visualize the implementation of the project. It should convince the reader that the faith community knows what it is doing, thereby establishing credibility. The Foundation Center suggests dividing this discussion of methods into the following: how, when, and why.

- *How:* the detailed description of what will occur from the time the project begins until it is completed; the methods should match the previously presented objectives.
- *When:* the order and timing for the tasks; it is visually helpful to the reader to provide this information in a GANTT chart format (Table 14-1).
- *Why:* the rationale for the methods chosen; this is especially important if the methods are innovative or unorthodox. (http://fdncenter.org/learn/shortcourse/prop2.html)

TABLE 14-1

GANTT Chart

OBJECTIVE	JUL	AUG	SEP	OCT	NOV	DEC	JAN	FEB	MAR	APR	MAY	JUN
Obj. 1.1—250 church members will be screened for diabetes by 6/30												
Purchase glucometer	X											
Train volunteer RNs	X											
Monthly post-worship service screening	X	X	X	X	X	X	X	X	X	X	X	
Referral to physician		X	X	X	X	X	X	X	X	X	X	
FCN follow-up with client			X	X	X	X	X	X	X	X	X	
Evaluation report							X					X

STAFF AND ADMINISTRATION

This section of the proposal will discuss the number and qualifications of staff needed to implement the program. It will clearly define the specific assignments of each staff member and state whether they will work full-time or part-time (hours per week). Each position should be described in narrative form with a position description provided. Biographical detail about each position and staff member may be required within this section or in the appendix. Figure 14-4 presents the biographical form used in federal proposals.

Staffing may refer to volunteers and consultants as well as to paid staff. The use of volunteers to complement a program underscores the value of the program to the faith community as well as its cost-effectiveness. Because salary costs are affected by the qualifications of the staff, describe the practical experience and educational credentials required of the staff.

For large-scale projects, the plans for administering the project should be discussed. If more than one agency is collaborating on the project, the proposal writer needs to be very clear about which agency has the fiscal responsibility.

Principal Investigator/Program Director (Last, First, Middle):

BIOGRAPHICAL SKETCH
Provide the following information for the key personnel in the order listed on Form Page 2.
Follow this format for each person. **DO NOT EXCEED FOUR PAGES.**

NAME	POSITION TITLE

EDUCATION/TRAINING *(Begin with baccalaureate or other initial professional education, such as nursing, and include postdoctoral training.)*

INSTITUTION AND LOCATION	DEGREE *(if applicable)*	YEAR(s)	FIELD OF STUDY

Figure 14.4 Biographical sketch.

Evaluation

Evaluation methodology is a critical piece to a successful proposal. Evaluation is an important management tool that helps refine and improve programs. Two types of formal evaluation are described:

Outcome (or summative) *evaluation* measures the outcomes, the program's effectiveness in achieving its objectives, and the program's impact on the need or problem it was designed to address. Outcome evaluation uses primarily quantitative methods, such as measures of pre- and post-intervention related to knowledge, skills, attitudes, and/or behavior changes. Outcome evaluation may also identify or uncover unexpected benefits of the program. Such information is useful in preparing future proposals.

Process (or formative) *evaluation* analyzes the process and provides corrective feedback to allow for program adjustments. It assists the organization to assess effectiveness, participant satisfaction, and staff efforts at specific points in time. Although both types of evaluation may be appropriate for a given project depending upon its nature, the funder will be most interested in the program outcomes. For both types of evaluation, one needs to explain the methods to be used to collect and analyze evaluative data. How the evaluation data will be used and to whom it will be presented should be discussed.

When designing an outcome evaluation plan, the stated measurable objectives provide the content. The evaluation methods to collect data—which measure how successfully each objective was met—might include pretesting and posttesting, follow-up surveys or actual observation of skill performance, or behavioral change. Accountability is an important responsibility when an organization accepts money from an external source.

Coley and Scheinberg (2000) state that from the funder's perspective, evaluation results may be used to:

1. Determine whether the funds were used appropriately and whether the stated objectives were accomplished.
2. Assess whether the program's benefits were worth the cost.
3. Assist in the development of future funding objectives related to the same need or problem.
4. Promote positive public relations through promotion of the benefits gained as a result of the program. (p. 56)

Coley and Scheinberg (2000) state that from the perspective of the organization (the faith community), evaluation has the following benefits:

1. It compels the organization to create measurable objectives.
2. It helps the organization to continually refine its approaches to service.
3. It provides feedback on the level of effort and cost required to accomplish objectives.
4. It increases the organization's capacity to meet the need through increased knowledge about both the group served and the effectiveness of the interventions.
5. It assists the organization to communicate the benefits of service.
6. It assists other organizations in program development through the dissemination of results. (p. 56)

Some funders provide very specific directions about how the evaluation section of the proposal should be structured. If no specific directions are provided, do include the following information:

- Indicate program objectives.
- Indicate evaluation method.
- Identify what will be measured.
- Describe what data will be collected and how they will be collected.

- Indicate the timetable for the evaluation process.
- Discuss data analysis.

Sustainability

Most funders want to know how an organization plans to fund the program after the grant money is no longer available. This presents somewhat of a "Catch 22" to faith communities that may never intend their health ministries to be revenue-producing. However, many of the proposals that faith communities write actually create programs that have a life well beyond the period of the grant. For example, funding attained for health screening equipment provides equipment that will be used for many years beyond the funding period, and the health ministry budget (or other identified means of fundraising) can assume the cost of consumable supplies (such as glucometer strips).

Federal/public grants usually require both internal and external evaluations at specific points in time during the life of a grant. Internal evaluation refers to the outcome evaluation discussed earlier, produced in a written report form. In external evaluation, a person from outside the organization reviews the program, its budget and spending and outcomes, and presents a formal report. External program evaluation should confirm internal evaluation. External evaluators are entitled to a fee, which should be included in the budget of the proposal.

Capacity

The capacity section of a proposal describes the organization's ability to get the job done as proposed. An important consideration is to be able to demonstrate to a prospective funder that the organization has the capacity to manage money effectively, to implement the program as designed, and to handle the reporting requirements. Karsh and Fox (2003) suggest that the following kinds of information be included to show capacity:

- The history and mission of the organization.
- Physical facilities.
- Size and demographics of the organization.
- The organization's budget.
- Organization's governance structure.
- Previous success(es) in program implementation.
- Any proposed collaborations.
- Management and staff experience, qualifications, awards.
- Availability of volunteer help.
- Letters of support from the community. (p. 194)

The Foundation Center cautions against overwhelming the reader with facts about your organization. It suggests that in two pages or fewer, tell the reader when your organization came into being, state its mission, being certain to demonstrate how the subject of the proposal fits within or extends that mission, and describe the organization's structure, programs, and special expertise. Provide information about the board and its level of participation and whether there is an active group of volunteers. Briefly describe the demographics of the organization and how many people will be served by the proposed program (http://fdncenter.org/learn/shortcourse/prop2.html).

Funding Preferences

Funding preferences are available in some federal grant programs. The funding preference awards additional points to those proposals that specifically address a stated specific need, in addition to meeting the broader eligibility requirements for the grant program. An example might be a grant program for health education in faith-based settings with a funding preference for the provision of health education about prostate cancer to African American men. If a proposal qualifies for a funding preference, it is awarded a fixed number of extra points in the scoring process. For example, if a grant program is established to provide funds to faith-based communities for health education, those faith communities that provide specifically designated programming to high-risk groups would be awarded extra points.

Checklist

Federal grant proposal packages provide a checklist that goes at the end of the proposal (Figure 14-5). The checklist helps ensure that all of the necessary parts of the proposal are included. Foundations usually do not provide a checklist; however, the Foundation Center has created a generic checklist form that is helpful to all proposal writers. This four-page form can be purchased from the Foundation Center.

Appendix

The appendix to a proposal provides additional and supplemental information to the reader. Some funders require that appendix pages be included in the total allowable page length of the proposal, some do not. Materials included in the appendix should be only those items that are highly *relevant* to the proposal.

Depending on the nature of the proposal (and the instructions), letters of support may be included in the appendix. Letters of support can be solicited from other faith communities or community agency directors who support the proposed program. When requesting a letter of support, it is both acceptable and helpful to provide the person with a sample (or boilerplate) of what the letter should say. If the content of the sample letter is acceptable, the person can easily transfer it to his or her own letterhead. A self-addressed and stamped return envelope should also be provided to anyone from whom you have requested a letter of support.

A Few Words About Presentation

Proposals should be neat, clean, and easy to read. They should be under the maximum pages in length, and they must be submitted on time. As discussed earlier in this chapter, the document should be word-processed on white, standard 8.5- $\times$ 11-inch paper with a standard font (such as Times New Roman) and font size no smaller than 12 points. Each page should be numbered. A proposal should always be backed up on floppy disks or CDs—do not trust a hard drive with a single copy of a proposal. The document should be carefully proofread for typographical errors. Do not rely solely on a spell-check feature. On one proposal the spellchecker consistently changed the word "underserved" to "undeserved," which greatly changed the meaning. Do not use jargon or abbreviations.

Proposals should not include any type of decorative materials or use color. The use of borders, clip art, and photos are generally unacceptable. Xeroxed copies of charts or graphs should be clear and readable.

Although all proposal writers are mindful of page limits, 1-inch margins, the use of consistent headings, diagrams, charts, and bulleting make for ease of reading. Many proposal readers will be reading many proposals in a short amount of time and need to have reader-friendly documents.

Proposals should be presented in the number of copies requested (one of which should be an original with signatures in ink). Some funders request that proposals not have staples and request, rather, the use of rubber bands. *Do not* ever use elaborate packaging.

Principal Investigator/Program Director (Last, First, Middle):

CHECKLIST

TYPE OF APPLICATION *(Check all that apply.)*

☐ NEW application. *(This application is being submitted to the PHS for the first time.)*

☐ SBIR Phase I
☐ STTR Phase I

☐ SBIR Phase II: SBIR Phase I Grant No. _____
☐ STTR Phase II: STTR Phase I Grant No. _____

☐ SBIR Fast Track
☐ STTR Fast

☐ REVISION of application number: _____

(This application replaces a prior unfunded version of a new, competing continuation, or supplemental application.)

☐ COMPETING CONTINUATION of grant number: _____

(This application is to extend a funded grant beyond its current project period.)

INVENTIONS AND PATENTS
(Competing continuation appl. and Phase II only)

☐ No   ☐ Previously reported

☐ SUPPLEMENT to grant number: _____

☐ Yes. If "Yes."   ☐ Not previously reported

(This application is for additional funds to supplement a currently funded grant.)

☐ CHANGE of principal investigator/program director.
Name of former principal investigator/program director. _____

☐ FOREIGN application or significant foreign component.

1. PROGRAM INCOME *(See Instructions.)*
All applications must indicate whether program income is anticipated during the period(s) for which grant support is requested. If program income is anticipated, use the format below to reflect the amount and source(s).

Budget Period	Anticipated Amount	Source(s)

2. ASSURANCE/CERTIFICATION *(See instructions.)*
The following assurances/certifications are made and verified by the signature of the Official Signing for Applicant Organization on the Face Page of the application. Descriptions of individual assurances/ certifications are provided in Section III. If unable to certify compliance, where applicable, provide an explanation and place it after this page.

• Human Subjects • Research Using Human Embryonic Stem Cells • • Research on Transplantation of Human Fetal Tissue• Women and Minority Inclusion Policy • Inclusion of Children Policy• Vertebrate Animals

•Debarment and Suspension; • Drug-Free Workplace *(applicable to new [Type 1] or revised [Type 1] applications only);•* Lobbying;• Non-Delinquency on Federal Debt• Research Misconduct• Civil Rights (Form HHS 441 or HHS 690); •Handicapped Individuals (Form HHS 641 or HHS 690); •Sex Discrimination (Form HHS 639-A or HHS 690); • Age Discrimination (Form HHS 680 or HHS 690); • Recombinant DNA and Human Gene Transfer Research;• Financial Conflict of Interest (except Phase I SBIR/STTR) •STTR ONLY: Certification of Research Institution Participation.

3. FACILITIES AND ADMINISTRATIVE COSTS (F&A)/INDIRECT COSTS. See specific instructions.

☐ DHHS Agreement dated: _____

☐ No Facilities And Administrative Costs Requested.

☐ DHHS Agreement being negotiated with _____ Regional Office.

☐ No DHHS Agreement, but rate established with _____ Date

CALCULATION* *(The entire grant application, including the Checklist, will be reproduced and provided to peer reviewers as confidential information.)*

a. Initial budget period: Amount of base $ _____ x Rate applied _____ % = F&A costs $ _____

b. 02 year   Amount of base $ _____ x Rate applied _____ % = F&A costs $ _____

c. 03 year   Amount of base $ _____ x Rate applied _____ % = F&A costs $ _____

d. 04 year   Amount of base $ _____ x Rate applied _____ % = F&A costs $ _____

e. 05 year   Amount of base $ _____ x Rate applied _____ % = F&A costs $ _____

TOTAL F&A Costs $ _____

*Check appropriate box(es):

☐ Salary and wages base   ☐ Modified total direct cost base   ☐ Other base *(Explain)*

☐ Off-site, other special rate, or more than one rate involved *(Explain)*
Explanation *(Attach separate sheet, if necessary.):*

4. SMOKE-FREE WORKPLACE   ☐ Yes   ☐ No *(The response to this question has no impact on the review or funding of this application.)*

PHS 398 (Rev. 05/01)   Page____

Figure 14.5 Federal grant proposal checklist.

Managing a Grant

The grant process does not end when the check has been delivered. Once the celebration is over, remember to write thank-you letters. If you have received funding from a foundation, direct the letter of thanks to the foundation's director (or to the person who signed the award letter). If it is appropriate, also thank any technical assistance that any foundation officer provided to you. For a federal grant, call or write your Congressional representative to thank him or her (if that is relevant) and to provide the courtesy of keeping their office informed.

Federal and government grant award letters will detail the conditions for which the grant is being made and will advise you of the nature and timing of any reports that are required. Most funders do not permit the grantee to move monies between discrete budget categories without their expressed permission and your clear documentation of the rationale for doing so. Grant management should be highly organized to attain the data required for adequate reporting to the funder. At the receipt of the award, the program staff should review the program implementation plan, timetable, and budget to be sure that all continue to be appropriate and achievable. If any problems or doubts occur about the ability of the organization to implement the grant according to the proposal, those concerns should be raised promptly with the funder. If problems arise during the implementation process, do keep the funder informed, as things occur, and provide an alternative plan of action. Do not wait until a report is due to report changes in the implementation of the grant.

Summary

This chapter has provided the reader with information and resources for finding grant funding in both the public and private sectors. The importance of matching the mission of the faith community to the mission of the funder was discussed as an issue critical to success in the grant writing process.

The single most important element of proposal writing is following the directions provided by the funder. The directions relate to the required components of the proposal, eligibility criteria, deadlines, and document length requirements and limitations. The directions are *not* negotiable and must be followed to the letter to even be *considered* for funding.

Grant management was addressed, and the importance of meeting reporting and accountability requirements was discussed. Web-based resources and publication resources have been provided throughout the chapter.

Reflect and Discuss

An FCN wants to implement an after-school program for disadvantaged school-age children. She wishes to provide tutoring services, health-screening services, snacks, recreation, and Bible study to 50 children. The program will operate Monday through Friday from 3:00 PM to 6:00 PM. The Board of Elders is very supportive of this plan but has no funds available to make it operational, and suggests that a proposal be written to request funds from an external source.

1. What data should the FCN collect prior to researching public and private funding sources?
2. Where should the FCN look to find funding sources for this type of project?
3. Does the provision of Bible study limit funding sources?
4. What resources does the FCN have to prepare the proposal?
5. What will be the sustainability of this project?

Case Study

Mary Ann is a faith community nurse at Calvary Church. In the electronic *IPNRC Notes* that she receives by e-mail she is made aware of Wheat Ridge Ministries. In investigating their Web site, she discovers that this group provides major grants from $5,000 to $50,000 (distributed over a 3-year period in declining amounts) and special short-term grants for 1 year or fewer in amounts below $5,000. The Web site tells her that grants have been awarded in several areas, including health and wellness ministries.

The Web site allows her to view current and previous major grants by state. The Web site also advises that requests will not be considered without prior conversation with a member of the Wheat Ridge Ministries staff. Mary Ann's immediate reaction is to pick up the telephone and call them, but at the last minute she decides to first have some conversations within her faith community.

First, Mary Ann reviews the list of previous and current grant awards made by Wheat Ridge Ministries. She reads their mission statement and believes that the mission of the organization and that of her church are congruent. Mary Ann then presents the information she has gathered at the next Health Ministry Team meeting. The thought of bringing in external funding to supplement their health ministry offerings is exciting to the members of the team. A great deal of meeting time is used to brainstorm about needs and priorities of the congregation. Mary Ann reminds the team of the findings of her congregational needs assessment. One of the identified needs was for education related to conflict resolution and violence prevention for school-age children and teens. Another was the need for transportation services to get elderly members to health care provider appointments. Another suggestion was to establish a Stephen's Ministry.

Although Mary Ann found the brainstorming helpful to consider the possibilities for programming, much of what was suggested was not based on any clearly documented faith community needs. She suggested that a small task force be established to consider data-based needs and to recommend priorities back to the health ministry team. Mary Ann also volunteered to follow up with the funder about particulars of the proposal writing process.

References

Coley, S. M., & Scheinberg, C. A. (2000). *Proposal writing* (2nd ed.). Thousand Oaks, CA: Sage Publications.

Foundation Center, The. (2004). Proposal writing short course. Available online at: http://fdncenter.org/learn/shortcourse/prop1.html.

Karsh, E., & Fox, A. S. (2003). *The only grant-writing book you'll ever need.* New York: Carol & Graf.

Kenner, C., & Walden, M. (2001). *Grant writing tips for nurses and other health professionals.* Washington, DC: American Nurses Publishing.

Additional Resources

Association for Healthcare Philanthropy. (2003). *Report on giving FY 2002 USA/Canada.* Falls Church, VA: Author.

Brinckerhoff, P. C. (1999). *Faith-based management: Leading organizations that are based on more than just mission.* New York: Wiley.

Brown, L. G. (2001). *Demystifying grant seeking.* San Francisco: Jossey-Bass.

Browning, B. A. (2001). *Grant writing for dummies.* New York: Dummies Books.

Carlson, M. (2002). *Winning grants step by step.* San Francisco: Jossey-Bass.

Fitzpatrick, J. J., & Deller, S. S. (2000). *Fundraising skills for health care executives.* New York: Springer Publishing.

Foundation Center, The. (2005). *National guide to funding in health* (9th ed.). New York: Author.

Gitlin, L. N., & Lyons, K. J. (2004). *Successful grant writing: Strategies for health and human services professionals.* New York: Springer Publishing.

Karber, B. A. (Ed.). (2004). *The health funds grants resources yearbook.* Manasquan, NJ: Health Resources Publishing.

Kastel, J. L. (2003). *Grant funding for elderly health services* (4th ed.). Manasquan, NJ: Health Resources Publishing.

Krath, D. (1990). *How to use the catalog of federal domestic assistance.* Los Angeles, CA: The Grantsmanship Center.

Laura, N., & Gitlin, K. J. (2003). *Successful grant writing: Strategies for health and human services proposals.* New York: Springer Publishing.

Queen, E. L. (Ed.). (2000). Serving those in need: A handbook for managing faith-based human service organization. San Francisco: Jossey-Bass.

Stuart, G. W. (2004). Raising $4 million in 4 months. *Journal of Professional Nursing, 20*(1), 5, 6. New York: Foundation Center.

U.S. Government. (2003). *2004 Essential guide to grant writing and federal grants: Proposal writing tips, resources, funding options for government money.*

van Maanen, J. (n.d.). *The process of program evaluation.* Los Angeles, CA: The Grantsmanship Center.

 ## Web Resources

http://www.ANF@ana.org   American Nurses Foundation

http://www.archstone.org   Archstone Foundation

http://www.gatesfoundation.org   Bill and Melinda Gates Foundation

http://www.cfda.gov   Catalog of Federal Domestic Assistance

http://www.philanthropy.com   Chronicle of Philanthropy

http://www.cof.org   Council on Foundations

http://www.dvg.org/grantseekers/index.html   Delaware Valley Grantmakers

http://www.donorsforum.org   Donors Forum

http://www.access.gpo.gov/su_docs/aces!40.html   Federal Register

http://www.fdncenter.org   The Foundation Center

http://www.foundations.org   Foundations On-Line

http://www.fdncenter.org/learn/bookshelf/grantseek/text.html   The Foundation Center's Guide to Grantseeking

http://www.granthelp.clarityconnect.com   Granthelp

http://www.grantsinfo@nih.gov   Grantsinfo

http://www.grantproposal.com   Grantproposal

http://www.grantselect.com   Grantselect

http://www.grantstech.com   Grantstech

http://www.grantsupdate.com   Grantsupdate

http://www.thegrantdoctors.com   Grant Doctors

http://www.library.wisc.edu   Grants Resources

http://www.infoserv.rttonet.psu.edu/gweb.htm   Grants Web

http://www.guidestar.org   Guidestar

http://www.idealist.org   Idealist

http://www.nonprofits.org   Internet Nonprofit Center

http://www.modimes.org   March of Dimes

http://www.pednurse.org/   Society of Pediatric Nursing

http://www.tgci.com   The Grantsmanship Center

http://www.wheatridge.org/grants/newgrant.html   Wheat Ridge Grant Programs

http://www.wkkf.org   W. K. Kellogg Foundation

Faith Community Nursing Practice Concepts

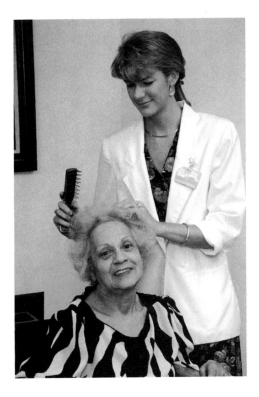

15

Faith Community Nursing Practice With Clients With Chronic Illness

Chronic illness and disability is a leading health care issue in the United States in all age groups (Potter & Perry, 2001). The number of people with chronic illness is staggering, with 105 million people coping with chronic illness in the United States in 2000, at an estimated cost of $503 billion (Smeltzer & Bare, 2000). Chronic illness is defined by Curtin and Lubkin as "the irreversible presence, accumulation, or latency of disease states or impairments that involve the total human environment for supportive care and self-care, maintenance of function, and prevention of further disability" (1995, pp. 6, 7). Chronic diseases are characterized by uncertain etiology, multiple risk factors, a long latency period, a prolonged course of illness noncontagious in origin, functional impairment, or disability; and incurable illness. The illness may also be progressive, resulting in complete or partial disability. Some of the more common chronic illnesses that the faith community nurse (FCN) will see in the community include heart disease, hypertension, cancer, diabetes, renal disease, mental illness, alcoholism, emphysema, and arthritis.

Physical, psychological, and cognitive reactions to chronic illness are likely to occur at any point in the disease process. A person recovering from a stroke might have impaired mobility and impaired speech. A person with cancer of the uterus is likely to find it difficult to cope with the knowledge that childbirth is no longer an option. A person diagnosed with a brain tumor may struggle with the changes in cognitive function. The challenge for the person with chronic illness is to cope with the limitations of the disease in the most positive manner possible.

Lubkin and Larsen (2002) describe the impact of chronic illness on the independence of people at each developmental level. "The very young child may be unable to work at self-sufficiency tasks; the school-age child may be unable to stay abreast of school work or participate in activities; adolescents and young adults may have obstacles that prevent them from reaching their goals and becoming independent; and the older adult, who may have been independent prior to a crisis, is unable to complete the developmental tasks of older age" (p. 10). The role of the faith community nurse becomes supporting each client to achieve the highest possible level of self-care.

Disease and Illness

Lubkin and Larsen (2002) remind us that the U.S. health care system is designed to identify diseases, to treat symptoms, and sometimes to produce cures. Designed for acute and episodic care, it generally provides this type of care effectively and efficiently. When this model of care is used for individuals with chronic disorders, a mismatch occurs. The authors identify *disease* as a problem viewed from a biomedical model, such as an alteration in structure and function (pp. 3, 4). *Illness*, however, is the human experience of symptoms and suffering and refers to how the disease is perceived, lived with, and responded to by individuals and their families. Although it is important to recognize the biomedical aspects of a disease, understanding the illness experience is more salient when caring long-term for chronically ill people. Helping individuals and families cope with the illness experience is a key element of FCN practice. The faith community nurse has a key role in the care of clients with chronic illness because the relationship between the faith community nurse and the client will also be long-term.

Glaser and Strauss (1968) first introduced the term *trajectory* when they were studying dying clients in hospital settings. "A *trajectory* is defined as a course of illness over time, and the actions taken by clients, families, and health professionals to manage or shape that course" (Corbin, 2001, p. 3). Using an illness trajectory framework is helpful for caring for clients on a long-term basis because it allows the nurse to understand where the client is on the continuum—in terms of both disease and illness. Health care professionals tend to focus on symptoms and treatment while the client and family manage the illness experience. This experience includes controlling symptoms and performing the necessary everyday tasks to manage the illness (Lubkin & Larsen, 2002). The FCN may serve as the interpreter between the professional disease-oriented model and the individual/family who is coping with the illness experience.

Living with a Chronic Illness

Living with a chronic illness is a unique challenge for the person with the disease. Despite this challenge, persons with chronic illness state that coping with the disease is definitely possible. Many people even view the diagnosis as an opportunity, living fuller lives than they ever have before. The role of the health care professional during the process of the disease progression often becomes one of facilitator, providing both information and suggestions for coping strategies that may be helpful during the experience.

Chronic illness is also a unique challenge for family members and friends close to the person with the disease. Chronic illness affects the entire family. Persons who have been diagnosed with chronic disease embark on a difficult journey, and the entire family dynamics may be disrupted. Each person in the family may experience different emotions. Sometimes family members require more support than the person with the disease. People with chronic illness often need assistance with activities of daily living and help with other adaptations in their daily lives. The family must often take on the role of caregiver, and this role reversal is a challenge for everyone in the family system. Without question, the challenge of a chronic illness can bring families closer together or drive them apart from one another (Smeltzer & Bare, 2000). Maintaining a degree of wellness or keeping symptoms in remission is a juggling act of balancing treatment protocols and regimens with quality of life issues (Lubkin & Larsen, 2002).

Adapting successfully to chronic illness assumes that a meaningful quality of life will be the result. Lubkin and Larsen (2002) state that the disease is only one factor that impacts a person's quality of life. Perception of the disease is a key piece of the difference between people on this issue. Christopher Reeve, the actor who played Superman in the movies, was paralyzed and confined to a wheelchair for several years before he died because of an equestrian accident, and yet he described his quality of life as good. The main character in the movie, *Whose Life Is It Anyway,* played by Richard Dreyfus, was also paralyzed, and yet he described his quality of life as nonexistent and expressed to everyone who would listen to him that he wanted to die.

Cultural Beliefs

Cultural beliefs also have an impact on a person's attitude toward chronic illness. Without question, different cultural groups view health and disease according to their own belief system. With the increased diversity present in today's society, it is important for health care professionals to be knowledgeable about the different cultural beliefs related to health and to be aware of the cultural diversity present in their faith community. Purnell and Paulanka (1998) offer information on 16 different cultural groups in their book on this subject. This text also includes *Purnell's Model for Cultural Competence,* which would be a valuable resource to the nurse in the faith community.

Chin (2000) describes three issues that are essential in providing culturally competent care: access, utilization, and quality of care. *Access* refers to the degree to which services are convenient and obtainable. Access also includes providing an interpreter for non-English-speaking clients or providing literature in different languages. *Utilization* refers to the availability of services and how often those services are used. *Quality of care* refers to the client's perception of whether culturally competent care is being provided. Addressing each of these issues is important for the FCN when providing care in the faith community.

Using Assessment Data

Congregational needs assessments can assist the FCN to become aware of the extent and types of chronic diseases that are present in the faith community. FCNs might be provided time during the announcements section of a church service to introduce the needs assessment and then be available at each exit to collect the information. This strategy is helpful for planning educational programming and for identifying individuals and families with needs related to their chronic conditions.

Holistic Assessment

A holistic assessment is an essential first step in working with people with chronic illness. The FCN has a key role in this part of the process because the nurse is often welcomed into the homes of the parishioners. The assessment must include gathering data that address the physiological, psychological, social, and spiritual aspects of this person's life. Taking time during the initial visit for this thorough assessment data can often pave the way to effective interventions that the client might use to help the family cope with the chronic disease. Each of these elements provides a framework from which to work toward this effort.

Education

Education is essential as a person copes with a chronic disease. The assessment data gathered by the FCN during the initial visit will be helpful in identifying the deficits in the person's knowledge. Once these deficits are identified, the nurse helps determine the educational needs of the person with the chronic disease and the family. Some faith community members may be referred to educational opportunities that are readily available in the community. Such programs might include lectures on topics that address different diseases like Coping with Cancer, Coping with Heart Disease, or Coping with Arthritis. Another avenue for an educational experience may be through the hospital in a Diabetes Education Series for people newly diagnosed with this chronic disease or Mental Illness Series. Support groups available in most communities may also have a component of educational programming during their sessions.

Referrals

Referrals are another important part of the role of the FCN. The holistic assessment can provide the data to determine the need for referrals. Families dealing with alcoholism might be referred to Alanon, AA, and/or Alateen for the various members of the family. A person with congestive heart failure with severe edema might be referred to the primary care physician for follow-up care on that issue. A family coping with the loss of a parent might be referred to a Bereavement Support Group to deal with the loss in a healthy way. A family member coping with a parent with Alzheimer's disease may need a referral to a home health agency that can provide occasional respite care to give the caregiver some relief or some time to do something just for herself.

Home Visits

The FCN in the faith community has an opportunity to make home visits. These visits help the nurse gain a holistic perspective on a person with chronic illness. Observing people in their home environment gives a more accurate assessment of the family process and behavior in their natural environment. The FCN can work with the client firsthand to identify interventions that will meet realistic goals that they may have (Stanhope & Lancaster, 2004). Meeting the family members on their home ground contributes to the family's sense of control and active participation in meeting the health care needs. If a home visit is going to be effective, appropriate planning must occur.

The FCN must always remember that the home visit occurs on the family member's "own turf." Scheduling the visit for a time that is convenient for the family is an important first step in establishing positive rapport with the family. Most families view the nurse as an invited guest in their home and it is important to honor that boundary. Sitting with the family to have a cup of tea while performing the assessment might help the client and family to be more relaxed and will increase the likelihood of collecting as much data as possible. Importantly, the nurse must communicate to the family that confidentiality will be maintained. Maintaining confidentiality is an important aspect of professional behavior and is part of the Nursing Code of Ethics and Professional Standards. Respect is demonstrated when the nurse maintains this essential privacy need. Faith community nurses within the team should only give the relevant information about a client's status. The Health Insurance Portability and Accountability Act of 1996 emphasizes this need for privacy.

Family caregivers are an important part of the health care team when planning care for the person with chronic illness. Maintaining persons with chronic illness in the home often requires that there be some family caregiver responsibility. "The unique characteristics of the caregiver and the care recipient, their relationship with each other, and the dynamics within a caregiving family make no two caregiving arrangements exactly alike" (Lubkin & Larsen, 2002, p. 233). The need for respite and for adult day care programs becomes essential as families try to balance their own lives and caring for family members with chronic illness.

Independent Nursing Interventions

Independent nursing interventions are those activities that the nurse is licensed to perform on the basis of knowledge and skills learned as a nurse. These activities include physical care, assessment, emotional support and comfort, teaching, counseling, making referrals, and so forth. Important to note is that the role of the FCN does not include physical care. Because complementary/integrative health care has become more common in the health care arena, several other examples of independent nursing interventions have presented themselves, including spiritual care or prayer, therapeutic touch, humor, and other nursing interventions.

> ## BOX 15-1
> ## How a Faith Community Nurse Can Provide Presence
>
> 1. Take the time to truly listen to one of your clients today.
> 2. Be sure that your schedule allows for enough time for "presence."
> 3. After all of the usual tasks are completed, sit in a comfortable position facing the person, maintain eye contact, and ask the person to share what the experience of chronic illness is for him or her. Try not to interrupt the person's thoughts and don't worry so much about taking notes as simply being attentive and "present" to the moment.

Presence

The concept of presence has been described in several nursing theories, including Watson, Parse, and Patterson and Zderad (Kelly & Johnson, 2002; Hickman, 2002; Praeger, 2002;). These theorists each talk about the nurse being attentive, truly present, authentic, being with a person, and expressing caring in their interactions with the clients and their families. The interest in presence within a caring relationship has clearly gained increasing attention in recent years.

Covington (2003) presents an excellent review of the literature on presence and places presence within the context of caring. Covington describes "a caring presence as a way of being or deeply connecting with another person in a relationship. Nurses come to this relationship with intentionality, are authentic and available, and provide a safe space for the patients to share suffering and find meaning in the illness experiences" (p. 313). Covington believes that this caring presence allows the nurse and patient to connect as one person to another, and this experience then promotes healing.

FCNs have numerous opportunities to be "fully present" with people who have chronic illness in the faith community. Important for the FCN is to be available and attentive during the visits to the home. Deep connections often occur, providing an emotional bond that is significant. Most people want to share their stories, and a nurse who is willing to listen without interruption is "a gift from God" (Box 15-1).

Creative Arts

The creative arts are an excellent adjunct to the healing environment. Cameron (1992) refers to creativity as a spiritual experience. She believes that when a person learns to recognize and nurture the creative process, confidence is strengthened and fear is resolved. A wide variety of activities is available in the repertoire of the FCN to help the person with chronic disease use creativity to enhance healing.

Expressive therapies use the creative arts to promote health and well-being (Keegan, 2001). Examples of expressive therapies include art therapy, music therapy, drama therapy, poetry therapy, and dance therapy. Each of these avenues of creativity offers persons with chronic disease an outlet for emotions that they may be feeling or a distraction from the daily challenges of chronic illness.

Art therapy has been used with various populations, including children with learning disorders, people with psychiatric disorders, people with substance abuse issues, and people with cancer. Moore and Schmais (2000) describe the use of creative arts at the Michael and Rose Assarian Cancer Center in Michigan. In that setting, the surroundings and programs promote emotional and spiritual healing, in addition to treating the physical illness. The center's art gallery displays paintings, crafts, and writings of patients with cancer. An art therapy room offers a beneficial outlet for patients at the center. Mauk and Schmidt (2004) talk about the wide use of art therapy and indicate that nurses can easily incorporate art therapy into their nursing care plans. Nurses might ask the patients with cancer to draw a picture of how they felt when they were first diagnosed with cancer and then spend some time discussing the picture. Music therapy is one of the easiest modalities to incorporate into the environment of a person with chronic disease. Music has been described as a universal language that many people enjoy. Music is a very subjective experience and everyone has his or her own favorite styles and taste in music (Libster, 2001). For one person it might be a country music song, for another an opera, and for another rock-and-roll. In the movie, *The Awakening,* the psychiatrist (played by Robin Williams) used different styles of music to trigger the patients who had Parkinson's disease. Some patients responded to classical music, and others responded to rock-and-roll. It became clear in the movie that choice of music must be individualized to each person.

Nurses who use music are often able to connect with patients in a different way than they might have in communicating orally. Keegan (1994) states that the arts have always served as a medium for bringing people closer to one another. She indicates that the benefit in healing with music is remarkable. Music therapists within the American Music Therapy Association are skilled in the use of music as a therapeutic modality and might be used as a resource for the FCN.

Writing has been shown to be an effective tool for expressing feelings about a disease. Slaninka (1995) had members of her cancer support group "write a letter to their cancer" and then share those letters with the group. Group members quickly realized that they were not alone and learned that others felt the same way they did. The support group was encouraged to continue to use the journal to express what they were feeling as the disease progressed.

Humor

The positive impact of humor therapy is becoming more accepted as an appropriate intervention to impact chronic disease (Mauk & Schmidt, 2004). The physiological benefits of laughter include increased oxygenation, increased energy levels, and the release of endorphins into the body. Humor has also been demonstrated to decrease stress, anxiety, and pain. Norman Cousins (1977) is credited with documenting one of the first cases of the benefits of humor. Cousins describes how he spent at least 10 minutes a day laughing, which was often triggered by shows on television, such as the Marx Brothers movies or *Candid Camera.* Cousins describes that he was able to sleep without pain from the inflammatory disease ankylosing spondylitis.

Humor has been incorporated into many acute health care facilities as volunteers circulate the halls with a "humor cart" filled with items designed to distract patients from the impact of their disease. These volunteers encourage patients, at least for a small portion of their day, to take things less seriously. The results are incredibly positive for all involved.

The movie *Patch Adams* depicts the life of a nontraditional-age medical student who is intent on incorporating humor into the lives of the patients on the units. One of the clips in the movie shows Patch on a children's cancer unit and as he performs for them, the energy levels increase and the smiles on the faces of the children are everywhere. Another clip shows medical students immersing a woman with a chronic illness in a huge vat of spaghetti for a "swim." What a difference this simple intervention made in the life of this woman. See Box 15-2 for interventions using humor.

Prayer

The expression of spirituality has been proposed as an important factor in quality of life. Brady, Perman, Gitchett, Mo, and Cella (1999) report that persons with chronic illnesses, such as AIDS and cancer, have described the value of spirituality in their lives. These researchers

> ## BOX 15-2
> ## Humor Therapy "Bag of Tricks"
>
> 1. Keep a clown nose with you at all times. Put it on when your client least expects it.
> 2. Begin to collect items that you believe might help someone laugh. This "humor bag" will become a ready source of things to make someone laugh.
> 3. Use humorous items to do your assessments in the home. A plastic hammer with a squeaker noise or a stethoscope with a funnel on the end to enhance hearing are just two examples of these items.
> 4. Share humorous cartoons that you have collected over the years with your client, especially cartoons about the health care system.
> 5. Drop off a copy of a funny movie with your client who is homebound. You might even pop some popcorn into the microwave and stay there for lunch.
> 6. Smile often during your time with the person.
> 7. Share funny anecdotes from your day that will liven up the day of the person.
> 8. Blow bubbles in the house.

identified spiritual well-being as an independent predictor of quality of life in their study. In fact, contentment with the quality of one's life correlated with spiritual well-being, emotional well-being, and physical well-being, as measured by the Functional Assessment of Chronic Illness Therapy System. Beery, Baas, Fowler, and Allen (2002) examined the role of spirituality as a dimension of quality of life in a group of people with heart failure. They used several scales in this research, including the Medical Outcome Survey Short Form 36, the Index of Well-being measures of quality of life, the Spiritual Well-being Scale, and the Relative Importance Scale. They concluded that spirituality had an important effect on quality of life in persons with heart failure.

Byrd (1988) is responsible for the landmark study on the therapeutic effects of intercessory prayer. Byrd used a prospective randomized double-blind protocol in a population of people in the coronary care unit (CCU). Over 10 months, 393 patients were randomly assigned to either an intercessory prayer group (192 patients) or to a control group (201 patients). The first group received intercessory prayer from participating Christians praying outside the hospital and the control group did not. The intercessory prayer group definitely had better outcomes during their stay in the CCU. The control group required ventilator-assistance, antibiotics, and diuretics more frequently than patients in the intercessory prayer group. Byrd concluded that intercessory prayer had a beneficial effect on the patients in the CCU.

Brown-Saltzman (1997) describes prayer as an important component of working with people with cancer. She identifies readings, reciting of prayers, reflective listening, conversing with God in a less formal way, and requesting something specific from God as different examples of prayer. This author suggests that guided imagery may be combined with prayer to effectively replenish the spirit. She believes that meditative prayer and guided imagery are two approaches that can be used to provide spiritual care to people with cancer and their families.

Robinson-Smith (2002) describes how eight patients used prayer after stroke as a coping strategy to improve self-efficacy and quality of life. This researcher used a qualitative methodology in her study. In a long interview format she asked the following questions 1 year after the person had the stroke. These questions were the format for the interview guide:

1. In what ways does prayer help you cope since the stroke?
2. What kind of prayers have you used to cope with the stroke?
3. Are there other ways that prayer has helped you since the stroke? (p. 357)

BOX 15-3
Serenity Prayer

God grant me the serenity
to accept the things I cannot change,
the courage to change the things I can,
and the wisdom to know the difference.

—Anonymous

BOX 15-4
The Lord's Prayer

Our Father, who art in heaven,
hallowed be thy name.
Thy kingdom come, thy will be done,
on earth as it is in heaven.
Give us this day our daily bread,
and forgive us our trespasses as we forgive
those who trespass against us.
And lead us not into temptation,
but deliver us from evil,
for thine is the kingdom, the power, and the glory,
forever and ever.
Amen.

BOX 15-5
Prayer for the Presence of Christ

O Living Christ, make us conscious now of Your
healing nearness.
Touch our eyes that we may see You.
Open our ears that we may hear Your voice.
Enter our hearts that we may know Your love.
Overshadow our souls and bodies with Your
Presence, that we may partake of Your
Strength, Your love and Your healing life.

—The International Order of
St. Luke the Physician

The researcher was able to identify four themes that focused on how prayer was used for coping after a stroke, including connecting to God, ways of praying now, reaching back to family life experience, and finding strength through prayer. See Boxes 15-3, 15-4, and 15-5 for sample prayers.

Use of Volunteers

The volunteers in your faith community offer a wide variety of opportunities for the person with chronic illness. Volunteers can provide services that the person with chronic illness may no longer be able to perform. Volunteers can do grocery shopping, provide transportation, rake the leaves in the fall, wash windows in the spring, do the wash and hang out the clothes outside to give them that fresh smell. In the parish nursing program at St. Joseph's Church in Somers Point, New Jersey, the teen group has been able to serve in this capacity, offering free labor to the elders in that community.

Faith community groups have been consistently known for providing meals when a member of the parish is sick or recovering from a hospital stay. Hall (2003) encourages the use of extended family, neighbors, or church members who can create a helping network for the family. She urges application of a holistic model to facilitate psychosocial-spiritual growth, thus enhancing the quality of life in the person with chronic illness.

Education for the volunteers is essential so that people can feel comfortable in their new roles as faith community volunteers. Elaine Kunigonis, RN, MSN, developed the volunteer training program at St. Joseph's Church in Somers Point, New Jersey, that has proven to be a huge success. The program included didactic information on basic assessment, the importance of confidentiality, and loss and grief issues. During the second portion of the volunteer training, volunteers participated in role-play experiences that they might anticipate in the home situation. After the training, volunteers stated that they believed they were more confident in the new roles they were about to assume. Volunteers were assured that the volunteer coordinator would be available by telephone to consult on any issue that might arise.

Matching volunteers with people in the faith community is a key part of the success of this program. If a family is coping with a loss related to a cancer diagnosis, it might be helpful to have a volunteer working with that family who has had a similar experience and who can truly empathize with what they may be feeling. For families dealing with alcoholism in a family member, matching that family with a person who is a member of Alcoholics Anonymous or Alanon might also be helping in paving the way to coping for that member.

Volunteers definitely have a need for their own support mechanism as they cope with the challenges within the faith community. Having volunteers meet once a month to address these issues is helpful as they work through the challenges they face and gain different perspectives from their fellow volunteers. The volunteer coordinator serves as a resource for this group as well and can often provide a helpful idea for the volunteer to try on the next visit to the member of the parish.

Support Groups

Social isolation is one of the most difficult outcomes of chronic illness, and the FCN must manage this issue. Social isolation is identified as the number, frequency, and quality of contacts that a person has (Lubkin & Larsen, 2002). People with chronic disease may find themselves isolated because of the disabilities associated with the disease, or they may choose to isolate themselves rather than cope more effectively with this disease.

People who have been diagnosed with chronic illness embark on a difficult journey. Adaptations by the whole person are necessary on all levels: physical, psychological, social, and spiritual. Nurses have long recognized the overwhelming effects of chronic illness on the patient, family members, and significant others. The establishment of community support groups in several settings has been effective in supporting people with various diseases, during what is often the most difficult time of their lives. Support groups exist for people with cancer, diabetes, Parkinson's disease, arthritis, heart disease, and for just about any other illness you can imagine. Support groups are also available for the caregivers because we know that the family is impacted by the illness as well.

Spiegel (1992) reviewed evidence that found that participation in a cancer support group not only improved quality of life in the women with breast cancer that attended the meetings, but also actually increased their survival times. These researchers suggested that social support could accelerate recovery and protect people in crisis against the health consequences of life stress. The members of the group were less phobic, had better coping responses, and had reduced pain.

Isolation and loneliness are common issues for people with chronic illness. Social support is vital and can help people accept and cope with the losses associated with the illness that they have. Acknowledging the need for a support group is an important first step in acknowledging the impact of the illness in their lives. Many support groups offer educational programs as a strategy to open the door to those needing support without requiring an admission of weakness. In fact, reaching out for help can be a sign of strength.

Kinney, Rodgers, Nash, and Bray (2003) report on the results of an integrated mind-body-spirit self-empowerment program (MBSSP) that they introduced to a group of women who were at various stages of coping with breast cancer. Fifty-one women completed a series of lessons offered in a support group format that helped them to adjust to their changed lives and to develop ways to use resources for survival, recovery, and healing. Strategies included journaling, meditation, and imagery. Throughout the program, the support group members came together to share their feelings and discovered they were not alone in this experience. Members grew to become advocates for themselves and each other during this process.

One of the best strengths of the support group is that the people attending can truly understand like no one else what it is to have this disease. Support group members are able to share their fears and frustrations with people "who have been there." Members learn to help each other and no longer feel alone in coping with their illness.

Mauk and Schmidt (2004) caution that not everyone finds support groups to be helpful. Some people view such groups as an invasion of privacy and not at all helpful as a coping mechanism. They state that people must be allowed to decide for themselves whether a support group would be a helpful strategy for them.

Summary

Large numbers of people in the United States are coping with the effects of chronic illness. Many people have more than one diagnosis of different chronic illnesses adding to the burden that they feel. Parish nurses serve an important role in supporting these clients to remain as independent as possible. Various independent nursing functions are available for the nurse to draw upon in helping these clients. The use of prayer, music therapy, art therapy, and humor are a few of the interventions discussed in this chapter. Volunteers are also viewed as a positive addition to serve the needs of the faith community.

Reflect and Discuss

1. What is the role of the faith community nurse in the case study?
2. What are some of the cultural issues that the faith community nurse might anticipate for this family?
3. Discuss a health teaching plan that might work for this family.
4. What referrals might the faith community nurse make that would assist this family in coping with this chronic illness?
5. Identify some alternative measures that might be helpful for Mr. Robinson as he copes with the diabetes.

Case Study

The Robinson family is a typical family in the United States trying to cope with the impact of a chronic disease. Mr. and Mrs. Robinson are an elderly African American couple living in a Center City row home in Philadelphia. In the last few weeks, Mr. Robinson was diagnosed with diabetes and his treatment plan includes insulin injections and dietary changes. His wife thought that she could care for him at home after his discharge from the hospital, but his recovery process is more difficult than Mrs. Robinson imagined, and she admits it is hard to care for him at home. Mr. and Mrs. Robinson have two daughters, one who lives in the area and has a full-time job. The other daughter lives several states away and is frustrated that she is unable to be available to help her parents as much as she would like during this crisis. They also have a son, but he is in college and too busy to help out. The nurse in the faith community has been brought into the picture and is trying to assist this family with the effects of this disease on the family.

References

Beery, T., Baas, L., Fowler, C., & Allen, G. (2002). Spirituality in persons with heart failure. *Journal of Holistic Nursing, 20*(1), 5–26.

Brady, M. J., Perman, A. H., Gitchett, G., Mo, M., & Cella, D. (1999). A case for including spirituality in quality of life measurement in oncology. *Psycho-Oncology, 8,* 417–428.

Brown-Saltzman, K. (1997). Replenishing the spirit by meditative prayer and guided imagery. *Seminars in Oncology Nursing, 13*(4), 255–259.

Byrd, R. (1988). Positive therapeutic effects of intercessory prayer in a coronary care unit population. *South Medical Journal, 81,* 826–829.

Cameron, J. (1992). *The artist's way: A spiritual path to higher creativity.* New York: GP Putnam's Sons.

Chin, J. (2000). Culturally competent health care. *Public Health Reports, 115,* 25–33.

Corbin, J. (2001). Introduction and overview: Chronic illness and nursing. In R. Hyman and J. Corbin (Eds.), *Chronic illness: Research and theory for nursing practice* (pp. 1–15). New York: Springer Publications.

Cousins, N. (1977). *The healing heart.* New York: Bantam.

Covington, H. (2003). Caring presence: Delineation of a concept for holistic nursing. *Journal of Holistic Practice, 21*(3), 301–317.

Curtin, M., & Lubkin, I. (1995). What is chronicity? In I. Lubkin (Ed.), *Chronic illness: Impact and interventions* (3rd ed.). Sudbury, MA: Jones and Bartlett.

Glaser, B., & Strauss, A. (1968). *Time for dying.* Chicago: Aldine.

Hall, V. (2003). Applying holism in the home care environment for clients with advanced ALS: A toolkit for practice. *Topics in Advanced Practice Nursing eJournal, 3*(2), 1–19.

Hickman, J. S. (2002). Theory of human becoming: Rosemarie Rizzo Parse. In J. B. George, *Nursing theories: The base for professional practice* (5th ed., pp. 427–461).Upper Saddle River, NJ: Prentice Hall.

Keegan, L. (2001). *Healing with complementary and alternative therapies.* Albany, NY: Thomson Delmar Learning.

Keegan, L. (1994). *The nurse as healer.* Albany, NY: Thomson Delmar Learning.

Kelly, J. H. & Johnson, B. J. (2002). Theory of transpersonal caring: Jean Watson. In J. B. George, *Nursing theories: The base for professional practice* (5th ed., pp. 405–425). Upper Saddle River, NJ: Prentice Hall.

Kinney, C. K., Rodgers, D. M., Nash, K. A., & Bray, C. O. (2003). Holistic healing for women with breast cancer through a mind, body, and spirit self-empowerment program. *Journal of Holistic Nursing, 21*(3), 260–279.

Libster, M. (2001). *Demonstrating care: The art of integrative nursing.* Albany, NY: Thomson Delmar Learning.

Lubkin, I. M., & Larsen, P. D. (2002). *Chronic illness: Impact and interventions* (5th ed.). Sudbury, MA: Jones and Bartlett.

Mauk, K. L., & Schmidt, N. K. (2004). *Spiritual care in nursing practice.* Philadelphia: Lippincott Williams & Wilkins.

Moore, K., & Schmais, L. (2000). The ABCs of complementary and alternative therapies and cancer treatment. *Oncology Issues, 15*(6), 20–22.

Potter, P. A., & Perry, A. G. (2001). *Fundamentals of nursing.* St. Louis: Mosby.

Praeger, S. G. (2002). Humanistic nursing: Josephine G. Paterson and Loretta T. Zderad. In J. B. George, *Nursing theories: The base for professional practice* (5th ed., pp. 385–404). Upper Saddle River, NJ: Prentice Hall.

Purnell, L. D., & Paulanka, B. J. (1998). *Transcultural health care.* Philadelphia: FA Davis Company.

Robinson-Smith, G. (2002). Prayer after stroke: Its relationships to quality of life. *Journal of Holistic Nursing, 20*(4), 352–366.

Slaninka, S. C. (1995). Dear cancer. *Illness, Crises, and Loss: Multidisciplinary Linkages, 5*(1), 41–45.

Smeltzer, S., & Bare, B. (2000). *Brunner and Sudharth's textbook of medical-surgical nursing.* Philadelphia: Lippincott Williams & Wilkins.

Spiegel, D. (1992). Effects of psychosocial support on patients with metastatic breast cancer. *Journal of Psychosocial Oncology, 10*(2), 113–120.

Stanhope, M., & Lancaster, J. (2004). *Community health nursing: Process and practice for promoting health.* St. Louis: Mosby–Year Book.

Additional Resources

Brownson, R., Remington, P., & Davusm, H. R. (1998). *Chronic disease epidemiology and control.* Washington, DC: APHA.

Narayansamy, A. (1996). Spiritual care of chronically ill patients. *British Journal of Nursing, 5*(7), 441–456.

O'Neill, D. P., & Kenny, E. K. (1998). Spirituality and chronic illness. *Image, 30,* 275–280.

Pehler, S. R. (1997). Children's spiritual response: Validation of the nursing diagnosis spiritual distress. *Nursing Diagnosis, 8,* 55–66.

Riley, B. B. (1998). Types of spiritual well-being among persons with chronic illness: Their relation to various forms of quality of life. *Archives of Physical Medicine and Rehabilitation, 79,* 228–264.

Samuel-Hodge, C. D., Headen S. W., Skelly, A. H., Ingram, A. F., Keyserling, T. C., & Jackson, E. J., et al. (2000). Influences on day-to-day self management of type 2 diabetes among African American women: Spirituality, the multi-caregiver role and other social context factors. *Diabetes Care, 23*(7), 928–933.

→ Web Resources

http://www.ahcpr.gov   Agency for Health Care Policy and Research

http://www.cancer.org   American Cancer Society

http://www.americanheart.org   American Heart Association

http://www.lungusa.org   American Lung Association

http://www.ama-assn.org   American Medical Association

http://www.best4health.org   Best Practice Network

http://www.cancercareinc.org   Cancer Care, Inc.

http://www.cdc.gov   Centers for Disease Control and Prevention

http://www.head-info.org   G/Health Care Education Association

http://www.healthfinder.gov   Health Finder

http://www.oncolink.upenn.edu   Hospital of the University of Pennsylvania

http://www.mayohealth.org   Mayo Clinic Health Oasis Site

http://www.cancernet   National Cancer Institute

http://www.ncemch.org   National Center for Education in Maternal and Child Health

http://www.cdc.gov/nchswww/   National Center for Health Statistics

http://www.infcacares.org   National Family Caregivers Association

http://www.niddk.nih.gov   National Institute for Diabetes, Digestive, and Kidney Disease

http://www.nih.gov   National Institutes of Health

http://www.nlm.nih.gov   National Library of Medicine

16

Faith Community Nursing Practice and Palliative Care, Grief, and Loss

P alliative care focuses on the quality of life rather than on the progression of an injury or illness. In modern times, this focus on care rather than on cure began with the founding of St. Christopher's Hospice, the first modern hospice, by Dame Cicely Saunders, in 1967 in a London suburb (*History of hospice care,* par. 1). She was also responsible for introducing the concept in the United States, beginning in 1963, through her interactions with the School of Nursing at Yale University (par. 2). Hospice care is typically provided during the terminal stages of an illness.

At any stage in a life-threatening illness, from initial symptoms to the terminal stage, the patient and family are subject to experiencing a sense of loss. Loss of any sort is associated with grieving; grieving persons may be assisted through grief counseling. Faith community nurses (FCNs) minister to individuals and families through all stages of an illness experience. FCNs provide spiritual care, emotional support, education, advocacy, and serve as a referral resource for individuals and families who are experiencing illness as well as those who are coping with grief and loss.

History and Definitions of Palliative Care

What is palliative care, and how does it relate to hospice care? Essentially, palliative care is an extension of the principles of hospice care to a broader population. Hospice care is centered on the caring of the whole person rather than on curing the illness, with care usually occurring in the home and involving symptom control, pain management, and support for the family of the person in the terminal stages of illness. Palliative care is based on the same principles but is extended to those who are in an earlier stage of a life-threatening illness and could benefit from this approach. In palliative care, no form of therapy is specifically excluded (*What is hospice and palliative care?,* pars. 1–3.) See Box 16-1 for definitions of palliative care formulated by the World Health Organization (WHO) and by The National Hospice and Palliative Care Organization.

In palliative care, a family member is usually the primary caregiver with the support of an interdisciplinary team (Hospice and Palliative Nurses Association, HPNA, & American Nurses Association, ANA, 2002; The National Hospice and Palliative Care Organization, n.d.; Task Force on Palliative Care, 1997; Wheeler, 2004; WHO, 2003a). The team is likely to include the person's physician; possibly a medical director for the care program; nursing staff, including home health care aides, social workers, clergy; possibly therapists (physical, music, occupational); and program volunteers. The FCN is an ideal member of such a team and can provide coordination and knowledge about the person and family from a perspective other than that of the medical diagnosis.

BOX 16-1
World Health Organization's Definitions of Palliative Care

PALLIATIVE CARE FOR ADULTS

Palliative care is an approach that improves the quality of life of patients and their families who are facing the problem associated with life-threatening illness. This approach is achieved through the prevention and relief of suffering by means of early identification and impeccable assessment and treatment of pain and other problems, physical, psychosocial, and spiritual. Palliative care

- provides relief from pain and other distressing symptoms;
- affirms life and regards dying as a normal process;
- intends neither to hasten nor postpone death;
- integrates the psychological and spiritual aspects of patient care;
- offers a support system to help patients live as actively as possible until death;
- offers a support system to help the family cope during the patient's illness and in their own bereavement;
- uses a team approach to address the needs of patients and their families, including bereavement counseling, if indicated;
- will enhance quality of life and may also positively influence the course of illness; and
- is applicable early in the course of illness, in conjunction with other therapies that are intended to prolong life, such as chemotherapy or radiation therapy, and includes those investigations needed to better understand and manage distressing clinical complications.

PALLIATIVE CARE FOR CHILDREN

Palliative care for children represents a special, albeit closely related, field to adult palliative care. WHO's definition of palliative care appropriate for children and their families is included in the following:

- Palliative care for children is the active total care of the child's body, mind, and spirit, and also involves giving support to the family.
- It begins when illness is diagnosed and continues, regardless of whether or not a child receives treatment directed at the disease.
- Health providers must evaluate and alleviate a child's physical, psychological, and social distress.
- Effective palliative care requires a broad multidisciplinary approach that includes the family and makes use of available community resources; it can be successfully implemented, even if resources are limited.
- It can be provided in tertiary care facilities, in community health centers, and even in children's homes.

World Health Organization. (2003a). The National Hospice and Palliative Care Organization (n.d.).

Characteristics of Palliative Care

Although palliative care is a relatively recent focus for health care in modern society, some significant efforts have been made to identify precepts and provide guidelines for the provision of such care. In 1997, the Task Force on Palliative Care of Last Acts, a national coalition to improve care and caring at the end of life, developed five precepts of palliative care to be incorporated into all end-of-life care (see Table 16-1). These precepts were further delineated in relation to infants, children, and adolescents in 2003 (Last Acts, 2003). Using these precepts as well as materials from the National Hospice and Palliative Care Organization, the Joint Commission on Accreditation of Healthcare Organizations, and the Americans for Better Care of the Dying, the Minnesota Commission on End of Life Care developed the five guiding principles reflected in Table 16-1 (Norlander & Baines, 2003). An international example is

TABLE 16-1		
Principles of Palliative Care		
LAST ACTS PRECEPTS	**MINNESOTA'S FRAMEWORK FOR END-OF-LIFE CARE**	**UK'S GOLD STANDARD**
Respecting patient goals, preferences, and choices	Preferences for treatment and care will be discussed and respected.	Communication
Comprehensive caring	Every reasonable effort will be made to relieve pain and other undesirable physical symptoms; emotional, spiritual, and personal suffering will be identified, addressed, and discussed.	Controlling symptoms
Acknowledging and addressing caregiver concerns	Grieving will be acknowledged.	Care of the dying; caregiver support
Using the strengths of interdisciplinary resources		Coordination
Building systems and mechanisms of support		
	Appropriate and realistic information will be provided regarding prognosis and the expected course of events preceding death.	Continuity; continued learning

found in the Gold Standards Framework developed in the United Kingdom (Robinson, 2003). All of these efforts are aimed at improving the quality of care provided in life-threatening circumstances, especially in light of findings of lack of communication, poor coordination of care, challenging symptom control, and lack of adequate support for home caregivers as major problems in such caregiving situations (HPNA & ANA, 2002; Robinson, 2003).

Palliative Care Challenges

The challenges provided by palliative care occur as a result of both the personal characteristics of the ill person and of more universal problems typically associated with the need for palliative care.

Age

One of the personal characteristics is that of age. Kane, Barber, Jordan, Tichenor, & Camp (2000) argue that current models of care for children with life-threatening illnesses are inadequate and that palliative care should be introduced early in the treatment of any severe illness in children. With palliative care as a bridge between the scientific medical model of care and a person-oriented form of care, the whole child and family will more likely be included and have their needs met. At the other end of the age spectrum, Amella (2003) discusses the impact of the effects of aging on the provision of palliative care in the elderly. A major point is that geriatric palliative care must pay attention to the problems associated with aging, such as joint pain, changes in mental status, vague symptoms, decreased hearing and visual acuity, and fatigue, that may be present in addition to those problems directly associated with the identified life-threatening illness. She recommends that assessment of all elderly persons include data related to pain, mental status (confused or exhibiting signs of dementia?), fatigue, dyspnea, ability to perform activities of daily living, nutritional status, depression, anxiety, and, for the family, assessment of the burden being experienced by the caregivers.

In a challenging special report, Alvarez et al. (2002) point out two populations who are candidates for palliative care as they discuss the care of chronic wounds in the frail population. Their definition of frail refers not only to those who are subject to the wasting syndrome associated with advanced aging, but also to those who meet the acronym of For Recognition of the Adult Immobilized Life. Their report is intended to encourage the acceptance of "nonhealing endpoints as appropriate and in the best interests of many frail patients" (p. 5S). Covinsky et al. (2003), in a study of the functional trajectories of 917 frail older persons for the 2 years prior to their deaths, found that functional independence steadily decreased for at least a year prior to death, with only a slight acceleration in the loss of independence shortly before death. These findings suggest that because a sudden loss of functional independence does not occur in this population as a signal of impending death, the frail elderly should be considered for palliative care programs long before they are eligible for Medicare funded hospice care. Anna Mulgrew is an example of a person who fits this description (see Case Study at the end of this chapter).

Family Members

The family members who are the primary caregivers also present some special challenges. Taylor (2003) found that family caregivers expressed the need to be treated with kindness and respect, for communication that includes both talking and listening, to be connected through active presence, for sharing in prayer, for support in mobilizing faith-related resources, and to receive needed nursing care in a timely manner. Stajduhar (2003) found that caregivers who were family members reported varied experiences. Some found the caregiving experience to have enriched their lives; others felt pressured to provide home care and reported both a sense of obligation and of exploitation. The parish nurse can provide support across the range of these responses, through encouraging those who are feeling enriched and through helping those who feel pressured to identify and use available resources, such as respite care, to help relieve their burden.

In the case study presented at the end of the chapter, Mr. Mulgrew is able to provide some of the care that his wife needs but is not able to do dressing changes or to fix other than simple meals. The FCN introduces the concept of palliative care and the use of an interdisciplinary team to help the Mulgrews. The pastor of their church has also been in close touch with them. The interdisciplinary team will include, in addition to the pastor and the FCN, Mrs. Mulgrew's primary physician who will be in consultation with the surgeon as needed; Mr. and Mrs. Mulgrew; a nutritionist; a homemaker to clean, do laundry, and prepare the evening meal; a physical therapist; and a home health nurse to change dressings.

Comfort and Pain Management

The more universal problems that are expected to arise in palliative care include pain management and comfort, wound care, nutrition and hydration, elimination, and social isolation. A major focus of palliative care is the provision of comfort and management of pain to improve the quality of life. The position statement of the HPNA (2004) on pain includes that all people have a right to optimal pain relief, and health care providers have an obligation to believe the person's report of pain and to implement appropriate pain management in a culturally sensitive manner, with uncontrolled pain being considered an emergency. In addition, the health care provider is to be an advocate for pain relief, supporting the patient's active involvement in decisions about pain management and family members' observations of and efforts to relieve the patient's pain. Placebo use is inappropriate in palliative care, and the regulatory control of opioids must be balanced with the patient's need for access to opioids for pain management. The ANA Position Statement on Pain Management and Control of Distressing Symptoms in Dying Patients (2003) states "the patient should have appropriate and sufficient medication by appropriate routes to control symptoms, in whatever dosage, and by whatever route is needed to control symptoms as perceived by the patient" (par. 3).

Pain may be directly associated with the life-threatening illness, with another acute or chronic problem, or related to certain procedures or changes of position (Alvarez et al., 2002; Gibson & Schroder, 2001). Of importance is to know whether the pain is episodic or continual, because the interventions will vary. Episodic pain, especially when associated with certain procedures such as dressing changes or movements such as turning in bed, can be anticipated and medication administered prior to those activities. Pain that is more continual should be treated by medication given on a regular schedule. WHO's pain ladder suggests this schedule be every 3 to 6 hours (WHO, 2003b). In brief, the pain ladder recommends three levels for the prompt administration of medication for pain with level one being nonopioids, such as aspirin. If level one does not provide pain relief, level two is mild opioids, such as codeine and, if that is not successful, level three is strong opioids, such as morphine. At any of these levels, other drugs to calm fears and relieve anxiety may also be used. Also, Wootton (2004) points out that research is needed on the effectiveness of analgesics other than morphine, such as methadone, fentanyl, and ketamine, in treating difficult pain because current evidence on their effectiveness is anecdotal. Good nursing care would include other methods for comfort and relaxation, such as music, massage, warmth, positioning, imaging, as chosen by the individual patient.

The family may also be involved in helping with pain relief through any of the activities identified as helpful. Mehta & Ezer (2003) found that spouses felt helpless, afraid, and a sense of unfairness when they were aware of their loved one in pain, and described feeling at peace and relaxed once pain control was achieved. Being involved in helping control the pain could enhance the spouse's positive feelings. The FCN can encourage the spouse's involvement through education on how to assess the loved one's pain and how to administer the selected medications and comfort measures.

Anna Mulgrew reports that, other than phantom limb pain, her pain is no different than prior to her surgeries. Her usual routines of oral nonopioid analgesics and mentholated arthritis rub massaged into her hands are adequately meeting her pain relief needs.

In some situations, often as the person has moved from palliative care to hospice care, pain may become intractable with none of the previous methods of pain relief any longer providing adequate comfort levels. In this situation, palliative sedation may become the treatment of choice. The HPNA position paper (2003b) on palliative sedation defines it as "the monitored use of medications intended to induce varying degrees of unconsciousness, but not death, for relief of refractory and unendurable symptoms in imminently dying patients" (p. 235). This position statement also indicates that comfort must be the primary goal of care, and cardiopulmonary resuscitation is usually viewed as inconsistent with palliative sedation. The decision to use palliative sedation must be made with the patient and family because it is very much based upon their value systems and views of quality of life. The FCN can play a very important part of such discussions because the patient and family may be more comfortable discussing their value system with someone who is known to have at least some of the same values.

Lynch (2003) points out that the suffering associated with refractory or intractable pain involves the whole person and, thus, decisions about palliative sedation are congruent with the goal of palliative/hospice care to provide whole person care. Thorns (2002) explains how the doctrine of double effect provides a moral justification for palliative sedation—the double effect being the provision of comfort in the face of possibly shortening the person's life. The criteria that are met include that the relief of pain and distress (the intended effect) is a good one, the bad effect (death) may be foreseen but is not intended and is not the means of creating the good effect (that is, death is not the means of relieving pain), and the good effect (comfort) must outweigh the bad effect (possibly a shortened life in someone already identified as being in the dying phase). Again, the FCN can be an appropriate counselor in relation to the double effect principle of ethics, when palliative sedation is being considered.

Palliative sedation is not considered to be compatible with cardiopulmonary resuscitation. However, some people find it difficult to agree to "a do not resuscitate" or DNR order. An alternative to DNR could be an "allow natural death" or AND order. According to Salladay (2002), AND is proactive and involves talking with the dying patient about what a natural death means to that person. Such conversation allows for the development of a plan of palliative care that meets the patient's desires and is limited only by the creativity of those developing the plan. The plan will be individualized. One person may ask that there be no tubes inserted, another may want oxygen to ease shortness of breath.

Although Anna Mulgrew is not currently at a stage that can be considered terminal, this should be recognized as likely to occur in the fairly near future, based upon her age and her increasing frailty. When the FCN raises the question of a living will and the possibility of a DNR, Mrs. Mulgrew states she already has a will and everything will go to her husband. The nurse then explains about a living will and offers to leave the materials with the Mulgrews so they can read and discuss them before making any decisions. On the nurse's next visit Mrs. Mulgrew indicates that she is more than willing to sign a living will but that she is not ready to give up on living and walking again so she is not interested in signing a DNR request. They then discuss an AND and both Mr. and Mrs. Mulgrew agree to develop an AND order.

The goal of comfort is primary also in the management of wounds in palliative care. Rather than seeking to cure or close the wound as the primary effort, the focus of care is on providing comfort, including managing odors. Alvarez et al. (2002) point out that, in addition to the use of medically prescribed antibiotics, comfort and odor management can be accomplished through keeping wounds clean and covered with topical dressings, especially if drainage is a problem, and the use of odor absorbents such as charcoal, kitty litter, or used coffee grounds placed unobtrusively in the room or of deodorizers, such as vanilla, fresh coffee grounds, or vinegar as preferred by the patient and family. Odor neutralizer sprays may also be acceptable.

Although Anna Mulgrew's stump wound is not healing as well as anticipated, she is not reporting any particular pain associated with the wound itself. Also, the regular dressing changes performed by the home health nurse are taking care of the minor amount of drainage, and odor has not been a problem.

Artificial Nutrition and Hydration

An issue that is typically more difficult for the family than for the patient is the issue of artificial nutrition and hydration. The person with a life-threatening illness will characteristically lose weight and, as the illness progresses, experience decreases in appetite and interest in food or drink, even to the extent of no longer desiring favorite foods (ANA, 1992; Ersek, 2003; HPNA, 2003a). Food, and the provision of it, is frequently an emotionally laden topic that may be tightly linked to the family caregiver's perception of successful caring. The decision to implement or not to implement artificial forms of nutrition and hydration must be made in an environment of open communication among the patient, family, and the interdisciplinary palliative/hospice care team.

Mechanisms of artificial nutrition and hydration carry both potential benefits and potential harm. Many are associated with varying degrees of discomfort. Ersek (2003) states that the goals of artificial nutrition and hydration include prolonging life, preventing aspiration, and increasing comfort. However, she indicates that research does not consistently support that the mechanisms of artificial nutrition and hydration always accomplish these goals. For example, some studies have not supported that tube feedings prolong life in nursing homes, and others have not been able to equate prolonged life with an improved quality of living.

The position of HPNA (2003a) is that artificial nutrition and hydration should not be started as a routine but only after the decision has been made by a patient and family who have been provided with accurate, and nonjudgmental, information. HPNA also encourages that the interdisciplinary team, especially speech therapists and nutritionists, be involved with the nurses to explore and devise effective ways of offering oral intake. In addition, it is important to support the right of competent patients to request or refuse such therapy and to support the family or other surrogate decision maker when the patient is not competent to make the decision. Recommended is that discussions of such choices begin early in the palliative caregiving process.

Anna Mulgrew has indicated in her living will that she does not wish to have any means of artificial nutrition or hydration as a means of prolonging life. If she requires surgery, she is willing to have intravenous fluids necessary for the routine care but she does not want any extraordinary methods used. At the present time, she is able to eat and drink as needed, although she reports that she often does not feel hungry. The nutritionist comes to meet with her to explore what might "tantalize her taste buds." Anna Mulgrew indicates she would really like some of the bread pudding that Betty Wilkins at the church is well known for making. The FCN talks with Mrs. Wilkins, and the next day Mrs. Wilkins stops by with a warm pan of her bread pudding. Mrs. Mulgrew eats a small serving and says it is the tastiest thing she has had in a long time.

Elimination

Problems related to elimination may also arise in palliative care. Especially in the frail elderly, urinary incontinence often occurs. Multiple possible causes of urinary incontinence can occur, some of which may be treatable with medications. Nursing concerns include the person's ability to reach a toilet and the presence of any open wounds that may be irritated by exposure to urine. Although the use of a Foley catheter is not generally the preferred treatment for such incontinence because of the danger of urinary tract infection, in a fragile person whose pain is aggravated by turning, the use of such a catheter may help accomplish the goal of comfort. Fecal incontinence may also be of concern. The treatment of fecal incontinence mandates a thorough assessment of the underlying causes that may vary from constipation to inability to access a toilet in a timely fashion to a physical malfunction. The focus may be on prevention of the incontinence or on odor control, skin protection, and methods to contain the feces (Alvarez et al., 2002).

Presence

Because Mrs. Mulgrew is able to transfer herself from chair to wheelchair and wheelchair to toilet, she has been able to care for her own toileting needs. She reports no problems with incontinence or constipation.

Stanley (2002) discusses the importance of presence in palliative/hospice care. She points out that people with life-threatening illnesses frequently become socially isolated as friends and family drift away. Because the ill person is feeling increasingly vulnerable and lonely, family and friends are often feeling increasingly uncomfortable and demonstrate their lack of comfort through decreased eye contact and other forms of withdrawal from interaction with the ill person. This isolation, combined with dealing with a life-threatening situation, emphasizes a fear of abandonment. When all others have left, or decreased their contact, the nurse is one who often remains in contact. Stanley uses the definition of presence provided by Doona et al. (1997, p. 3):

> [Presence is] an intersubjective encounter between a nurse and a patient in which the nurse encounters the patient as a unique human being in a unique situation and chooses to spend her/himself on the patient's behalf.

Stanley describes presence as a mode of being that requires knowing and being comfortable with oneself, knowing the other, connection with the other, affirmation and valuing, acknowledgment of vulnerability, intuition, empathy, a willingness to be vulnerable, as well as sincerity and silence. The parish nurse needs to be present and to help the family understand the importance of presence, including the comfort of sitting silently with the patient or of being there to let the patient hear a familiar voice.

Anna Mulgrew indicates that she feels very much cared for and cared about. Her husband has been attentive and someone from the interdisciplinary team is either at the house or on the telephone on a daily basis.

P-A-I-N

Wheeler (2004) suggests the use of a P-A-I-N format for assessment in all areas of palliative care. All four aspects of this format involve helping the patient communicate his or her perception of the problem. *P* is for place—where does the problem occur and how is it perceived? Is it always there or sporadic and for how long? How does this problem affect the quality of life? *A* is for amount—on a scale of 0 to 10 with 0 being no problem and 10 being the worst possible problem, how great is this problem? *I* is intensity—again, using 0 to 10, when the problem is at its worst, what triggers it, and how long does it last? *N* is for negates—on the 0 to 10 scale, describe the problem at its least and identify what leads to feeling better and how long does this last?

An example of P-A-I-N assessment for Anna Mulgrew would be Problem: stump wound is not healing. *P*—the location of the problem is the stump wound and she perceives it as a barrier to being able to walk again. This has had a very negative impact on her quality of life. She is rather stoic about it but wonders if she will ever be able to fix a meal in her kitchen again. *A*—this problem is an 8; initially, it was a 5 but now seems to be the major reason she is not becoming more self-sufficient. *I*—the intensity of the problem is a 5 because she still hopes that the solution to wound healing will be found. *N*—the problem will only approach 0 when the wound is obviously healing and the incision has never completely closed.

Faith Community Nursing in Palliative Care

The FCN has two sets of nursing standards to guide palliative care practice: *Faith Community Nursing: Scope and Standards of Practice* (American Nurses Association & Health Ministries Association [ANA-HMA], 2005), discussed throughout this text, and the *Scope and Standards of Hospice and Palliative Nursing Practice,* developed by the HPNA. Although these standards of care have a great deal in common, and essentially nothing in conflict, the standards for palliative care are more specific in certain areas (HPNA & ANA, 2002, pp. 13–20). The areas include that, in palliative care, assessment involves the collection of basic individual and family data, with priorities established by the immediate needs of the patient and family. The measurement criteria for diagnosis specify that the nursing diagnosis will be communicated to the members of the interdisciplinary team. Outcomes are formulated with the individual, the family, the interdisciplinary team, and with other providers as appropriate. Outcomes must be realistic and focus on improving the quality of life and being attainable. The plan of care is developed in consultation with the same persons involved in formulating outcomes and is to be considered dynamic, needing to vary as patient and family priorities change. Implementations are tightly tied to available resources. Thus, the emphasis on individual needs and priorities, family, functioning in an interdisciplinary team, and communication found in the definitions of palliative care and in the guidelines for palliative care are also reflected in the standards of care for nurses.

The use of these standards by the FCN in the care of Anna Mulgrew, and her husband, is reflected in the previous discussions of how the challenges of palliative care are being met with this family.

Grief and Loss Counseling

Living and dying are filled with losses. Even positive experiences involve loss. For example, the excitement of beginning a long awaited new job may be diminished by the loss of frequent contact with good friends who will stay in the former workplace. Loss is associated with grief. Obviously, not every loss leads to a prolonged grieving process. However, situations that lead to palliative care, and probably eventually to hospice care, involve losses of such magnitude that grief counseling may be needed.

Definitions Related to Grief and Loss

Loss may be real or perceived, have already occurred, or be in the future. Many of the losses in palliative care settings are all too real—loss of function, loss of occupation, loss of social interaction, and loss of life may all occur. Some of these real losses may have already occurred, and some may be anticipated to occur in the future. Others may be in the perception of the patient only—the husband believing he has lost his wife's respect because he can no longer provide for the family at his previous level of income when the wife may be happy that he is still alive and that they can spend time together and make decisions about the future of their family together. Other losses may be apparent to all—for example, the loss of function associated with a below-the-knee amputation, as we have seen with Anna Mulgrew.

No matter the degree of reality or perception of the loss, any loss can lead to grief. Grief is a whole-body experience associated with loss; the magnitude of grieving will be determined on an individual basis, influenced at least to some extent by the importance of the loss to the person. Cowles and Rodgers (2000) conducted a concept analysis of grief and initially identified five attributes of grief. The first attribute is that grief is dynamic and occurs in a nonlinear fashion of fluctuating thoughts, feelings, and behaviors. The second attribute is that grief is a process in which work occurs to reconcile the loss or to progress beyond the impact of the loss. No identified time limit is known for this process. The third attribute is that grief is individualized, both in the experience and in how the response is made apparent to others. Factors influencing this individual response include the relationship between the person and the lost object, the nature of how the loss occurred (suddenly or over a period of time, surprise, or anticipated), past experiences with loss, cultural expectations, religious beliefs, and support systems. The fourth attribute is that grief is pervasive and can potentially impact every aspect of the person's being and doing. In the original study, the fifth attribute was that grief is normative; that there is something that can be identified as normal grieving. In Cowles' (2000) expanded concept analysis, she reported that she could not identify any discussion of normative grief by the study participants. Thus, we can identify grief as a dynamic process that is pervasive for those who are grieving and is experienced and expressed in an individualized manner.

Anna Mulgrew is not verbal about her grieving the loss of her lower right leg. However, the plaintiveness of her nonverbal communication when she wonders whether she will ever get to fix a meal in her kitchen again reflects her grief.

Two terms that are sometimes used essentially interchangeably with grieving are *bereavement* and *mourning*. These terms refer to more specific aspects of grieving. They were differentiated as early as the 1980s. Demi and Myles (1986) defined bereavement as being associated with the loss of a significant other through death. Parkes (1985) defined mourning as the rituals and activities associated with the public demonstration of grief.

Approaches to Helping

Having some information is useful for anticipating who may have the greatest difficulty in dealing with grieving, or who might be the most amenable to being helped with grieving. Ellifritt, Nelson, and Walsh (2003) found that the most significant risks for a complicated bereavement were a perceived lack of social support, a personal history of alcohol or drug abuse or of mental illness, poorly developed coping skills, and when the person who died was a child. Thus, Janet Jonas, a widow who is a member of AA and describes herself as having only one friend and not being able to handle unexpected events, is likely to have greater difficulty dealing with the death of a 10-year-old granddaughter than is Mary Morrow who describes herself as being in a happy marriage, a member of Mothers Against Drunk Driving and is described by others as the rock to whom they turn in times of trouble. Although both are grieving the loss of a child, Janet Jonas appears to have all of the other significant risks described by Ellifritt, Nelson, and Walsh, whereas Mary Morrow appears to have only the one risk.

Cowles (2000) found that grieving, bereavement, and mourning are all strongly influenced by culture. Clements et al. (2003) provide a perspective of the death, grief, and bereavement customs of Latino, African American, Navajo, Jewish, and Hindu groups. Even as they discuss the differences between the groups, they also point out that there are individual variations within each group. Although faith may influence the process of grieving, Mystakidou et al. (2003) reported that the rituals related to grieving and burial in Greece have changed very little since before Christianity was introduced in Greece, supporting that culturally established traditions may not be strongly influenced by religious beliefs introduced after the traditions were established. Fletcher (2002) discussed the importance of being aware of one's own sense of time and space in relation to communicating with a grieving other, especially when cultural diversity is present. As in all situations, it is appropriate to be alert to cultural diversities, and individual variations within those diversities, when seeking to assist a grieving person.

Methods to help those who are grieving will vary according to the age of the griever. A special concern of the FCN may be the children in a grieving family. It is not unusual for family members to exclude children from the family grieving rituals in the belief that children should be protected from such activities. Hames (2003) states that shutting children out of such family gatherings, including memorial rituals, denies them access to activities that can facilitate the formation of memories and a healthy integration of grief. Such exclusion also keeps children from learning about how the family expresses bereavement.

Riely (2003) points out that excluding children from information about the loss leads to their regarding death as always frightening and traumatic. These children are denied permission to grieve.

Developmentally, it is expected that the child's behavior will change in some way when there is a significant loss, particularly the loss of the major caregiver, in the family. Hames (2003) recommends that very young children have one person who is the primary caregiver, that routines be maintained, questions be answered in a straightforward manner, using correct words and avoiding euphemisms such as "sleeping" or "lost." She also indicates that including even the very young in a short memorial or graveside service can provide experiences that will become cherished memories and have a positive effect on the child's grieving.

Families need to be aware that the young child's grieving process is not quickly completed, although it is not always apparent. The child is likely to continue to explore the meaning of the loss as he or she continues to develop. As the child ages, participation in a children's bereavement group could become appropriate. Children's bereavement centers can be identified through the National Center for Grieving Children and Families (http://www. grievingchild.com). Riely (2003) emphasizes that school-age children also need a sense of stability and security as well as a supportive atmosphere that encourages them to ask questions and to exhibit grieving behaviors, such as crying or being angry. She suggests storytelling, play, art, reminiscence, books, music, and letter writing as some activities for school-age children who are grieving.

Kirk and McManus (2002) focus on children within the family and have developed a program for therapeutic group work for grieving families that includes all of the family members, based upon the need for open communication among family members. They used drama and other creative media for 2-day-long workshops, "When Someone In Your Family Dies" and "Listening and Telling Bereavement Stories." Their experience demonstrates the importance of including all willing family members, the universal nature of grief, and that having families with varying lengths of grieving time (from 4 months to 3 years at the beginning of the program) was therapeutic in itself. Those for whom the grief was newer realized that the rawness of the pain could be alleviated and those who had been grieving longer were able to recognize how far they had come from their initial grief reactions.

The use of groups has been reported to be also helpful for widowed seniors. Stewart et al. (2001) conducted face-to-face groups for widowed seniors for a maximum of 20 weeks. The groups were developed based upon the belief that the widowed have lower levels of social support than do married couples and that seniors, by nature of having outlived many of their friends, are particularly susceptible to lowered social support. The results of these groups demonstrated more positive affect, fewer reported support needs, and more satisfaction with support for those who participated.

The FCN may be involved with various grieving clients. The client could be an individual of any age, a family, or the faith community itself. Any of the implementations presented throughout this text may be useful. The key factors include that doing something is better than doing nothing in a situation where people tend to feel isolated and that in working within a faith community, there are some common values from which to start. Remembering that grief is individual is vital. Helping someone understand that what he or she is experiencing may well not be the same as what others are experiencing, even within the same family or faith community, may be one of the most useful actions that can occur. Also, it is important to reinforce with those who are grieving that this is a dynamic process that can pervade all aspects of life. Feelings of sorrow may occur at totally unexpected times with the person being unable to identify what triggered these feelings. No time frame exists for grieving—one person may come to a high degree of resolution of the grief fairly quickly, whereas another may continue to experience grief for years. Anticipating the need to provide support around the times of anniversaries is important—the birthday of the one who died, holidays, the anniversary of the death, and/or of the funeral or memorial service. For the first anniversaries, this may be especially true but may continue to be true for longer than the first year.

Just as the response is individual, so will the care need to be adjusted to the response. Some will prefer to grieve privately; others will find solace in a support group. Some may seek private time for Scripture reading and prayers, others may want to share these activities with someone such as the parish nurse, and still others may seek out a group for studying Scripture. Hugs and touching are comforting to most but may be distasteful to some. When feelings of sorrow and sadness need to be worked through, various mechanisms occur that might be useful. These include exercise—ranging from a quiet walk around the block to intensive training to run a marathon (again, the key is what works for the individual)—journaling, engaging in various forms of art, and talking with others.

Whether dealing with an individual, a family, or a faith community, the primary activities for the FCN are to be there, to ask about what would be helpful, and to watch for responses to efforts made to be helpful so that the help offered can be useful. With Anna Mulgrew, providing her with the opportunity to talk about what her loss means to her, when she is ready to discuss it, is one approach to helping her deal with the grief. If she does not wish to discuss how she feels, she should not be pressured to talk about it; but members of the interdisciplinary team, especially the FCN, should continue to be present for her.

Summary

In summary, palliative care is a fairly recent addition to our health care scene. Palliative care is an extension of the precepts of hospice care to include those in earlier stages of life-threatening illnesses. The hallmarks of palliative care include symptom control, maintaining function, support for the whole person, inclusion of family, and an interdisciplinary team. The inclusion of the patient and family as decision makers and caregivers places importance on their values and right to be informed. Challenges associated with pain control, nutrition and hydration, and wound care are more satisfactorily met when the choices and values of the patient and family are paramount.

Palliative care is closely associated with loss, and loss is associated with grief and grieving. Grief has been described as a dynamic process that occurs in an individualized manner that involves the whole person.

The FCN has an important role to play in palliative care and in assistance with grieving. Within the interdisciplinary team, the FCN is in an ideal position to serve as the link between the faith community and the health care providers and can function as a two-way interpreter when needed. When a death occurs, the FCN may provide support to individuals, families, and the faith community.

Palliative care can be challenging and may not be an appropriate area of practice for all. However, Webster and Kristjanson (2002) found that palliative care workers who find satisfaction in this work described it as a way of living and demonstrated vitality as the core meaning for their work. Even with vitality at the core, the experience of palliative care provision is perhaps best illuminated by Lamendola's (1996) phrase of "burning brightly, burning dimly." The FCN burns brightly on those days when the patient and family have received the best the nurse has to give. The nurse burns dimly during those times of fatigue and struggle to give of oneself. Fortunately, working with an interdisciplinary team provides the opportunity to have backup during the times of burning dimly, and the core vitality of palliative care feeds the flames to burn brightly.

Reflect and Discuss

1. How are the nursing theories of Neuman, Parse, and Watson, discussed in Chapter 1, consistent with, or in conflict with, palliative care?
2. Most of the research related to palliative care has been conducted within the qualitative paradigm. Why do you believe this is the case?
3. Discuss the relationship between palliative care and hospice care.
4. How would your personal grief experiences influence your approach to grief counseling with an individual? A family? Within the faith community?
5. How can the FCN best respond to a member of the church who says, "I just don't understand what is going on with Mary. She still won't come to a memorial service at church. After all, it's been more than a year since her son died. Isn't it about time she got over it?"

Case Study

Anna Mulgrew is an 82-year-old woman who is at home after a below-the-knee amputation of her right leg. This was her second major surgery in 6 months. The first was a femoral-popliteal bypass to improve circulation to her right leg after a medical diagnosis of severe peripheral vascular disease, with 90% impairment of circulation to the right leg. The circulation to the lower portion of her leg and her foot was still inadequate to prevent tissue breakdown, so the decision was made to amputate above the area of poorest circulation.

She is on medication for high blood pressure and for respiratory allergies. She has some residual pain from an episode of shingles on her left shoulder 1 year ago. She is no longer able to take care of her home, fix meals, or do laundry, all of which she was doing prior to the first surgery. Her stump wound keeps breaking open, so she is not able to use a prosthesis. Arthritis in her hands and arms make it difficult for her to use a walker. She has had a physical therapist visit her home regularly but has not been able to gain enough strength to get about other than with a wheelchair. She is able to do bed-to-chair, chair-to-chair, and chair-to-toilet transfers.

Her 87-year-old husband is at home and able to fix light meals and care for himself.

References

Alvarez, O. M., Meehan, M., Ennis, W., Thomas, D. R., Ferris, F. D., & Kennedy, K. L., et al. (2002). Chronic wounds: Palliative management for the frail population. *Wounds: A Compendium of Clinical Research and Practice, 14*(8), 4S–27S.

Amella, E. J. (2003). Geriatrics and palliative care: Collaboration for quality of life until death. *Journal of Hospice and Palliative Nursing, 5*(1), 40–48.

American Nurses Association. (1992). *Position statement on foregoing nutrition and hydration.* Retrieved July 3, 2004, from http://www.nursingworld.org/readroom/position/ethics/etnutr.htm.

American Nurses Association. (2003). *Position statement on pain management and control of distressing symptoms in dying patients.* Retrieved July 3, 2004, from http://www.nursingworld.org/readroom/position/ethics/etpain.htm.

American Nurses Association and Health Ministries Association. (2005). *Faith community nursing: Scope and standards of practice.* Silver Springs, MD: ANA.

Clements, P. T., Vigil, G. J., Manno, M. S., Henry, G. C., Wilks, J., & Das, S., et al. (2003). Cultural perspectives of death, grief, and bereavement. *Journal of Psychosocial Nursing and Mental Health Services, 41*(7), 18–26, 42–43.

Covinsky, K. E., Eng, C., Lui, L-Y, Sands, L. P., & Yaffe, K. (2003). The last 2 years of life: Functional trajectories of frail older people. *Journal of the American Geriatrics Society, 51*(4), 492–498.

Cowles, K. V. (2000). Grief in a cultural context: Expanding concept analysis beyond the professional literature. In B. L. Rodgers & K. A. Knaft (Eds.), *Concept development in nursing: Foundations, techniques, and applications* (2nd ed., pp. 119–128). Philadelphia: WB Saunders.

Cowles, K. V., & Rodgers, B. L. (2000). The concept of grief: An evolutionary perspective. In B. L. Rodgers & K. A. Knaft (Eds.), *Concept development in nursing: Foundations, techniques, and applications* (2nd ed., pp. 103–117). Philadelphia: WB Saunders.

Demi, A. S., & Myles, M. G. (1986). Bereavement. *Annual Review of Nursing Research, 4,* 105–123.

Doona, M. E., Haggerty, L. A., & Chase, S. K. (1997). Nursing presence: An existential exploration of the concept. *Scholarly Inquiry for Nursing Practice, 11,* 3–16.

Ellifritt, J., Nelson, K. A., & Walsh, D. (2003). Complicated bereavement: A national survey of potential risk factors. *American Journal of Hospice and Palliative Care, 20*(2), 114–120.

Ersek, M. (2003). Artificial nutrition and hydration: Clinical issues. *Journal of Hospice and Palliative Nursing, 5*(4), 221–230.

Fletcher, S. N. (2002). Cultural implications in the management of grief and loss. *Journal of Cultural Diversity, 9*(3), 86–90.

Gibson, M. C., & Schroder, C. (2001). The many faces of pain for older, dying adults. *American Journal of Hospice & Palliative Care, 18*(1), 19–25.

Hames, C. C. (2003). Helping infants and toddlers when a family member dies. *Journal of Hospice and Palliative Nursing, 5*(2), 103–112.

History of hospice care. (n.d.). Retrieved July 6, 2004, from http://www.nho.org/i4a/pages/index.cfm?pageid=3285&openpage=3285.

Hospice and Palliative Nurses Association. (2003a). HPNA position paper: Artificial nutrition and hydration in end-of-life care. *Journal of Hospice and Palliative Nursing, 5*(4), 231–234.

Hospice and Palliative Nurses Association. (2004). HPNA position paper: Pain. *Journal of Hospice and Palliative Nursing, 6*(1), 62–64.

Hospice and Palliative Nurses Association. (2003b). HPNA position paper: Palliative sedation at the end of life. *Journal of Hospice and Palliative Nursing, 5*(4), 235–237.

Hospice and Palliative Nurses Association & American Nurses Association. (2002). *Scope and standards of hospice and palliative nursing practice.* Washington, DC: American Nurses Publishing.

Kane, J. R., Barber, R. G., Jordan, M., Tichenor, K. T., & Camp, K. (2000). Supportive/palliative care of children suffering from life-threatening and terminal illness. *American Journal of Hospice and Palliative Care, 17*(3), 165–172.

Kirk, K., & McManus, M. (2002). Containing families' grief: Therapeutic group work in a hospice setting. *International Journal of Palliative Nursing, 8*(10), 470–480.

Lamendola, F. (1996). Keeping your compassion alive. *American Journal of Nursing, 96*(11), 16R–16T.

Last Acts. (2003). *Precepts of palliative care for children, adolescents, and their families.* Retrieved June 9, 2004, from http://www.lastacts.org.

Lynch, M. (2003). Palliative sedation. *Clinical Journal of Oncology Nursing, 7*(6), 653–657.

Mehta, A., & Ezer, H. (2003). My love is hurting: The meaning spouses attribute to their loved ones' pain during palliative care. *Journal of Palliative Care, 19*(2), 87–94.

Mystakidou, K., Tsilika, E., Parpa, E., Katsouda, E., & Vlahos, L. (2003). A Greek perspective on concepts of death and expression of grief, with implications for practice. *International Journal of Palliative Nursing, 9*(12), 534–537.

The National Hospice and Palliative Care Organization. (n.d.). *Palliative care.* Retrieved July 3, 2004, from http://www.nho.org/i4a/pages/index.cfm?pageid=3657.

Norlander, L., & Baines, B. K. (2003). The five guiding principles for end of life care: Minnesota's framework. *Home Health Care Management & Practice, 15*(2), 110–115.

Parkes, C. M. (1985). Determinants of outcome following bereavement. *Omega, 6,* 303–323.

Riely, M. (2003). Facilitating children's grief. *The Journal of School Nursing, 19*(4), 212–218.

Robinson, F. (2003). New roles for practice nurses in palliative care: Practice nurses across the UK are working to improve care of terminally ill patients. *Practice Nurse, 25*(12), 10–12.

Salladay, S. A. (2002). Making plans to "allow natural death." *Nursing, 32*(5), 24, 25.

Stajduhar, K. I. (2003). Examining the perspectives of family members involved in the delivery of palliative care at home. *Journal of Palliative Care, 19*(1), 27–35.

Stanley, K. J. (2002). The healing power of presence: Respite from the fear of abandonment. *Oncology Nursing Forum, 29*(6), 935–940.

Stewart, M., Craig, D., MacPherson, K., & Alexander, S. (2001). Promoting positive affect and diminishing loneliness of widowed seniors through a support intervention. *Public Health Nursing, 18*(1), 54–63.

Task Force on Palliative Care, Last Acts. (1997). *Precepts of palliative care.* Retrieved June 9, 2004, from http://www.lastacts.org.

Taylor, E. J. (2003). Nurses caring for the spirit: Patients with cancer and family caregiver expectations. *Oncology Nursing Forum, 30*(4), 585–590.

Thorns, A. (2002). Sedation, the doctrine of double effect and the end of life. *International Journal of Palliative Nursing, 8*(7), 341–343.

Webster, J., & Kristjanson, L. J. (2002). But isn't it depressing? The vitality of palliative care. *Journal of Palliative Care, 18*(1), 15–24.

What is hospice and palliative care? (n.d.). Retrieved July 3, 2004, from http://www.nho.org/i4a/pages/index.cfm?pageid=3281&openpage=3281.

Wheeler, M. S. (2004). Palliative care is more than pain management. *Home Healthcare Nurse, 22*(4), 251–255.

Wootton, M. (2004). Morphine is not the only analgesic in palliative care: Literature review. *Journal of Advanced Nursing, 45*(5), 527–532.

World Health Organization. (2003a). *WHO definition of palliative care.* Retrieved July 3, 2004, from http://www.who.int/cancer/palliative/definition/en/.

World Health Organization. (2003b). *WHO's pain ladder.* Retrieved July 9, 2004, from http://www.who.int/cancer/palliative/painladder/en/.

Additional Resources

Cameron, M. E. (2002). Older persons' ethical problems involving their health. *Nursing Ethics, 9*(5), 537–556.

Diver, F., Molassiotis, A., & Weeks, L. (2003). The palliative care needs of ethnic minority patients: Staff perspectives. *International Journal of Palliative Nursing, 9*(8), 343–351.

Ferrell, B. R., & Borneman, T. (2002). Community implementation of home care palliative care education. *Cancer Practice: A Multidisciplinary Journal of Cancer Care, 10*(1), 20–27.

Gaydos, H. L. (2004). The living end: Life journeys of hospice nurses. *Journal of Hospice and Palliative Nursing, 6*(1), 17–26.

Goodwin, D. M., Higginson, I. J., Edwards, A. G., Finlay, I. G., Cook, A. M., & Hood, K., et al. (2002). An evaluation of systematic reviews of palliative care services. *Journal of Palliative Care 18*(2), 77–83.

Halstead, M. T., & Hull, M. (2001). Struggling with paradoxes: The process of spiritual development in women with cancer. *Oncology Nursing Forum 28*(10), 1534–1544.

Harstde, C. W., & Andershed, B. (2004). Good palliative care: How and where? The patients' options. *Journal of Hospice and Palliative Nursing, 6*(1), 27–35.

Harvey, S. A. (2001). Hospital information services. S. C. A. L. E.—spiritual care at life's end: A multidisciplinary approach to end-of-life issues in a hospital setting. *Medical Reference Services Quarterly, 20* (4), 63–71.

Hayes, C. M. (2003). Surrogate decision-making to end life-sustaining treatments for incapacitated adults. *Journal of Hospice and Palliative Nursing, 5*(2), 91–102.

Kabel, A., & Roberts, D. (2003). Professionals' perceptions of maintaining personhood in hospice care. *International Journal of Palliative Nursing, 9*(7), 283–289.

Lyons, M., Orozovic, N., Davis, J., & Newman, J. (2002). Doing-being-becoming: Occupational experiences of persons with life-threatening illnesses.

American Journal of Occupational Therapy, 56(3), 285–295.

Nåden, D., & Eriksson, K. (2004). Understanding the importance of values and moral attitudes in nursing care in preserving human dignity. *Nursing Science Quarterly 17*(1), 86–91.

Nightingale, E., Kristjanson, L. J., Toye, C., & Aranda, S. (2003). Evaluating the Navigate Care Model: Clinical palliative care pathways based on anticipated care outcomes. [Commentary by S. Aranda]. *International Journal of Palliative Nursing, 9*(7), 298–307.

Ryan, A., Carter, J., Lucas, J., & Berger, J. (2002). You need not make the journey alone: Overcoming impediments to providing palliative care in a public urban teaching hospital. *American Journal of Hospice and Palliative Care, 19*(3), 171–180.

→ Web Resources

http://www.abcd-caring.org   Americans for Better Care of the Dying

http://www.nursingworld.org/readroom/position/ American Nurses Association, position statements

http://www.cancersourcern.com   Cancer Source for Nurses

http://www.griefloss.org   Center for Grief

http://www.christiancaregivers.com   Christian Caregivers

http://www.cityofhope.org/prc   City of Hope Pain/Palliative Care Resource Center

http://www.hpna.org   Hospice and Palliative Nurses Association

http://www.stoppain.org   Department of Pain Medicine and Palliative Care, Beth Israel Medical Center

http://www.grief.net   The Grief Recovery Institute

http://www.griefresourcescatalog.com/catalog/ The Grief Resources Catalog

http://www.lastacts.org   Last Acts (a national coalition to improve care and caring near the end-of-life care)

http://www.minnesotapartnership.org/cgi-bin/index.cgi Minnesota Palliative Care Partnership

http://www.mournerspath.com   Mourners Path

http://www.grievingchild.com   National Center for Grieving Children and Families (includes listing of children's bereavement centers worldwide)

http://www.nho.org   The National Hospice and Palliative Care Organization

http://www.palliativecarenursing.net   Nurses Leadership Academy for End-of-Life Care

http://www.palliative.org   Regional Palliative Care Program, Edmonton, Alberta, Canada

17

Vulnerable Populations

This chapter will address definitions and characteristics of vulnerable populations. The potential roles of faith community outreach ministries and the faith community nurse (FCN) will be discussed in relation to assisting these vulnerable persons.

Concept of Vulnerability

Dr. Lu Ann Aday is a sociologist and an expert on vulnerable populations in America. She conducts research that frames the issues related to health disparities and recommends public policy change(s) to address these multifaceted issues. Dr. Aday eloquently begins her book, *At Risk in America,* with the following paragraph:

> Both the origins and remedies of vulnerability are rooted in the bonds of human communities. The parentheses that inscribe our lives (its beginnings and endings, as well as the passages within it) take form in the arms of those who care for us when we are most in need of physical help, spiritual solace, or warm companionship. Their presence supports and strengthens us, and the blessings of their caring seek to salve the wounds of body, mind and spirit that accompany the odyssey of our lives. (2001, p. 1)

Aday goes on to say that, "To be vulnerable is to be susceptible to harm or neglect, that is, acts of commission or omission on the part of others that can wound. The word *vulnerable* is derived from the Latin verb *vulnerare* (to wound) and the noun *vulnus* (wound). . . . As members of human communities, we are all potentially vulnerable" (2001, p. 1).

Vulnerability results from the combined effects of limited resources for living. These resources can be biological, psychological, spiritual, environmental, economic, and educational. Some of these resources are intrapersonal and some are environmental. Deficits in one area may create deficits in another and a cycle perpetuates itself. Living in a cycle of vulnerability also results in living with chronic stress. Vulnerable persons have a higher *risk* for disease and adverse health events. Risk is an epidemiological term that means that one has a higher probability of having a disease.

The vulnerable populations conceptual model (VPCM) was developed by Flaskerud and Winslow (1998). It proposes that resource availability, relative risk, and health status are related (Figure 17-1). Koniak-Griffin, Flaskerud, and Nyamathi (2005) state that *resource availability* refers to human capital [income, jobs, education, housing, health insurance, social status (power), social connection (integration into society, societal networks), and environmental resources (health care access and quality)]. *Relative risk* is the ratio of the risk of poor health among groups having fewer resources and exposed to increased risk factors compared with those having more resources and exposed to fewer risk factors. Risk factors may be behavioral (e.g., lifestyle choices; availability, access to and use or nonuse of screening and health promotion services; exposure to violence or abuse) or biological (e.g., physiological and genetic predisposition). Disease prevalence and morbidity and mortality rates indicate the

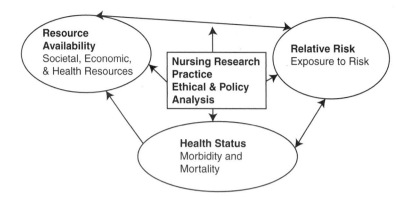

Figure 17.1 Vulnerable population conceptual model. Adapted from Flaskerud, J. H., & Winslow, B. J. (1998). Conceptualizing vulnerable populations health related research. *Nursing Research, 47*(2), 69–78. Used with permission.

health status of a community. These authors propose three relationships among the major constructs of the model:

1. Resources and risks
2. Risks and health status
3. Health status and resources

Lack of community resources increases exposure to risk, and increased risk factors can reduce resource availability. Increased exposure to risk factors leads to decreased health status, which may increase further exposure to risk factors and affect resource availability by further depleting them. Nursing research, practice, and ethical and policy analysis are presented in the model and are seen as having the potential to affect resources, relative risk, and health status, both directly and indirectly. The VPCM is supported by extensive research (Koniak-Griffin, Flaskerud, & Nyamathi, 2005).

Vulnerable persons experience health disparities, which means that they have worse health outcomes than more advantaged persons in terms of both morbidity and mortality (Sebastian, 2004). Vulnerable groups have a higher prevalence of chronic diseases, such as hypertension, and high levels of communicable diseases, such as tuberculosis (TB), sexually transmitted diseases (STDs), hepatitis B virus (HBV), and upper respiratory illnesses. Vulnerable people also have higher mortality from crime and violence, including domestic violence.

The term *human capital* refers to the strength, knowledge, and skills that enable people to be healthy. *Resilience* is an element of human capital strength that allows some people to cope with conditions of great adversity. Aday (2001) also relates the concept of human capital to communities. She states that the investments that communities make (or choose not to make) in jobs, schools, and housing, and the resulting payoffs to individuals and families, in terms of working, getting a good education, and having adequate housing, all directly affect vulnerability. The decrease in manufacturing jobs and declining tax base for support of public education in urban neighborhoods, coupled with urban regentrification and the federal housing policy, have resulted in fewer low-income housing available. This has, in turn, resulted in the emergence of a hardcore, extremely socially and economically disadvantaged underclass, many of whom are likely to be vulnerable.

Poverty is considered to be the primary cause of vulnerability because poverty limits resources in so many areas of life. Bezruchka (2000, 2001) argues that the economic structure of a country is the single most powerful determinant of the health of its people. He advocates redistribution of wealth as a solution to health disparities. Vulnerability also results from being very young or very old, or being a teenager, regardless of income. Vulnerability can also result from a disease process. It can be real or perceived—again, regardless of income. The absence of caring for others in people's lives increases their likelihood of being vulnerable.

Persons who are vulnerable are characterized by feelings of powerlessness, lack of control over one's life, hopelessness, depression, victimization, disadvantage, and disenfranchisement. From a public health perspective, a population is vulnerable by virtue of status, that is, some groups are at risk at any given point in time relative to other individuals or groups (de Chesnay, 2005). Although anyone can be vulnerable at any given time as a result of life circumstances, illness, or events, the following specific groups are labeled "vulnerable" as a result of their limited life resources:

- Persons living in poverty
- Homeless persons
- Pregnant teens
- Frail elderly
- Mentally ill persons
- Persons with HIV/AIDS
- Migrant workers
- Substance abusers
- Persons with disabilities
- Victims of violence

Several university nursing research centers focus on improving the health of vulnerable populations. Research in these centers is supported by funding from the National Institute of Nursing Research. Web addresses for these centers are presented in Box 17-1.

Poverty

Overview

The U. S. Census Bureau reports that the official poverty rate in 2003 was 12.5%, up from 12.1% in 2002. In 2003, 35.9 million people were in poverty, up 1.3 million from 2002. As defined by the Office of Management and Budget and updated for inflation using the consumer price index (CPI), the average poverty threshold for a family of four in 2003 was $18,810. Important to note is that persons who earn just a little more than the official threshold are ineligible for financial assistance programs, yet they are unable to manage their living expenses. This population of "near-poor" people is not reflected in the numbers presented here. The official poverty rates remained unchanged for Hispanics, non-Hispanic whites, and blacks, although it rose for whites and Asians. For children under age 18, both the poverty rate and the number in poverty rose between 2002 and 2003,

---

BOX 17-1
Nursing Research Centers

Center for Health Outcomes and Policy Research
http://www.nursing upenn.edu/chopr

Center for Health Promotion and Disease Prevention Research in Underserved Populations
http://www.utexas.edu/chpr2000/chpr.html

Center for Health Promotion and Risk Reduction in Specific Populations
http://www.sc.edu/nursing/center/index.html

Center for Vulnerable Population Research
http://www.nursing.ucla.edu/cvpr/

from 16.7% to 17.6% and from 12.1 million to 12.9 million, respectively. The poverty rate of children under age 18 remained higher than that of those ages 18 to 64 and that of seniors age 65 and over (10.8% and 10.2%, respectively, both unchanged from 2002) (http://www.census.gov/hhes/povert/poverty03/pov03hi.html).

The U.S. Census reports that real median household income remained unchanged between 2002 and 2003 at $43,318 (2004). At the same time, the number of people without health insurance rose by 1.4 million to 45 million. The percentage of the nation's population without coverage grew from 15.2% in 2002 to 15.6% in 2003 (http://www.census.gov/Press-Release/www/releases/archives/income_wealth/002484.html).

In 2003, Arkansas, New Mexico, Mississippi, Louisiana, West Virginia, and the District of Columbia had the highest poverty rates (18.5%), whereas New Hampshire and Minnesota had the lowest poverty rates (6%). The following states had increases in their poverty rates: Illinois, Michigan, Nevada, North Carolina, South Dakota, Texas, and Virginia; whereas two states, Mississippi and North Dakota, showed decreases (http://www.census.gov/hhes/povert/poverty03/pov03hi.html).

Effects of Poverty

Poverty is a primary cause of vulnerability, and living in poverty decreases access to resources. It increases the likelihood that one will experience adversity related to physical, psychological, and social health as well as inadequate or substandard housing, nutrition, health care services, and education. More years of formal education and higher incomes are directly associated with better health. Persons of lower socioeconomic status (less education, lower incomes, or employed in low-status jobs) are more likely to have serious chronic physical or mental health problems. Aday (2001) states that economic factors play a major role in family abuse and neglect, and that the vast majority of homeless people are extremely poor.

Homelessness

Overview

A person is considered homeless who "lacks a fixed, regular, and adequate night-time residence and . . . has a primary night-time residency that is: (a) a supervised publicly or privately operated shelter designed to provide temporary living accommodations . . . (b) an institution that provides a temporary residence for individuals intended to be institutionalized, or (c) a public or private place not designed for, or ordinarily used as, a regular sleeping accommodation for human beings" [Stewart B. McKinney Act, 42 U. S. C. 11301, et seq. (1994)].

The National Coalition for the Homeless (2004) reports two trends that are largely responsible for the rise in homelessness over the past 20 to 25 years: a growing shortage of affordable rental housing and a simultaneous increase in poverty. The actual number of homeless persons is difficult to measure because of the mobility of this population. Most studies show that single homeless adults are more likely to be male than female. The U.S. Conference of Mayors' survey found that single men comprised 41% of the urban homeless population and single women comprised 14% (2003). Of this group, 23% suffer from some form of severe and persistent mental illness and 30% suffer from substance addiction. This study also reports that families with children make up the fastest growing segment of the homeless population. With their 2003 survey of 25 American cities, the Conference of Mayors found that families comprised 40% of the homeless population. On a national level, the Urban Institute (2000) found that 39% of the homeless population are children. These figures are likely to be higher in rural areas where research indicated that families, single mothers, and children make up the largest group of homeless persons (Vissing, 1996).

In its 2003 survey of 25 American cities, the U.S. Conference of Mayors' survey found that the homeless population was 49% African American, 35% Caucasian, 13% Hispanic, 2% Native American, and 1% Asian. Like the U.S. population, the ethnic makeup of homeless populations varies according to geographic location. For example, rural homeless are more likely to be white, Native American and migrant, whereas urban homeless are more likely to be African American.

The National Coalition Against Domestic Violence reports that approximately half of all women and children who are experiencing homelessness are fleeing from domestic violence (Zorza, 1991).

Effects of Homelessness

Homelessness adversely affects all people; however, homelessness has unique effects on each age group. Homeless pregnant women are at higher risk for complex health problems and poorer pregnancy outcomes, such as low-birth weight babies and preterm births. These women have higher rates of sexually transmitted and other communicable diseases, higher incidence of substance abuse, poorer nutrition, and less access to prenatal care (Sebastian, 2004).

Weinreb (1998) reports that homeless children experience more symptoms of acute illness, such as fever, ear infection, diarrhea, and asthma than children who are housed. Menke and Wagner (1998) report that homeless children demonstrated higher levels of anxiety, were significantly more depressed, and were at higher risk for physical and mental health problems and abuse than poor children who were not homeless. Homeless children are more likely to experience inadequate nutrition, with resulting developmental delays, failure to thrive, or obesity. Homeless children also have higher rates of school absences, academic failure, and emotional and behavioral adjustment problems.

Adolescents who are homeless exhibit greater risk-taking behaviors, poorer health status—both mental and physical—and decreased access to health care services (Ensign & Santelli, 1997). They are also at higher risk for sexually transmitted and other communicable diseases, such as HIV and hepatitis B and C, and for substance abuse. Teenage women who exchange sex for survival are at risk for pregnancy.

Recent research on factors influencing homelessness in women (Anderson & Rayens, 2004) demonstrates the significance of families of origin and learning how to develop and use support systems in preventing and reducing homelessness. They report that the homeless group scored significantly lower on support and reciprocity scales and significantly higher in conflict than the never-homeless groups. The never-homeless, never-abused group scored significantly higher on autonomy and intimacy scales than the homeless and abused groups.

Pregnant Teens

The United States has the highest teen pregnancy rate in the world. Thirty-five percent of girls get pregnant at least once by age 20—nearly 850,000 in 2003. The vast majority of these pregnancies (78%) are unintended. Teen childbearing costs taxpayers at least $7 billion each year in direct costs associated with health care, foster care, criminal justice, and public assistance as well as lost tax revenues. Although the overall teen pregnancy rates declined 24% between 1992 and 2000, 25% of teen mothers have a second baby before age 20 (National Campaign to Prevent Teen Pregnancy, 2004). Kirby (2001) reports that between 2000 and 2010, the population of teen girls ages 15 to 19 is expected to increase by nearly 10%, which means that even with declining rates, there will be increased actual numbers of teen pregnancies and births.

Teen pregnancy has important implications for the health and development of babies. The babies of teen mothers are more likely to be born at low-birth weight. Low-birth weight raises the probabilities of infant death, blindness, deafness, chronic respiratory problems, mental retardation, mental illness, and cerebral palsy. Low-birth weight doubles the chance that a child will later be diagnosed with dyslexia, hyperactivity, or another disability. Children of teen mothers

- perform less well in school than children born to older mothers;
- suffer higher rates of abuse and neglect;
- are 13% more likely to be imprisoned; and
- are 22% more likely to become teen mothers themselves. (National Campaign to Prevent Teen Pregnancy, 2004)

Teen pregnancy in America is closely tied to poverty with 66% of families begun by a young mother living in poverty. Almost half of all teen mothers and over three-quarters of unmarried teen mothers began receiving welfare within 5 years of the birth of their first child. The reduction in the number of teen births in the past 10 years accounts for a 26% decrease in the number of children under age 6 living in poverty.

Faith Community Initiatives for Teens

Whitehead, Wilcox, and Rostosky (2001) report that teens are religious, with over 90% of teens reporting a religious affiliation. As teens get older, they are less likely to participate in formal religious activities but are just as likely to say that religion is important to them. Girls are more likely to participate in religious activities than boys, and black teens are more likely to participate than white teens. Regardless of gender and race, teens who attend religious services are frequently less likely to have permissive attitudes about sexual activity. However, important to note is that attitudes are only moderately predictive of behavior.

Whitehead et al. (2001) state that faith communities contribute to teenagers by helping them to develop spiritually and morally. Faith communities transmit the teachings and observances of their faith, by guiding and protecting teens through the passage of adolescence, and some faith communities directly address the issue of teen sexuality. Regardless of conservative and liberal stances, the common denominator is that people of faith believe that God has something to say about the way that they, as his created beings, express their sexual natures and desires.

In 1998, the National Campaign to Prevent Teen Pregnancy and its Religion and Public Values (RPV) Task Force developed a reader-friendly pamphlet that offers faith leaders and their communities nine tips to help address teen pregnancy. These tips are presented in Box 17-2. In 1999, this organization conducted a series of regional and local meetings with faith leaders nationwide, and they continue to advocate for collaborations between the public health community and faith communities.

Again, depending upon the congregation and its resources, the faith community nurse or a youth minister may provide sexuality education to teens. The True Love Waits Program, a teen abstinence program, was originally developed by the Southern Baptists, but it is not exclusively church- or denomination-based. Its Web site lists over 88 Christian entities as cooperating ministries. Information about this program is available at http://www.truelovewaits.com. The Unitarian Universalist Association and the United Church of Christ joined together to develop a sex education program for youth in their congregations. After 7 years of work, the resulting program is called Our Whole Lives (OWL), a curriculum described as lifespan sexuality education. Information is available at http://www.uua.org/owl/roots.html.

BOX 17-2
Nine Tips to Help Faith Leaders and Their Communities Address Teen Pregnancy

1. Address the need teens have for spiritual fulfillment, and help them find answers to the many challenging problems they face.
2. Encourage parents to talk with their children about sex and morality within the context of their faith tradition.
3. Enlist adults in your faith community to help young people.
4. Make sure that the children and teenagers in your faith community understand what your faith tradition says about sex, love, and marriage in general and teen pregnancy, in particular. Use clear and unambiguous language.
5. Learn about contemporary youth culture—what your young people are reading, listening to, watching, and doing.
6. Organize supervised group activities for teenagers in your faith community.
7. Reach out to teenagers who are not involved in any faith community.
8. Celebrate achievement and excellence.
9. Reach out to other faith communities, neighborhood organizations, and institutions that work with young people.

The National Campaign to Prevent Teen Pregnancy. (2002). Available online at: http://www.teenpregnancy.org.

Frail Elderly

People over 65 years of age represented 24% of the population in the year 2000. By 2030, this group will comprise 20% of the population (Administration on Aging, 2002). These numbers are projected to nearly double by 2030 (Health United States, 2002). Frail elderly adults represent the largest group of consumers of both health care and as recipients of nursing care. They have a higher frequency of primary care visits, consume 50% of all hospital care, use over 80% of home care services, and occupy 90% of all nursing home beds (Mezey & Fulmer, 1998).

Zisberg and Young (2005) discuss frail elderly adults as a vulnerable population. Their working definition of frailty is the potential for functional threats to independence or demonstrated reduced reserve capacity based on physical evaluation tests.

Markle-Reid and Browne (2003) identified six major conceptual models explaining the nature and occurrence of frailty. Three models are biologically/physiologically based. In these, frailty may result from a loss of skeletal muscle mass (Walston & Fried, 1994), reduction in aerobic capacity and metabolic changes (Campbell & Buchner, 1997), and dysfunction resulting from disuse (Bortz, 1993). Two additional models include psychological and personal factors related to attitudes about health, cognition, and

spirituality (Raphael et al., 1995). The last model asserts that frailty is a social by-product of the interaction of the persons and their caregivers, as determined by roles, norms, and beliefs (Kaufman, 1994).

Medicare data over a 7-year period identified frailty as an antecedent of death in 47% of the cases. The typical trajectory of frailty is described as a steady progression of disability, with eventual complications, such as pneumonia. Frailty is a substantial indicator of functional deterioration and often results in a progressive process ending in death (Lunney, Lynn, & Hogan, 2002; Young, 2003).

Zisberg and Young (2005) report that nursing is taking a more central role in alleviating functional decline in older adults by introducing novel interventions. They describe specialized, nurse-managed geriatric units that emphasize early rehabilitative services (Francis, Fletcher, & Simon, 1998) and the transitional care model (Naylor, 2000) in which geriatric clients are carefully case managed. These interventions occur at the tertiary level of prevention.

FCNs are positioned well in the congregational community to be a resource for primary prevention of frailty by promoting healthy and successful aging. Health counseling and health education about immunizations (flu and pneumonia), exercise, socialization, and whole-health education provide primary prevention of frailty to the growing elderly population.

Mental Illness

Overview

Mental health is defined by *Healthy People 2010* (USDHHS, 2001) as the ability to engage in productive activities and fulfilling relationships with other people, to adapt to change and to cope with adversity. Mental health is integral to personal well-being. *Healthy People 2010* defines mental disorders as conditions that are characterized by alterations in thinking, mood, or behavior, which are associated with distress and/or impaired functioning. Mental illness refers to all diagnosable mental disorders.

Mental illnesses are equal opportunity diseases. They occur across the life span and affect persons of all genders, races, educational, and socioeconomic groups. About 40 million adults (ages 18 to 64), or 22% of the American population, have a mental illness. The most serious and disabling conditions affect 5 to 10 million adults. By 2020, major depressive illness will be the leading cause of disability in the world for women and children. At least one in five children (ages 5 to 17) has a diagnosable mental disorder in a given year, and about 5% to 9% of children are extremely impaired by mental disorders. An estimated 25% of older persons experience mental illness, such as depression, anxiety, and substance abuse. Alzheimer's disease is the primary cause of dementia and affects between 8% and 15% of people over age 65 (USDHHS, 2001; NAMI, 2004).

Effects of Mental Illness

The impact of mental illness is underrecognized. Dr. Thomas Insel, the director of the National Institute of Mental Health (NIMH) (2004), reports that the cost of direct (treatment-related) and indirect (productivity loss) expenses may exceed $150 billion per year, with rapid annual increases. Mental illnesses account for four of the top six causes of disability among those ages 15 to 44 in the Western world. In addition to morbidity, mental illnesses are a substantial source of mortality. Of the 30,000 Americans who die by suicide each year, 90% have a mental illness. Deaths from suicide outnumber deaths from homicide (18,000), as well as AIDS-related deaths and most forms of cancer. Suicide incidence is high among several ethnic minority groups, though it remains highest in older, white men. Between 1952 and 1992, the incidence of suicide among adolescents and young adults nearly tripled; currently, suicide is the third leading cause of death in adolescents (NIMH, 2004).

In spite of the prevalence of mental illness, *Healthy People 2010* reports that only 25% of the persons with a mental disorder obtain *any* medical treatment for their condition, and even a smaller percentage actually receive specialized mental health services (USDHHS, 2001), a clear reflection of the lack of insurance to cover treatment for mental illness. Even persons with "excellent" health insurance benefits have considerably less coverage for mental health treatment than for other medical conditions. The politics of mental health care in America is a subject too complex for the purposes of this chapter, but clearly the political system has consistently ignored the mental health treatment needs of the nation.

As a result of these huge unmet needs, advocacy groups have become a first line of support for consumers and their families. The National Alliance for the Mentally Ill (NAMI) is a consumer group that advocates for better mental health services and provides mental health

---

BOX 17-3
Web Resources About Mental Health

American Association of Suicidology
http://www.suicidology.org

Anxiety Disorders Association of America
http://www.adaa.org

Attention Deficit Information Network
http://www.addinfonetwork.com

Bazelon Center—legal advocacy
http://www.bazelon.org.

Children and Adults with Attention Deficit Disorders
http://www.chadd.org

Depression and Bipolar Support Alliance
http://www.ndmda.org

Learning Disorders Association of America
http://www.ldanatl.org

National Alliance for the Mentally Ill
http://www.nami.org

National Center for Post-traumatic Stress Disorders
http://www.ncptsd.org

National Center for Learning Disabilities
http://www.ld.org

National Eating Disorders Association
http://www.openmind.org

National Institute of Mental Health
http://www.nimh.nih.gov

National Mental Health Association
http://www.nmha.org

Obsessive Compulsive Foundation
http://www.ocfoundation.org

Overeaters Anonymous
http://www.overeatersanonymous.org

Schizophrenics Anonymous
http://www.nsfoundation.org

education and self-help services for individuals and families. Political action efforts by NAMI created the establishment of the Community Support Program (CSP), which is funded by the NIMH. This program provides grant funds to states to develop comprehensive mental health services for persons who are discharged from psychiatric institutions. Box 17-3 provides Web-based resources for information about mental health and illness.

Faith Community Nursing and Mental Health

A large, vulnerable population that the FCN will become very involved with are persons with mental diseases and/or substance abuse, and their family members. As discussed earlier in this chapter, the sheer numbers of persons affected by mental illness and the scarcity of adequate and affordable services is daunting. The majority of major mental disorders are long-term chronic situations, with recurring acute episodes.

Family resources may be stretched both emotionally and financially for long periods of time. The FCN is often the only support person available to these individuals, and they can easily take over an FCN's ministry time and personal time. Such a situation is described in the case study at the end of the chapter.

To assist in the care of this population, and to maintain a balance of service to the rest of the congregation, the FCN will need excellent counseling skills and must be familiar with both community mental health resources and resource people. If the FCN does not have a background in psychiatric nursing (and most do not), the FCN may feel both uncomfortable and inadequate working with these clients. Where possible, the FCN should use professional resource persons within the congregation and the community. The FCN should be very familiar with the support services that NAMI provides in the local community.

HIV/AIDS

Human immunodeficiency virus (HIV) is the virus that causes AIDS. This virus may be passed from one person to another when infected blood, semen, or vaginal secretions come in contact with an uninfected person's broken skin or mucous membranes. In addition, pregnant women can pass HIV to their baby during pregnancy and delivery, as well as through breast-feeding.

The estimated number of diagnoses of AIDS through 2002 in the United States is 886,575. Adult and adolescent AIDS cases total 877,275, with 718,002 cases in men and 159,271 cases in women. During the same time period, 9,300 AIDS cases were estimated in children under age 13 (CDC, 2004).

Each year, approximately 40,000 new HIV infections occur in the United States. By gender, 70% of new HIV infections occur among men. By risk, men who have sex with men represent the largest proportion of new infections, followed by men and women infected through heterosexual sex and injection drug use. By race, more than half of the new HIV infections occur among blacks (54%), though they represent only 13% of the U.S. population. Hispanics, who make up about 12% of the population, are also disproportionately affected, with 19% of the new cases (CDC, 2004). The 10 leading states or territories reporting the highest number of cumulative AIDS cases among residents as of December 2002 are as follows: New York, California, Florida, Texas, New Jersey, Illinois, Pennsylvania, Puerto Rico, Georgia, and Maryland.

During the mid- to late 1990s, advances in HIV treatment led to dramatic declines in AIDS deaths and slowed the progression from HIV to AIDS. In recent years, however, the rate of decline for both cases and deaths has begun to slow, and, in 1999, the annual number of AIDS cases appears to be leveling, whereas the decline in AIDS deaths has slowed. Better treatments have also led to an increasing number of people living with AIDS in this country (322,856 in 2000). This growing population represents an increasing need for continued HIV prevention services for HIV-infected individuals and for treatment and care services.

AIDSinfo, a service of the U.S. Department of Health and Human Services, has developed a set of fact sheets titled, *HIV and Its Treatment: What You Should Know* (2004), which is available free of charge at http://aidsinfo.nih.gov/guidelines/adult/brochure. Web resources about HIV/AIDS are presented in Box 17-4.

Migrant Workers

Migrant farmworkers are a diverse population, and their numbers and composition vary from region to region. Between 3 and 5 million people leave their homes every year to follow the crops. An estimated 85% of all migrant workers are Hispanic (including Mexican Americans, Mexicans, Puerto Ricans, Cubans, and workers from Central America and South America). The migrant population also includes black/African Americans, Jamaicans, Haitians, Laotians, Thais, and other racial and ethnic minorities.

Most migrant farmworkers are American citizens or are working in the country legally (National Center for Farmworker Health, NCFH, 2004). Some migrant workers live apart from their families and travel with groups of men. Other workers, particularly the Midwestern migrant stream, travel with their families.

BOX 17-4
Web Resources About HIV/AIDS

Advancing HIV Prevention
http://www.cdc.gov/hiv/partners/AHP-brochure.htm

AIDS Statistics
http://www.cdc.gov/hiv/stats.htm

Guide to NIH HIV/AIDS Information
http://aidsinfo.nih.gov/guidelines/adult/brochure

HIV/AIDS Treatment
http://www.aidsinfo.nih.gov

HIV/AIDS Clinical Trials
http://www.aidsinfo.nih.gov/clinical_trials/

Findings of the National Agricultural Workers Survey (NAWS) 1997–1998 include the following demographic data:

- Eighty-one percent of all farmworkers were foreign born. Of these, 95% were born in Mexico.
- The average age is 31 years with 50% under age 29, 31% between ages 25 and 34, 21% between ages 20 and 24, and 18% between ages 35 and 44.
- Eighty percent of migrant workers were men and 20% were women.
- One half of the migrant workers were married, and slightly less than half were parents. Among those who were parents, one half were not accompanied by their children when they migrated.
- Farmworker women were more likely to live with their families than men (74% versus 27%), and 91% of farmworker mothers lived with their children as compared to 42% of farmworker fathers.
- Eight-four percent of farmworkers spoke Spanish only, 12% English as a second language, and 4% other languages.
- The median education completed was 6th grade, and 85% would have difficulty processing written information, regardless of language.
- Three quarters had incomes less than $10,000 per year; three of five families had incomes below the poverty level. (U.S. Department of Labor, 1999)

Migrant farmworkers' housing is substandard—overcrowded, lacks sanitation and working appliances, and contains severe structural defects. The housing is often located adjacent to fields that have been treated with pesticides. Under these conditions, workers are unable to store food safely, prepare a warm meal, or even shower (NCFH, 2004).

The health status of migrant workers is poor. Unsanitary working and housing conditions make workers vulnerable to health conditions no longer considered threats to the general public. Farmworkers are at increased risk for communicable diseases because of living conditions. Poverty, frequent mobility, low literacy, language, cultural, and logistical barriers impede access to health services. Farmworkers are not protected by sick leave and are reluctant to risk job loss if they miss a day of work.

The Migrant Health Act of 1962 provides primary and supplemental health services to over 600,000 migrant workers and their families in 360 sites. However, these centers provide care to fewer than 29% of the nation's farmworkers.

Napolitano and Jones (2004) report that migrant farmworkers are at high risk for the following health problems:

- Chronic pesticide exposure resulting in cancer, blindness, Parkinson's disease, infertility, liver damage, polyneuropathy, and neurobehavioral problems
- TB incidence (higher in the migrant worker population; mobility of the workers makes treatment difficult)
- Chronic respiratory problems
- Domestic violence

Napolitano and Jones (2004) report that children of migrant farmworkers often suffer from health care deficits, including malnutrition, infectious diseases, dental caries, inadequate immunizations, pesticide exposure, and injuries. The number of children of migrant farmworkers who are workers themselves is not known. Children ages 12 and 13 can work on a farm with their parent's consent, if the parent works on the same farm, and children younger than age 12 can work on a farm that has fewer than 7 workers (Davis, 2001).

Victims of Domestic Violence

The National Domestic Violence Hotline reports that 31% of American women report being physically or sexually abused by a husband or boyfriend at some point in their lives. Estimates range from 960,000 to 4 million incidents of physical abuse annually. Although women are less likely than men to be victims of violent crime overall, women are five to eight times more likely than men to be victimized by an intimate partner. This accounts for 21% of violent crimes experienced by women and about 2% of the violence experienced by men. Ninety-two percent of all domestic violence incidents are committed by men against women. Studies show that child abuse occurs in 30% to 60% of family violence cases, and that a child's exposure to a father who abuses the mother is the strongest at risk for transmitting violent behavior from one generation to the next (http://www.ndvh.org/dvInfo.html).

Domestic violence is an equal opportunity event. It cuts across lines of race, nationality, language, economics, sexual orientation, culture, religion, and educational level. Racism, sexism, ableism, homophobia, and other forms of oppression influence how people experience domestic violence in their lives and how they are able to cope and to get help. Substance abuse problems and/or mental illnesses, although not responsible for domestic violence, can change a family's experience of violence and the kind(s) of treatment needed (http://www.ndvh.org/dvInfo.html). The National Domestic Violence Hotline reports that 40% of teenage girls ages 14 to 17 report knowing someone their age who has been hit or beaten by a boyfriend, and that one in five high school students reports being physically or sexually abused by a dating partner (http://www.ndvh.org/dvInfo.html).

Mortality and morbidity statistics are chilling. In 1996, among all female murder victims in the United States, 30% were slain by their husbands or boyfriends. Between 1976 and 1996, 31,260 women were murdered by an intimate partner. Females accounted for 39% of the hospital emergency department visits for violence-related injuries, and 84% of these women were treated for injuries inflicted by intimate partners. Box 17-5 provides Web-based resources for information, prevention, and assistance related to domestic violence.

Substance Abusers

Overview

The 2003 National Survey on Drug Use and Health (NSDUH) is the primary source of statistical information on the use of illegal drugs by the U.S. population. The Substance Abuse and Mental Health Services Administration (SAMHSA) of the U.S. Department of Health and Human Services is its annual sponsor, and the NSDUH is conducted by SAMHSA's Office of Applied Studies (OAS). Because of important methodological changes in the survey design, only data from 2002 and 2003 can be compared for trend measurements. Selected highlights of the findings of the 2003 survey are as follows (Substance Abuse and Mental Health Services Administration, 2004):

ILLICIT DRUG USE

- In 2003, an estimated 19.5 million Americans, or 8.2% of the population ages 12 and older, were current illicit drug users.
- No change occurred in the overall rate of illicit drug use between 2002 and 2003.
- The rate of current illicit drug use among youths ages 12 to 17 did not change significantly between 2002 (11.6%) and 2003 (11.2%).
- Marijuana is the most commonly used illicit drug, with a rate of 6.2% (14.6 million) in 2003. An estimated 2.3 million persons (1.0%) were current cocaine users, 604,000 of

BOX 17-5
Web Resources on Domestic Violence and Faith-based Organizations

http://www.findthegood.org/faithcomm/index.htm
A positive path to end violence: What faith communities can do

http://www.cpsdv.org
Center for Prevention of Sexual and Domestic Violence; an interreligious educational resource addressing issues of sexual and domestic violence. Provides training opportunities, links, publications.

http://www.jewishwomen.org
Provides resources on domestic violence in Jewish homes as well as resource guides for rabbis and other links to family violence resources.

http://www.familytrefugecenter.com
Provides articles about family violence through a faith perspective. Also provides guides and suggestions for clergy dealing with abusive men within their congregations.

ADDITIONAL WEB RESOURCES

http://www.aidv-usa.com
American Institute on Domestic Violence

http://www.aworc.org
Asian Women's Resource Exchange

http://www.atask.org
Asian Task Force Against Domestic Violence

http://www.usda.gov/da/shmd/aware.htm
Domestic Violence Awareness Handbook

http://www.endabuse.org
Family Prevention Fund

http://www.ilj.org/dv/index.htm
Initiatives Related to Domestic Violence

http://www.dvinstitute.org
Institute on Domestic Violence in the African American Community

http://www.ncadv.org
National Coalition Against Domestic Violence

http://www.ncjrs.org
National Criminal Justice Reference System

http://www.ndvh.org
National Domestic Violence Hotline

http://www.ncvc.org
National Center for Victims of Crime

http://www.dvalianza.org
National Latino Alliance for the Elimination of Domestic Violence

http://www.now.org
National Organization for Women

http://www.tribalresourcecenter.org
National Tribal Justice System

http://www.nnvawi.org
Nursing Network on Violence Against Women International

http://www.TEAMCares.org
TEAMCares Inc.

http://www.rosefund.org
The R.O.S.E. (Re-gaining One's Self-Esteem) Fund

http://www.ojp.usdoj.gov/vawo
Office of Violence Against Women

whom use crack. Hallucinogens were used by 1 million persons, and an estimated 119,000 were current heroin users. All of these estimates are similar to the estimates for 2002.

- The number of current users of Ecstasy decreased between 2002 and 2004 from 676,000 (0.3%) to 470,000 (0.2%).
- An estimated 6.3 million persons were current users of psychotherapeutic drugs taken nonmedically. This represents 2.7% of the population ages 12 and older. An estimated 4.7 million used pain relievers, 1.8 million used tranquilizers, 1.2 million used stimulants, and .03 million used sedatives.
- A significant increase occurred in the lifetime nonmedical used pain relievers between 2002 and 2003 among persons ages 12 and older, from 29.6 million to 31.2 million. Drugs included: Vicodin, Lortab, Lorcet, Percocet, Percodan, Tylox, Hydrocodone, OxyContin, and Tramadol.
- Rates of current illicit drug use were highest among Native Americans and Alaskan Natives (12.1%), persons reporting two or more races (12.0%), and Native Hawaiians/Pacific Islanders (11.1%). Rates were 8.7% for blacks, 8.3% for whites, and 8.0% for Hispanics.

ALCOHOL USE

- An estimated 119 million Americans (50.1%) ages 12 and older were current drinkers of alcohol in 2003. About 54 million (22.6%) participated in binge drinking at least once in the 30 days prior to the survey, and 16.1 million (6.8%) were heavy drinkers. These 2003 numbers are all similar to the 2002 estimates.
- The highest prevalence of binge and heavy drinking was for young adults ages 18 to 25 (41.6%).
- An estimated 13.6% of persons ages 12 and older drove under the influence of alcohol at least once in the 12 months prior to the survey (a decrease from 14.2% in 2002).

SUBSTANCE DEPENDENCE OR ABUSE

- An estimated 21.6 million Americans in 2003 were classified with substance dependence or abuse (9.1%) of the total population ages 12 and older. Of these, 3.1 million were classified with dependence on or abuse of both alcohol and illicit drugs, 3.8 million were dependent on or abused illicit drugs but not alcohol, and 14.8 million were dependent on or abused alcohol but not illicit drugs.
- Serious mental illness (SMI) was highly correlated with substance dependence or abuse. Among adults with SMI in 2003, 21.3% were dependent on or abused alcohol or illicit drugs, whereas the rate among adults without SMI was only 7.9%.
- Between 2003 and 2003 there was no change in the number of persons with substance dependence or abuse.

TREATMENT FOR SUBSTANCE PROBLEMS

- An estimated 3.3 million people ages 12 and older (1.4% of the population) received some kind of treatment for a problem related to alcohol or illicit drug use in the 12 months prior to the survey. Treatment settings included in- and out-patient rehabilitation facilities, hospitals, physician's offices, mental health centers, emergency departments, and prisons.
- In 2003, the estimated number of persons needing treatment for an alcohol or illicit drug problem was 22.2 million (9.3%) of the total population.

Effects of Substance Abuse

Substance abusers use alcohol and/or other chemicals that impair cognition. In 2000, approximately 85,000 deaths were attributable to alcohol use, making alcohol the third leading cause of death (Mokdad, 2004). Alcohol use is associated with motor vehicle accidents, unintentional injury, violence (40% of crimes are committed under the influence of alcohol), fetal alcohol syndrome, risky sexual behaviors, hepatitis C and chronic liver diseases, and cancer (CDC, 2004).

In 2003, 44.9% of 9th through 12th graders reported drinking alcohol on one or more of the past 30 days (CDC, YRBS, 2003). Youth ages 12 to 17 reporting higher levels of religiosity were less likely to have used cigarettes, alcohol, or illicit drugs in the past month than youths reporting lower levels of religiosity. Alcohol use is a leading risk factor in three leading causes of death among youth—unintentional injuries (including motor vehicle crashes and drowning), suicides, and homicides. Other adverse consequences include risky sexual behavior and poor school performance (CDC, YRBS, 2003). Box 17-6 provides Web resources about substance abuse.

BOX 17-6
Web Resources About Substance Abuse and Treatment

Alcoholics Anonymous
http://www.alcoholics-anonymous.org

Alanon/Alateen
http://www.al-anon.alateen.org

American Council on Alcoholism
http://www.aca-usa.org

Center for Substance Abuse Research
http://www.cesar.umd.edu

Drug Abuse Resistance Education (D.A.R.E.)
http://www.dare.com

For Young Adults 17 to 25
http://www.strugglingyoungadults.net

Mothers Against Drunk Driving
http://www.madd.org

Narcotics Anonymous
http://www.na.org

National Center on Addiction and Substance Abuse (CASA)
http://www.casacolumbia.org

National Council on Alcohol Abuse and Alcoholism
http://www.ncadd.org

National Institute on Alcohol Abuse and Alcoholism
http://www.niaa.nih.gov

National Institute on Drug Abuse
http://www.nida.nih.gov

National Organization on Fetal Alcohol Syndrome
http://www.nofas.org

NIDA for Teens
http://www.teens.drugabuse.gov

Persons with Disabilities

Overview

The U.S. Census reports that 49.7 million, or 19.3%, of the 257.2 million civilians ages 5 and over who were not living in prisons, nursing homes, or other institutions, have some type of long-lasting condition or disability. This represents nearly one in five Americans. Disability rates rose with age for both sexes, but significant differences existed between genders. For persons under age 65, the prevalence of disability among men and boys was higher than among women and girls. In people over age 65, this reversed, with women having 43% and men 40% (U.S. Census, 2003).

According to the 2000 Census, people who indicated that they were white (and no other race) and were not of Hispanic or Latino origin, had a low overall disability rate (18.3% versus 19.3% overall), despite their median age being higher than other racial and ethnic groups. People who reported themselves as black or American Indian/Native Alaskan shared the highest disability rate of 24.3%. Asian Americans who reported only one race had the lowest overall disability rate of 16.6%. People reporting two or more races had the lowest median age but a high disability rate (21.7%). The overall disability rate for Hispanics was also high (20.9%) (U.S. Census, 2003).

In 2000, 8.7 million people with disabilities were poor—a substantially higher proportion (17.6%) than was found among people without disabilities (10.6%). The highest poverty rates in both cases were found among children ages 5 to 15. Young people with disabilities had a 25.0% poverty rate, compared with 15.7% for those without disabilities (U.S. Census, 2003).

The 2000 Census also reported that two of every five people with a disability lived in the South, whereas one in five lived in each of the other three regions of the country. West Virginia, the state with the highest median age also had the highest disability rate (24.4%) for 2000. Counties with very high disability rates were clustered in the coal mining areas of Kentucky, West Virginia, and Virginia. Alaska and Utah had the lowest rates, each at 14.9% (U.S. Census, 2003).

The National Center for Health Statistics, *Summary Health Statistics for the U.S. Population: National Health Interview Survey*, 2002, provides the following information about noninstitutionalized adults and children:

- The number of persons with limitation(s) in usual activities because of chronic conditions is 33.7 million or 12.2% of total population.
- Number of adults with hearing trouble: 30.8 million, or 15%.
- Percent of adults with vision trouble: 19.1 million, or 9.3%.
- Number of adults unable (or very difficult) to walk a quarter mile: 14.2 million, or 6.2%.
- Number of adults with any physical functioning difficulty: 28.3 million, or 13.8%.
- Number of children ages 3 to 17 years ever told had a learning disability: 4.9 million, or 8.1%.

Effects of Disabilities

Disabilities affect major life activities, which include self-care, receptive and expressive language, learning, mobility, self-direction, capacity for independent living, and financial sufficiency. The three major categories of causes of disabilities are injuries, developmental disabilities, and chronic diseases. These conditions can occur at different ages and stages of development and with varying degrees of severity. Disabilities affect individuals in relation to related health problems, self-esteem, life expectancy, and ability to assume roles. Disabilities affect families in relation to the stress that they cause to the family unit, the need for external resources to help the family meet its tasks, the related financial responsibilities, and the social stigma. Disabilities affect communities by the need and demand for more resources and the need to comply with legislation related to persons with disabilities (McClellan, 2004). Web resources about disabilities are provided in Box 17-7.

Faith Communities and Outreach Ministries

All faith communities believe in providing assistance and care to people who are in need. Faith communities reach out to nurture and to provide social support for the well-being of those who share their faith, and they reach out to those in need within their communities. Many faith communities maintain food and/or clothing banks, provide meals to homeless shelters, provide meeting rooms to service organizations, such as Alcoholics Anonymous, and provide visits by clergy and/or ministry staff or volunteers to homebound and hospitalized members.

Dr. David Satcher states, "At the heart of all faith organizations are places of worship where people come together to practice their faith. Through these special places, be they cathedrals, chapels, mosques, pagodas, synagogues, tabernacles, temples, or other meeting places, the health of individuals, families, and communities can be improved" (CDC-ATSDR Forum, 1999, p. 2). Rev. Gary Gunderson of the Carter Center's Interfaith Health Program,

BOX 17-7
Web Resources About Disabilities

ADA Technical Assistance Program
http://www.adata.org

American Association of People with Disabilities
http://www.aapd-dc.org

American Council of the Blind
http://www.acb.org

American Diabetes Association
http://www.diabetes.org

American Foundation for the Blind
http://www.afb.org

Christian Council in Persons with Disabilities
http://www.ccpd.org

Christopher and Dana Reeve Paralysis Resource Center
http://www.paralysis.org

Coalition for Citizens with Disabilities
http://www.ccd-life.org

Guide Dogs for the Blind
http://www.guidedogs.com

National Association for the Deaf
http://www.nad.org

National Catholic Partnership on Disability
http://www.ncpd.org

National Center for Birth Defects and Developmental Disabilities
http://www.cdc.gov/ncbddd/

National Federation of the Blind
http://www.nfb.org

National Limb Loss Information Center
http://www.amputee-coalition.org/

OPA-Office of Protection and Advocacy for Persons with Disabilities
http://www.ct.gov/opapd

People with Disabilities Foundation
http://www.pwdf.org

World Institute on Disability
http://www.wid.org

described the alignment of religion and health assets as a faith-health movement that can change communities. He defined a movement as a fundamental thing moving in the social structure that has the power to change policies and to change the way we relate to each other. He described the faith and health movement as having the following four aspects:

- The relationship between individual spirituality and individual health.
- Religious structures acting in communities for the expressed purpose of improving and contributing to the health of those communities.
- A broad-scale realignment of social responsibilities and a new understanding of enduring accountability for community structures.
- Congregational vitality, occurring in a strong, active minority of congregations—a revitalization of the social structure, the root from which the faith community's involvement with public health must be generated (CDC-ATSDR Forum, 1999).

Rev. Gunderson also speaks of the basic strengths that faith congregations have that are valuable in community health initiatives. These ideas are developed in-depth in his book, *Deeply Woven Roots: Improving the Quality of Life in Your Community*. Briefly, these strengths of congregations include the following:

- The strength to *accompany,* to be present in the lives of others.
- The strength to *convene,* to convene interests that would not otherwise come together around specific problems or opportunities.
- The strength to *connect* people to resources that exist in the membership of the congregation and in their connections with one another.
- The power to *frame,* providing a framework of meaning around experience and data.
- The power of *sanctuary*, providing a safe place to gather.
- The power to *bless,* to sanction.
- The power to *pray,* to find meaning between the holy and the human.
- A very different *sense of time.* Congregations are enduring institutions that have the power to persist and see the community produce change (1997).

Ammerman states that congregations are the most pervasive voluntary organizations in our society. As such, they are instruments in the generation of what sociologists call *social capital*. She states that congregations are often the only voluntary organization to which the most disadvantaged in our society have access, including access to learn civic skills, such as chairing a meeting or speaking in public (CDC-ATSDR Forum, 1999).

The type and need for community outreach ministries will differ depending on the location of the faith community. A rural faith community will have different needs than a suburban or an inner city congregation. A community assessment is an invaluable tool in identifying vulnerable populations, both within the congregation and in the larger community. Community assessment data analysis is also helpful to the health ministry team in prioritizing the needs of the community and in determining what other agencies or groups provide services to vulnerable populations. How, and to what extent the faith community addresses the needs of vulnerable populations, will depend on its personnel, time, and financial resources. Ministry workforces may cover the spectrum from seminary-trained clergy to small groups of dedicated volunteers, some of whom have "found faith" after struggling with substance abuse or being in trouble with the law (Whitehead, 2001). Community outreach ministries are labor intensive. Fiscal resources need to be available to support staff, and volunteers will need training to work with vulnerable populations. Compared to many health organizations, congregational fiscal resources are modest. More than 70% of the nation's religious congregations have fewer than 400 members and average revenues under $100,000 per year (Steinfels, 1995). More to the point, some ministries closest to the street operate with part-time pastors, church memberships between 50 and 200, and resources from their leader's pockets (Truclear, 2000). Congregations can create collaborative networks to work together to share resources and to provide outreach services to vulnerable populations.

In recent years, new political and policy interest has supported funding for faith-based answers to social problems. The welfare reform act, as well as domestic services block grants, include provisions that allow public funding for faith-based organizations. President Bush charged the White House Office of Faith-based and Community Incentives to lead a broad faith-based initiative. This initiative focuses on the following priority areas: at-risk youth, ex-offenders, homeless and hungry, substance abusers, persons with HIV/AIDS, and welfare-to-work families. Agency centers for faith-based and community initiatives have been established in five cabinet departments. Technical assistance activities are offered free of charge and include planning, financial management, board development, fundraising, and outcome measurement (White House, 2004). Depending on community needs, faith communities may do outreach in homeless shelters or migrant worker camps. If resources allow, a primary health clinic might be provided in these types of settings.

Whitehead et al. (2001) report that 75% of Americans polled supported the idea of government funding to faith-based organizations. However, much less consensus occurred about details. For example, only 38% of those polled supported funding Muslim mosques or Buddhist temples, and 59% opposed funding groups that promote religious conversion.

Wuthnow (2004) states that religion is fundamentally social about the relationships among people and within communities and between individuals and organizations and therefore contextual; it is given life and meaning through the concrete settings in which it is expressed. Religion is embedded in social norms, in cultural values, and in the resource and power arrangements that cause it to be the way it is. In Wuthnow's book, *Saving America: Faith-based Services and the Future of Civil Society* (2004), he suggests that the most extensive ways in which congregations provide services do not occur through formal programs (on which most political discussions have focused), but rather through the informal activities, the fellowship circles, Bible studies, classes, and worship services, that constitute what congregations themselves refer to as the "caring community" (p. xvi). He contends that the faith-based service organizations that are *most* effective *are* effective for reasons that probably disqualify them for receiving government funding under the prevailing understandings of separation of church and state.

Faith Community Nurses and Vulnerable Populations

The Scriptures of the world's religions direct people to provide for those in need. Faith communities respond in many ways to the needs of vulnerable people. Many faith communities maintain or participate in community food and clothing banks and participate in fund-raising efforts for organizations that provide services and housing for vulnerable people. Whitehead et al. (2001) report that 80% of congregations offer food and cash assistance to families in their communities.

The vulnerable population conceptual model (VPCM) presented at the beginning of this chapter diagrams the negative effect that decreased resources and increased risks have on health status. FCNs can provide assistance to vulnerable persons and families, using all of the roles and functions of faith community nursing practice. In living the role of integrator of faith and health, the FCN promotes wholeness and healing of both the spirit and the body by providing the vulnerable individual with unconditional acceptance.

Carson and Koenig (2004) suggest three overlapping categories of spiritual interventions: the ministry of presence, ministry of word, and ministry of action. They state that the ministry of presence is more than just showing up. It involves active listening and hearing both oral and nonverbal messages. It also requires empathy, vulnerability, humility, and commitment. Empathy involves using the mind and heart to understand another person's story. When we open ourselves to others, we are vulnerable to rejection or criticism. Humility involves realizing one's strengths and weakness as well as being open to learning from those we care for. Commitment is the last aspect of the ministry of presence; it is the willingness to go the distance—to maintain the relationship for as long as it is needed. Carson and Koenig state that the ministry of presence is what God provides to each person, and that each person has both a responsibility and a privilege of extending that ministry to God's people.

The second intervention described by Carson and Koenig (2004) is the ministry of the word. This intervention requires great sensitivity to the client's belief system. Included in this ministry are a willingness to discuss spiritual/religious issues; verbal support and encouragement of spiritual beliefs; making a referral to a chaplain; using Scripture or other religious literature; and using prayer. The third intervention is the ministry of action, how you do, and what you do. The authors caution that the simplest acts are capable of conveying a powerful message of love, and at the heart of spiritual care is a ministry of love.

The FCN uses the role of health counselor and educator to help the vulnerable client make healthy choices and learn basic life skills. Often the FCN is the one who listens to vulnerable persons, advocates for them, connects them to community resources, and orchestrates effective approaches to meet their needs. The FCN roles of advocate and referral agent include assisting the person/family to access medical, social, and spiritual care services. This may involve activities, such as providing transportation and/or assisting with reading and completing forms. Vulnerable persons are distrustful of the health care system and may need the FCN to be with them as they negotiate new resources. Using all of the roles or functions of the FCN, vulnerable populations can be connected with additional resources to reduce their risk factors for poor health.

Summary

This chapter provides a discussion of the concept of vulnerability and describes the groups that are traditionally labeled "vulnerable," with the caveat that any person or group can be vulnerable at a given time. A demographic overview of each vulnerable group is provided, and the effects of each type of vulnerability are discussed.

A community assessment will be valuable in identifying the needs within both the faith community and the surrounding community, and in assessing both needs and what resources currently exist. Responses and strategies that a faith community/health ministry may implement to assist vulnerable persons are discussed. The types of outreach health ministries that a congregation can implement will be dependent on the resources—people, time, and money—that are available.

Reflect and Discuss

1. Mrs. Jay, a 45-year-old member of your congregation, shares that she believes that her son-in-law is physically abusing her daughter. In what ways can the FCN assist this mother?
2. Mr. Wright, a 31-year-old new member, discloses to the FCN that he was hospitalized for schizophrenia in the past. He tells the FCN that because he accepted the Lord he is cured. What response should the FCN make?
3. Mrs. Keane tearfully tells the FCN that she has been diagnosed as HIV positive and does not deserve to live. How should the FCN respond?
4. Mr. Samuel is a poor, elderly gentleman whose hearing has become so limited that he is shouting responses during the worship service. A number of congregants have complained. In what way can the FCN respond?

Case Study

Linda has been the FCN for a small congregation for 5 years. She has enjoyed her health ministry in most aspects. Of late, Linda has become frustrated with a female congregant who has a long history of depression. This individual calls Linda's home at all hours of the day and night with requests, concerns, and, at times, she verbalizes that she wants to harm herself.

In response, Linda has sought consultation from a psychiatric clinical nurse specialist who advised her to refer the congregant to the crisis hotline. The next time this woman verbalized suicidal ideas on the telephone, Linda referred her to the crisis line and gave her the number to call.

About a week later, Linda received another call from this client. Linda asked her if the crisis line was helpful to her. The client admitted that she did not call the crisis line.

She then proceeded to tell Linda that she was again very depressed and felt as if she might harm herself. Linda again directed her to call the crisis line and she confronted the client about seeking advice from her and then not acting on the advice given. The client apologized for not following through but would not commit to making a call to the crisis line.

1. What should Linda do next?
2. With whom should she share this information?
3. What resources are available in the community?
4. What documentation should occur?

References

Aday, L. A. (2001). *At risk in America: The health and health care needs of vulnerable populations in the United States* (2nd ed.). San Francisco: Jossey-Bass.

Administration on Aging. (2002). *A profile of older Americans, 2002.* Available online at: http://aoa.gov/prof/Statistics/profile/2.asp.

Anderson, D. G., & Rayens, M. K. (2004). Factors influencing homelessness in women. *Public Health Nursing, 21*(1), 12–23.

Bezruchka, S. (2000). Culture and medicine: Is globalization dangerous to our health? *Western Journal of Medicine, 172,* 332–334.

Bezruchka, S. (2001). Societal hierarchy and the health Olympics. *Canadian Medical Association Journal, 164,* 1701–1703.

Bortz, W. M. (1993). The physics of frailty. *Journal of the American Geriatric Society, 41*(9), 1004–1008.

Campbell, A. J., & Buchner, D. M. (1997). Unstable disability and the fluctuations of frailty. *Age and Aging, 26*(4), 315–318.

Carson, V. B. & Koenig, H. G. (2004). *Spiritual caregiving: Healthcare as ministry.* Radnor, PA: Templeton Foundation Press.

Centers for Disease Control and Prevention–ATSDR Forum. (1999). *Engaging faith communities as partners in community health.* Atlanta, GA: CDC.

Centers for Disease Control and Prevention (CDC). (2004). General alcohol information. Available online at: http://www.cdc.gov/alcohol/factsheets/general_information.htm.

Centers for Disease Control and Prevention (CDC). (2003). Youth risk behavior surveillance system survey data. Atlanta, GA: Department of Health and Human Services. Available online at: http://www.cdc.gov/HealthyYouth/yrbs/index.htm.

Centers for Disease Control–National Center for HIV, STD, and TB Prevention. (2004). Basic statistics. Available online at: http://www.cdc.gov/hiv/stats.htm.

Davis, S. (2001). *Child labor: Migrant health monograph series.* Buda, TX: National Center for Farmworker Health.

de Chesnay, M. (Ed.). (2005). *Caring for the vulnerable: Perspectives in nursing theory, practice, and research.* Sudbury, MA: Jones & Bartlett.

Ensign, J., & Santelli, J. (1997). Shelter-based homeless youth: Health and access to care. *Archives of Pediatric Medicine, 151*(8), 817.

Flaskerud, J. H. & Winslow, B. J. (1998). Conceptualizing vulnerable population-health related research. *Nursing Research, 47*(2), 69–78.

Francis, D., Fletcher, K., & Simon, L. J. (1998). The geriatric resource nurse model of care: A vision for the future. *Nursing Clinics of North America, 33,* 481–496.

Gunderson, G. (1997). *Deeply woven roots: Improving the quality of life in your community.* Minneapolis, MN: Fortress Press.

Healthy United States. (2002). *Healthy, health care and disability: A profile of older Americans: 2001.* Available online at: http://www.aoa.gov/prof/Statistics/profile/profiles.asp.

Kaufman, S. R. (1994). The social construction of frailty: An anthropological perspective. *Journal of Aging Studies, 8,* 45–58.

Kirby, D. (2001). *Emerging answers: Research findings on programs to reduce teen pregnancy.* Washington, DC: National Campaign to Prevent Teen Pregnancy.

Koniak-Griffin, D., Flaskerud, J. H., & Nyamathi, A. (2005). Vulnerable populations research: A center for excellence. In M. de Chesnay (Ed.), *Caring for the vulnerable: Perspectives in nursing theory, practice, and research.* Sudbury, MA: Jones & Bartlett.

Lunney, J. R., Lynn, J., & Hogan, C. (2002). Profiles of older Medicare decedents. *Journal of American Geriatric Society, 50,* 1108–1112.

Markle-Reid, M., & Browne, G. (2003). Conceptualizations of frailty in relation to older adults. *Journal of Advanced Nursing, 44*(1), 58–68.

McClellan, M. A. (2004). The physically compromised. In M. Stanhope & J. Lancaster (Eds.), *Community and public health nursing* (6th ed., pp. 720–743). St. Louis: Mosby.

Menke, E. M., & Wagner, J. D. (1998). A comparative study of homeless, previously homeless, and never homeless school-aged children's health. *Issues in Comprehensive Pediatric Nursing, 20*(3), 153.

Mezey, M., & Fulmer, T. (1998). Quality care for the frail elderly. *Nursing Outlook, 46*(6), 291, 292.

Mokhad, A., Marks, J., Stroup, D., & Gerberding, J. (2004). Actual causes of death in the United States. *JAMA, 291,* 70–75.

Napolitano, M., & Jones, K. D. (2004). Migrant health issues. In M. Stanhope & J. Lancaster (Eds.), *Community and public health nursing* (6th ed.). St. Louis: Mosby.

National Alliance for the Mentally Ill. (2004). About mental illness. Available online at: http://www.nami.org/Content/NavigatioMenu/Inform_Yourself/About_Mental_Illness.

National Campaign to Prevent Teen Pregnancy. (2004). Available online at: http://www.teenpregnancy.org.

National Center for Farmworker Health. (2004). *Fact sheets.* Available online at: http://www.ncfh.org.

National Center for Health Statistics. (2002). *Summary health statistics for the U.S. population: National health interview survey, 2002.* Washington, DC: Author.

National Coalition for the Homeless. (2004). Who are the homeless? Available online at: http://www.nationalhomeless.org/who./html.

Naylor, M. (2000). A decade of transitional care research with vulnerable elders. *Journal of Cardiovascular Nursing, 14*(3), 1–14.

Raphael, D., Cava, M., Brown, I., Renwick, R., & Heathcote, K., et al. (1995). Frailty: A public health perspective. *Canadian Journal of Public Health, 86*(4), 224–227.

Sebastian, J. G. (2004). Vulnerability and vulnerable populations: An overview. In M. Stanhope &

J. Lancaster (Eds.), *Community and public health nursing* (6th ed.). St. Louis: Mosby.

Steinfels, P. (1995, October 28). Beliefs. *The New York Times* (p. 11).

Substance Abuse and Mental Heath Services Administration. (2004). *Overview of findings from the 2003 National Survey on Drug Use and Health.* Rockville, MD: Office of Applied Studies, NSDUH Series H-24, DHHS Publication No. SMA 04-3963.

Truclear, H. D. (2000). *Faith-based institutions and high-risk youth: First report to the field.* Philadelphia: Public/Private Ventures.

Urban Institute. (2000). *A new look at homelessness in America.* Available online at: http://www.urban.org.

U.S. Census. (2003). FactFinder: Disability. Available online at: http://factfinder.census.gov/jsp/saff/SAFFInfo.jsp?_pageId=tp4_disability.

U.S. Conference of Mayors. (2003). *A status report on hunger and homelessness in America's cities.* Washington, DC: Author.

U.S. Department of Health and Human Services. (2001). *Healthy people 2010: Understanding and improving health and objectives for improving health* (2 vols.). Washington, DC: U.S. Printing Office.

U.S. Department of Labor. (1999). National Agricultural Workers Survey 1979–1998. Washington, DC: Author.

Vissing, Y. (1996). *Out of sight, out of mind: Homeless children and families in small town America.* Lexington, KY: The University Press.

Walston, J., & Fried, L. P. (1994). Frailty and the older man. *Medical Clinics of North America, 83*(5), 1173–1194.

Weinreb, L., Goldberg, R., Bassuk, E., & Perloff, J. (1998). Determinants of health and service use patterns in homeless and low-income housed children. *Pediatrics, 102*(3 Pt 1), 554.

Whitehead, B. D., Wilcox, B. L., & Rostosky, S. S. (2001). *Keeping the faith: The role of religion and faith communities in preventing teen pregnancy.* Washington, DC: National Campaign to Prevent Teen Pregnancy.

White House Office of Faith-Based and Community Initiatives. (2004). President Bush's faith-based initiative.

Wuthnow, R. (2004). *Saving America: Faith-based services and the future of civil society.* Princeton, NJ: Princeton University Press.

Young, H. M. (2003). Challenges and solutions for care of frail older adults. *Online Journal Issues in Nursing, 8,* 5.

Zisberg, A., & Young, H. M. (2005). Vulnerability among hospitalized older adults. In M. de Chesnay (Ed.), *Caring for the vulnerable: Perspectives in nursing theory, practice, and research* (pp. 303–311). Sudbury, MA: Jones & Bartlett.

Zorza, J. (1991). Woman battering: A major cause of homelessness. *Clearinghouse Review, 25*(4). Qtd. in National Coalition Against Domestic Violence, "The importance of financial literacy," Oct. 2001.

Additional References

Abernathy, J. V. (2002). Relationship between poverty and health among adolescents. *Adolescence, 37*(145), 55–67.

Amarasingham, R., Spalding, S. H., & Anderson, R. J. (2001). Disease conditions most frequently evaluated among the homeless in Dallas. *Journal of Health Care for the Poor and Underserved, 12*(2), 162–176.

Ameling, A., & Povilonis, M. (2001). Spirituality: Meaning, mental health, and nursing. *Journal of Psychosocial Nursing, 39*(94), 15–20.

American Association of Colleges of Nursing. (1999). *Position statement: Violence as a public health problem.* Washington, DC: Author.

American Nurses Association. (1998). *Cultural competence assessment for family violence.* Washington, DC: Author.

Appel, S. J., Harrell, J. S., & Deng, S. (2002). Racial and socioeconomic differences in risk factors for cardiovascular disease among Southern rural women. *Nursing Research, 51,* 140–147.

Bearman, P. S., & Bruckner, H. (2001). Promising the future: Virginity pledges and first intercourse. *American Journal of Sociology, 106*(4), 859–912.

Blonna, R., & Watter, D. (2005). *Health counseling: A microskills approach.* Sudbury, MA: Jones & Bartlett.

Boland, C. S. (1998). Parish nursing: Addressing the significance of social support and spirituality for sustained health promoting behaviors in the elderly. *Journal of Holistic Nursing, 16*(3), 355–368.

Camphina-Bacote, J. (2002). The process of cultural competence in the delivery of health care services: A model of care. *Journal of Transcultural Nursing, 13*(3), 180–184.

Campolo, T. (2000). *Revolution and renewal: How churches are saving our cities.* Louisville, KY: Westminster John Knox Press.

Champion, J. D. (19998). Family violence and mental health. *Nursing Clinics of North America, 33*(1), 201–215.

Chaves, M. (2004). *Congregations in America.* Cambridge, MA: Harvard University Press.

Claus-Ehlers, C. S., & Levi, L. L. (2002). Violence and community, terms in conflict: An ecological approach to resilience. *Journal of Social Distress and the Homeless, 11*(4), 265–278.

Craft-Rosenberg, M., Powell, S. R., & Culp, K. (2000). Health status and resources of rural homeless women and children. *Western Journal of Nursing Research, 22*(8), 863–878.

Davis, T. (2005). *Sacred work: Planned parenthood and its clergy alliances.* New Brunswick, NJ: Rutgers University Press.

Deaton, A., & Lubotsky, D. (2003). Mortality, inequality and race in American cities and states. *Social Sciences and Medicine 56,* 1139–1153.

DiBenedetto, D. V. (2003). Finding disability-related information on the Web. *AAOHN Journal: Official Journal of American Association of Occupational Health Nurses, 51,* 10–12.

Diez Roux, A. V. (2001). Investigating neighborhood and area effects on health. *American Journal of Public Health, 91*(11), 1783–1789.

DiNapoli, P. P. (2003). Guns and dolls: An exploration of violent behavior in girls. *Advances in Nursing Science, 26*(2), 140–148.

Dixon, L., Lucksted, A., Stewart, B., & Delahanty, J. (2000). Therapists' contacts with family members of persons with severe mental illness in a community treatment program. *Psychiatric Services, 51*(4), 1449.

Doornbas, M. M. (2002). Family caregivers and the mental health system: Reality and dreams. *Archives of Psychiatric Nursing, 16*(1), 2.

Drevdahl, D. (2002). Social justice or market justice? The paradoxes of public health partnerships with managed care. *Public Health Nursing, 19*(3), 161–169.

Drevdahl, D., Kneipp, S., Canales, M., & Dorcy, C. (2001). Reinvesting in social justice: A capital idea for public health nursing. *Advances in Nursing Science, 24,* 19–31.

Ebersole, P. (2002). Situational vulnerability. *Geriatric Nursing, 23*(2), 4.

Elliot, B., Beatrtie, K., & Kaitfors, S. (2000). Health needs of people living below poverty. *Family Medicine, 33*(5), 36–366.

Fickenscher, A., Lapidus, J., Silk-Walker, R., & Becker, T. (2001). Women behind bars: Health needs of inmates in a county jail. *Public Health Reports, 116,* 191–196.

Flaskerud, J. H., Lesser, J., Dixon, E., Anderson, N., Conde, F., & Kim, S., et al. (2002). Health disparities among vulnerable populations: Evolution of knowledge over five decades in nursing research publications. *Nursing Research, 51*(2), 74–85.

Flaskerud, J. H., & Winslow, B. J. (1998). Conceptualizing vulnerable populations' health related research. *Nursing Research, 47*(2), 69–78.

Flaskerud, J. H., & Nyamathi, A. M. (2002). New paradigm for health disparities needed. *Nursing Research, 51,* 139.

Flynn, B. (1997). Partnerships in healthy cities and communities: A social commitment for advanced practice nurses. *Advanced Practice Nursing Quarterly, 2*(4), 1–6.

Flynn, L. (1997). The health practices of homeless women. *Nursing Research, 46*(2), 72–77.

Freudenberg, N. (2000). Health promotion in the city: A review of current practice and future prospects in the United States. *Annual Review of Public Health, 21,* 473–503.

Funk, M., Ostfeld, A. M., Chang, V. M., & Lee, F. A. (2002). Racial differences in the use of cardiac procedures in patients with acute myocardial infarction. *Nursing Research, 51,* 148–157.

Goff, P., & Harvey, P. (Eds.). (2004). *Themes in religion and American culture.* Chapel Hill, NC: University of North Carolina Press.

Grady, P. A. (2000). NINR and health disparities. *Nursing Outlook, 48,* 150.

Green, P. M., & Adderley-Kelly, B. (1999). Partnership for health promotion in an urban community. *Nursing & Healthcare Perspectives, 20*(2), 76–81.

Hahn, E. A., & Cella, D. (2003). Health outcomes assessment in vulnerable populations: Measurement challenges and recommendations. *Archives of Physical Medicine and Rehabilitation, 84*(Suppl 2), S35–S42.

Health Resources Services Administration. (2004). A plan of action for improving the health of migrant and seasonal farm workers. Available online at: http://www.hrsa.gov/migrant/migrant.html.

Hildebrandt, E. (1999). Focus groups and vulnerable population: Insight into client strengths and needs in complex community health environments. *Nursing and Health Care Perspectives, 20*(5), 256–259.

Hines-Martin, V., Malone, M., Kim, S., & Brown-Piper, A. (2003). Barriers to mental healthcare access in an African-American population. *Issues in Mental Health Nursing, 24,* 237–256.

Hofferth, S. (2003). The American family: Changes and challenges for the 21st century. In H. Wallace, G. Green, & K. Jaros (Eds.), *Health and welfare for families in the 21st century.* Sudbury, MA: Jones & Bartlett.

Humphreys, J., & Campbell, J. C. (2004). *Family violence and nursing practice.* Philadelphia: Lippincott Williams & Wilkins.

Institute for Research on Poverty. (2002). *Who is poor?* Available online at: http://www.ssc.wisc.edu/irp.

Institute of Medicine, National Academy of Sciences. (2003). *Unequal treatment: Confronting racial and ethnic disparities in health care.* Available online at: http://www.nap.edu.

Jacobs, B. B. (2001). Respect for human dignity: A central phenomenon to philosophically unite nursing theory and practice through consilience of knowledge. *Advances in Nursing Science, 24*(1), 17–35.

Karpati, A., Galea, S., Awerbuch, T., & Levins, R. (2002). Variability and vulnerability at the ecological level: Implications for understanding the social determinants of health. *American Journal of Public Health, 92*(11), 1768–1772.

Kelleher, L., & Johnson, M. (2004). An evaluation of a volunteer-support program for families at risk. *Public Health Nursing, 21*(4), 297–305.

Kissman, K. (1999). Respite from stress and other service needs of homeless families. *Community Mental Health Journal, 35*(3), 241–249.

Kneipp, S., & Snider, M. (2001). Social justice in a market model world. *Journal of Professional Nursing, 17*(3), 113.

Kotlowitz, A. (1991). *There are no children here.* New York: Doubleday.

Kozol, J. (1995). *Amazing grace.* New York: Crown Publishers.

Kozol, J. (1988). *Rachel and her children: Homeless families in America.* New York: Fawcett Columbine.

Kramer, A. (2002). Domestic violence: How to ask and how to listen. *Nursing Clinics of North America, 37*(1), 189–210.

Lantz, P. M., Lynch, J. W., House, J. S., Lepkowski, J. M., Mero, R. P., & Musick, M. A., et al. (2001). Socioeconomic disparities in health change in a longitudinal study of US adults: The role of health risk behaviors. *Social Science and Medicine, 53*, 29–40.

Leight, S. B. (2003). The application of a vulnerable populations conceptual model to rural health. *Public Health Nursing, 20*(6), 440–448.

Leung, W. (2002). Why the professional-client ethic is inadequate in mental health care. *Nursing Science Quarterly, 14*(4), 298–303.

Locsin, R. C., & Purnell, M. J. (2002). Intimate partner violence, culture-centrism, and nursing. *Holistic Nursing Practice, 16*(3), 1–4.

Loeb, S. J., Penrod, J., Falkenstern, S., Gueldner, S. H., & Poon, L. W. (2003). Supporting older adults living with multiple chronic conditions. *Western Journal of Nursing Research, 25*, 8–23.

Lutenbacher, M. (2002). Relationships between psychosocial factors and abusive parenting attitudes in low-income single mothers. *Nursing Research 51*(3), 158–167.

Lutz, B. J., & Bowers, B. J. (2003). Understanding how disability is defined and conceptualized in the literature. *Rehabilitation Nursing, 28*, 74–78.

Maternal and Child Health Bureau. (1992). *Violence: The impact of community violence on African American Children and Families*. Washington, DC: HHS.

Meisenhelder, J. B. (2002). Terrorism, posttraumatic stress, and religious coping. *Issues in Mental Health Nursing, 23*, 771–782.

Miles, A. (1999). When faith is used to justify abuse. *American Journal of Nursing, 99*(5), 32–35.

Moran, J. P. (2000). *Teaching sex: The shaping of adolescence in the 20th century*. Cambridge, MA: Harvard University Press.

Mundt, M. H. (1998). Exploring the meaning of "underserved": A call to action. *Nursing Forum, 33*(1), 5–10.

Neugebauer, R. (1999). Mind matters: The importance of mental disorders in public health's 21st century mission. *American Journal of Public Health, 89*(9), 1309–1311.

Nyamathi, A., Leake, B., & Gelberg, L. (2000). Type of social support among homeless women: Its impact on psychosocial resources, health and health behaviors, and use of health services. *Nursing Research, 49*, 318.

Owens, S. (2003). African-American women living with HIV/AIDS: Families as sources of support and of stress. *Social Work, 48*(2), 163–172.

Pickett-Shenk, S. (2002). Church-based support for African American families coping with mental illness: Outreach and outcomes. *Psychiatric Rehabilitation Journal, 26*(2), 173–180.

Place, M., Reynolds, J., Cousins, A., & O'Neill, S. (2002). Resilience: Where does it come from? *Early Childhood Today, 17*(2), 24, 25.

Rankin, D. T., & Ross, R. (1999). *When true love doesn't wait*. Nashville, TN: Lifeway Press.

Richardson, L. A. (2001). Seeking and obtaining mental health services: What do parents expect? *Archives of Psychiatric Nursing, 15*(5), 223.

Russell, K. (2002). Silent voices. *Public Health Nursing, 19*(4), 233, 234.

Sebastian, J. G., Bolla, C. D., Aretakis, D., Jones, K. D., Schenk, C. P., & Napolitano, M., et al. (2002). Vulnerability and selected vulnerable populations. In M. Stanhope & J. Lancaster (Eds.), *Foundations of community health nursing: Community oriented practice* (pp. 349–364). St. Louis: Mosby.

Sebastian, J. G., & Bushy, A. (1999). *Special populations in the community*. Gaithersburg, MD: Aspen Publishers.

Shi, L., & Stevens, G. (2004). *Vulnerable populations in the United States*. Indianapolis, IN: Jossey-Bass.

Sidel, R. (1992). *Women and children last*. New York: Penguin Books.

Spiers, J. (2000). New perspectives on vulnerability using etic and emic approaches. *Journal of Advanced Nursing, 31*(3), 715–721.

Stein, J. A., Lu, M. C., & Gelberg, L. (2000). Severity of homelessness and adverse birth outcomes. *Health Psychology 19*(6), 524–534.

Strehlow, A. J., & Amos-Jones, T. (1999). The homeless as a vulnerable population. *Nursing Clinics of North America 34*(2), 261–274.

Subramanian, S., Blakely, T., & Kawachi, I. (2003). Income inequality as a public health concern: Where do we stand? *Health Services Research, 38*, 153–167.

Veenema, T. G. (2001). Children's exposure to community violence. *Journal of Nursing Scholarship, 33*(2), 162.

Vezeau, T., Peterson, J., Nakao, C., & Ersek, M. (1998). Education of advanced practice nurses serving vulnerable populations. *Nursing and Health Care Perspectives, 19*(1), 124–131.

Walker, C. (1998). Homeless people and mental health. *American Journal of Nursing, 98*(11), 26–32.

Wallace, H. M., Green, G., Jaros, K. J., Paine, L. L., & Story, M. (1999). *Health and welfare for families in the 21st century*. Boston: Jones & Bartlett.

Walsh, F. (2003). Family resilience: A framework for clinical practice. *Family Process, 42*(1), 1–18.

Ward, L. S. (2003). Migrant health policy: History, analysis, and challenge. *Policy, Politics, and Nursing Practice, 4*(1), 45–52.

Watters, E. K. (2003). Literacy for health: An interdisciplinary model. *Journal of Transcultural Nursing, 14*(1), 48–54.

Weinstein, L. B. (2002). People in crisis: Clinical and public health perspectives. *Family and Community Health, 25*, 86, 87.

Weist, M. D. (2001). Toward a public mental health promotion and intervention system for youth. *Journal of School Health, 73*, 101–104.

White House Office of Faith-Based and Community
  Initiatives. (2004). President Bush's faith-based
  and community initiative. Available online at:
  http://www.whitehouse.gov/government/fbci/mis-
  sion/html.
Wilson, M. (2005). Health-promoting behaviors of shel-
  tered homeless women. *Family and Community
  Health, 28*(1), 51–63.
Young, C., & Koopson, C. (2005). *Spirituality, health
  and healing.* Thorofare, NJ: Slack Inc.
Zerwekh, J. V. (2000). Caring on the ragged edge:
  Nursing persons who are disenfranchised.
  Advances in Nursing Science, 22, 71.

 ## Web Resources

http://www.acog.org   American College of Obstetrics
  & Gynecology
http://www.aapc.org   American Association of
  Pastoral Counselors
http://www.aoec.org   Association of Occupational and
  Environmental Clinics
http://www.at-risk.com   Bureau for At-Risk Youth
http://wwww.cmwf.org   Commonwealth Fund
  Program on Quality of Care for Underserved
  Populations
http://www.docsfortots.org   Docs for Tots
http://www.frac.org   Food Research and Action Center
http://www.FoodStamps-Step1.usda.gov   Food Stamp
  Program/Prescreening Tool

http://www.healthliteracymonth.com   Health Literacy
  Month
http://www.hmassoc.org   Health Ministry Association
http://wwww.ihs.gov   Indian Health Service
http://www.ihpnet.org   Interfaith Health Program
http://www.elca.org/   Lutheran Church in America
  Health Ministries
http://www.migrantclinician.org   Migrant Clinicians
  Network
http://www.hispanichealth.org   Migrant Health
  Promotion
http://www.teenpregnancy.org   National Campaign to
  Prevent Teen Pregnancy
http://www.ncfh.org   National Center for Farmworker
  Health, Inc.
http://ncfy.com   National Clearinghouse on Families
  and Youth
http://www.nationalhomeless.org   National Coalition
  for the Homeless
http://www.nrscrisisline.org   National Runaway
  Switchboard
http://www.fns.usda.gov/fns   Nutrition Assistance
  Programs USDA
http://www.omhrc.gov   Office of Minority Health
  Resource Center
http://www.education-options.com/articles/Runaway
  Prevention.htm   Runaway Prevention
http://www.census.gov   U. S. Census
http://www.volunteersinhealthcare.org   Volunteers in
  Health Care
http://www.fbci.gov   White House Faith-based and
  Community Initiatives

Index

*Page numbers followed by *b* indicate boxed copy; page numbers followed by *f* indicate a figure.